Leaving Psychiatry

Leaving Psychiatry

J. R. Ó'Braonáin. M.D.

Published by Tablo

TABLE OF CONTENTS

INTRODUCTION

Custom would dictate that a book such as this should proceed from an introduction, though it is with some trepidation I write this as it remains to be seen if the book of my intention becomes a book in fact, much less a successful one. It may come to be a pamphlet little longer than the introduction preceding it, or rambling stream of consciousness which will make a good doorstop. Each of the chapters could easily be elaborated into books themselves, were they each to be developed. Yet insomuch as the book is a personal catharsis of my angst with psychiatry, better out than in one might say, and why prolong a birth that is past it's term of confinement. The affective urgency is simply too great to cast down on paper what you are gracious enough as to read, and finally be done with it. If I fail, it shan't be on account of either brevity or pleonastic fury.

Moreover, the introduction is the part of the book I'm usually least likely to read. After all, what of substance is within it save for as a summary of what is to come, the introduction being inadequate in itself? That having been said, the introduction of this pamphlet/book is perhaps the most important part, as it will lay out in advance the mode and method of argument I'll be following, what rules I intend to not to observe, and why. Hopefully this will dispel much criticism before it comes my way. Though logically sound where logic is employed, it is not intended to be a complete piece of analytical philosophy. Rather it is an unavoidably polemical personal reflection of my own career in the world of clinical psychiatry, very much an experienced view from the inside of the machine and the frontline of the so called war against so called mental illness. As such it is remotely possible my own experiences (technically speaking a large collection of mere anecdotes) are an aberration, with hospitals and clinics and other practitioners outside of my own experience practicing something entirely different, altogether orientated towards the truth and altogether corrosive to my argument. This is to be doubted, as I have practiced far and wide and also vicariously made use of stories told by others, along with availing myself of the rubbish that is regularly published and perpetuated in the literature endorsed by the international psychiatric intelligentsia.

Secondly, there is no pretence to this autoethnography being a piece of so called science, research or even good journalism. It is not the shadow of an adaptation of a doctoral thesis and I don't intend to fetter the book with footnotes, references and statistics ad nauseum, if for no other reason than my own laziness and fervent love of informality. A caveat to any would be critic would be this; should I make a statement taken as a matter of fact of the world as it is, or fact of history of something said or done open to challenge, I have the confidence that it will be all too easy to locate my vindication in a journal article under a pile of another papers under a further pile of papers. It all becomes a fatuous poker game of seeing the opponents piece of research and raising the stakes with a journal article conducive to one's own side of the argument, when the matter of debate is something ultimately philosophical anyway and something hermeneutical, i.e. related to the interpretation of data. Many works of so called psychiatric research are heavily bias, ghost-written by pharmaceutical companies, contrary to common or good sense, not successfully replicated and have data uncoupled from the interpretation of the data that is placed in the conclusion, this being especially the case with works that necessarily impact upon the philosophy of mind and what maketh a man (or woman) and their place in the world, which is essentially everything within the world of psychiatry come the end of the day. I'll even be using an example of a major article that employs references that even have nothing to do with the text citing them. I'm additionally reminded by what the great statistician and father of clinical trials Sir Austin Bradford Hill said of treatment effects

"you need neither randomisation, nor statistics, to analyse the results, unless the treatment effect is very small".

The spirit and implication of such a comment is simply that some facts are obviously the case or not (meaningful facts anyway), and much sophist mischief can be made with what one wishes to hide in, or conjure out of, mere numbers, invocations of "peer review", "science", "evidence base" and other spells and incantations, and window dressing a piece of writing into ostensive impressiveness with a litany of references will not save a poor argument from the ruin it deserves. Needless to say, treatment effects are predicated on a certain "x" being treated. What this "x" is, or if it is, is a serious can of worms assumed to have been adequately opened and answered by psychiatry as a basis for praxis. But has it been answered or can it be answered? I would say "no" to both questions. Now I shan't be making any claims controversial to my own experience and to those of thousands of other persons in the world. Is it not it enough to say "read this book", or "read that author" or "go out in the world and see as I have"? Why waste your time with more, and besides, whether you be friend or foe I'm preaching mostly to the converted already.

Neither will this book be an exhaustive critique of the prevailing, dare I say it, delusion in psychiatry that mental illnesses such as schizophrenia, ADHD and major depressive disorder are brain diseases, "neuro-genetic diseases" and the like. Many others have taken these myths to task and many books written, though these voices of truth are utterly dwarfed by the psychiatric machine. Though I can only claim to have personally read from a couple of these gadfly's, here and there this text will provide links to authors said to be critical of psychiatry for the reader to explore more widely and make up their own mind.

Neither will I claim to have thought of anything original, for there is nothing new under the sun. Occasionally what enters the mind might be an original thought to me, accompanied first by some blush of hubris soon supplanted by that dark cloud of doubt that someone must have thought or said the same thing before, and thought and said it better. As a prolific collector of books I almost never read beyond the second chapter, when I do read other works this deflationary intuition almost always empirically crashes one's ego back down to Earth. Moreover, usually the one taken to be the author of an original thought is not the first. Even my admissions of unoriginality will surely be unoriginal itself, and so on ad infinitum. But let's not make a pretence to mysticism here. The very assertion of my admission to unoriginality is part of the case in point. For if others share my conclusions, perhaps we share an anti-psychiatric delusion or an iconoclastic destructive "paranoid" personality. Or alternatively perhaps I'm onto something else good, and true and beautiful, and so are they. Sometimes one needs many years of education to discover deep truths. Sometimes we receive many years of ideology masquerading as education, the resultant being a trenchant disbelief in the obvious as our egos vainly leap to the defence of endless hours of wasted study. My experience and argument is my greatest weapon, the medical and other qualifications useless before the fact. Let the best argument win I say. All are welcome into the arena, and the argument with appeal to authority will not save you from harm.

Though it might seem otherwise, neither will this book be a chapter by chapter expansion and critique of the "disorders" as per DSM and ICD 11 (i.e. the American Psychiatric Associations Diagnostic and Statistical Manual and the World Health Organizations International Classification of Disease). For such an approach would, in some sense, give the disorders legitimacy and fail to escape the categorical and medicalized frame. These disorders will be addressed aplenty for sure, yet addressed incidentally within the chapters discussing other issues wider than the fiction of the disorders or disorder groups as natural categories, or deconstructing the successful work of fiction that is the DSM. The attack is "meta" to the DSM, specific psychiatric disorders merely illustrative of a larger argument which is epistemological and political, even moral, in nature. Mine is an attack not simply against the bible of the church of psychiatry whose scripture I cast aside years ago, but against it's very cannon and creed.

The audience for this book is everyone whose interest or personal experience falls within the orbit of what is called psychiatry or mental health, where mental health is paradoxically in practice a synonym for mental illness. Therefore, the audience includes the orthodox majority psychiatrists I'd like to foil yet who are immune from the voice of reason, the various minority heterodox spanners in the psychiatric wheel who call themselves critical psychiatrists (though curiously not critical enough to leave the profession and the comforts a qualification), junior doctors in psychiatry, nurses and allied health practitioners, and students of all the above. To budding trainees in psychiatry who pilgrim towards the good, the beautiful and the true through a road of free thinking and Socratic or scientific dialectic I'd plant this book as a sign alongside the path, a sincere plea that states "Go back. You will not find what you are looking for in psychiatry, and they are most definitely not looking for you either". This is the sign I wish someone had given me all those many years ago, or rather the sign I gave myself and failed to read at the time. Finally, this book is also aimed at members of the lay public who might have sat across from this species of secular priest who might in turn have pronounced them sane or insane, of good cheer or bad. To you patients I would simply say some emperors are finely clothed in wisdom, this despite of their apprenticeship and career in psychiatry. Evaluate them as any person would another. I am very blessed to have known and been mentored by a few who have taken their wisdom and placed it in peril of moral and intellectual famine by the profession they have chosen. In refraining from providing personal acknowledgment, I will offer the highest of compliments by dissociation from heresy. Sadly however, the vast majority of psychiatrists are as naked in wisdom as the day they were born.

As if it wasn't obvious, I'm using a nom de plume. In the fullness of time if the title of the book becomes a matter of past tense, i.e. having left psychiatry, I'll be tempted use my real name. Apart from the tradition amongst some doctors to write in pseudonym so as to protect the anonymity of patients discussed, anonymity also protects me. For I continue to practice behind enemy lines as it were, and have seen firsthand what happens to the careers of others who dare question too far mainstream psychiatry and the professional guilds from which it draws its power. I should very much like to continue to pay the bills, whilst seeking to quieten a whispering conscience lest it become a scream that will trouble me from sleep. On this point I wish to apologize to the reader for not revealing more of myself, for I would contend that one cannot really cannot understand why a thinker formulates the thought and arguably the quality of the thought itself without understanding the thinker his/herself in all his or her foibles and biases. Every creation carries the stain of its creator. Ergo caveat emptor.

Two of many questions haunt me into writing this book, and haunt me they do as mine is not a captious critique. These are the topics of the final two respective chapters. The first is the degree to which I might find it possible to identify with philosophy of the late psychiatrist Thomas Szasz (some would say anti-psychiatrist, I would say he was neither). I invite the reader to review the works of Szasz first, and also others critical of psychiatry. These include Peter Breggin, Paula Caplan, James Davies, Peter Gøtzsche, David Healy, Niall McLaren, Joanna Moncrief, John Read, Jeffrey Schaler, and Robert Whitaker et al.

The final chapter is more radical still, as if it were conceivably possible to be more radical than Szasz, i.e. what if psychiatry, as opposed to other medical/surgical specialities, simply went away. Would it matter in the same way the maimed would stay maimed if the orthopaedists were to vanish? The answer, cutting to the proverbial chase and making friends and enemies before the first word is read is this; the world does not need psychiatry. Nothing would happen of necessity were it to vanish, nothing bad anyway.

ONTOGENY. ENTERING SEMINARY.

"Ideally a book would have no order in it, and the reader would have to discover his own."
   Raoul Vaneigem

   "Education no longer has a humanist end or any value in itself; it only has one goal, to create technicians"
   Jacques Ellul

In the beginning, or in this beginning anyway, was the medical student. Only the medical student is far from being without form or void. Quite the contrary. By the time the medical student has their first encounter with psychiatry they are thoroughly encultured in a way of approaching whatever subject matter comes their way, and these cognitive (if not ideological) schemata have gathered such a powerful momentum that it can quite easily launch them into their psychiatric term and spit them out the other side without them having the faintest idea just how alien and even mythical was the species that passed into view for those 10 or so weeks. I include amongst them even the medical student who rejects psychiatry at the outset, for they know not what they reject. They are the ones whom, later as physicians and (especially) surgeons will politely describe their clerkship in mental health as "interesting' and "valuable but not for me", this being the most charitable descriptor they will offer to the psychiatrists face. What is said behind the psychiatrists back is, as usual in human nature, another matter entirely.

Broadly speaking, medical students pass through two pedagogical pathways nowadays, both reaching a considerable convergence in the latter phase of studies. The first is a more traditional form, starting with the basic medical sciences of anatomy, physiology, biochemistry and the like. If not stated explicitly, what is certainly taken up implicitly is the notion that one's vocation is as an applied engineer of a biological machine and, post Virchow, the fundamental patient is the cell, if not some subcellular molecular unit below cellular life or some organ system above it. Granted there will be plenty of lectures from plenty of health sociologists and public health physicians restating endlessly and to the point of tedium various definitions of "health" and "illness" and UN charters of this and that human right (and rite), all the while the student sits there yawning in the most justified assumption that their intuition as a human being informs them when they are well and when they are sick, and when they are making a mess of themselves qua a multicellular ship of Theseus as their soul voyages from birth to death. Granted there will be plenty of lectures and reminders of lectures that we are treating a whole person with whom we must communicate "empathically". Yet even these lectures on communication are, if to be honest, part of a micro-social engineering strategy. How do I get to the cell and physiological system "through", as it were, the person? How I might gather the data their body wants to tell me through what might otherwise be a brick wall of personality, should I not first gain "rapport" by uttering some comments here and there "that pain must have been hard for you" as we lean in a little, chair placed adjacent to the patient as we were taught in the class on proxemics (as opposed to on the other side of a desk). How might I charm the patient to take the pills if I don't empathize with their "lived experience" of side effects and "stigma" whilst pointing out the inevitably (or so it would seem inevitably) higher risks should they flush those very same pills down the toilet. It can be very disconcerting being a physician patient of another physician communicating in taught empathy. It's just too predictable and quasi-robotic and leaves the doctor who is patient looking in turn to find the person through, as it were, the physician who "cares for" the doctor who is the patient. Thankfully most patients live in blissful ignorance of feigned caring, and many a physician has first deceived themselves that they care. These will be the physicians taking the greatest umbrage at my analysis. No, the patient is the machine that is the body, and more to the point, an abstraction constructed from the machine, for even the body eventually is ignored in the age of information. Psychiatry is no different, though the castle it builds on the body is a castle built on sand.

Returning to the more traditional model of medical education; in learning by rote the almost endless list of facts of the basic medical sciences, which are of their very nature philosophically materialist, for there is never a hint of a mention of mind or telos or value in the cells that constitute the body let alone the body as a whole, the student hopefully acquires the raw materials to appreciate the clinical problem when they take up their stethoscope and are unleashed upon the hospital. An example of the clinical problem might be the matter of chest pain. The student has learned from basic anatomy that the heart

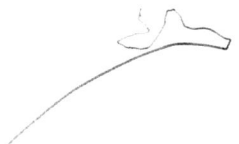

is in the centre (more or less) of the chest, the lungs either side, all enveloped in a sheath of muscle, bone, skin etcetera. They learn this in great detail, or at least they did when anatomy was taught properly. By the mid 2000's even the best medical schools had replaced long hours of expensive invaluable dissection with very limited "dissection experiences", for flesh and blood and time gets in the way of abstraction and assembly, and corporatized universities have become a business or mass production factory churning out as many medical students as the hierarchy will allow, whist specialty guilds pull up the drawbridge that might otherwise challenge the exclusivity of their own little clique. The student will have learned from basic physiology and cellular biochemistry to appreciate that the heart is a (kind of) muscle, and as such requires a constant supply of oxygen or lactate will accumulate, this triggering certain nerves to a state of activation that eventually be followed by the conscious phenomena of pain. The clever student may adduce from first principals what might be the cause of the pain, and from this what might be the remedy. To elaborate; the clever student may conclude that given the pain oscillates with a periodicity of breathing and is phenomenologically experienced as a pain spatially located to the chest wall, then it may relate to some structural pathology or inflammation of the chest wall itself. On the other hand, the pain may be steady and central, varies with exercise intensity and by extension the demands placed upon the heart. And so they may conclude the pain is that of angina of the cardiac variety. The really clever student who excelled in embryology might infer from first principles why the chest pain is perhaps also experienced as pain referred down the arm, or why pathology about the diaphragm (the muscle essentially dividing chest from abdomen) might be experienced in, of all places, the neck also. But these clever students are, believe it or not, very much the exception. In the majority of cases, the prior study of the basic medical sciences simply provides the raw materials from which to understand the reasoning and evidence behind vast lists of diseases and diagnostic reasoning that they are not expected to generate by their own synthetic cognitive devices, as opposed to simply remember and apply in a kind of algorithm/flow chart. Nowadays they are not even expected to generate the algorithm themselves from studying multiple sources. One will have already been published for them. They will learn that chest pain can be a manifestation of X, Y or Z pathology. They will memorize which signs (what can be seen/heard etc) and what symptoms (i.e. what the patient reports) correspond to narrowing the differential diagnosis from X, Y or Z to a single explanation of X (OR Y OR Z). And from the diagnosis of, say, angina what will follow is another memorized algorithm or pathway of what to do next, a treatment pathway. To this end the basic medical sciences are nothing more than lubricant to move through a pathway.

The same pedagogical journey towards pathway/algorithm arises from the more contemporary method of medical education known as problem based learning. Only in this case the student is confronted from the outset with the clinical problem (e.g. chest pain), perhaps in some cases with no prior learning of the basic medical sciences whatsoever, much less the basic or first order sciences of chemistry, physics and so on. What follows, without either word of an exaggeration, let alone a lie, is for the medical student to first learn what the chest is precisely, what is within it and so on. Often the student is almost expected to teach themselves, with lectures and such renamed as "learning resources" and the very structure of the students learning plan left to the devices of the student themselves. They may even be placed in "problem based learning" groups, with a facilitator at the helm who is explicitly instructed not to instruct, and rather sit there as the blind lead the blind, much like the marriage counsellor who sits, listens and asks each spouse what they think, all the while gagged from telling anyone what they (i.e. the counsellor) thinks or what they (the couple) ought to think, much less what they ought to do, though it may well be blindingly obvious. The hope of such a model of education is to cultivate an internal locus of self-organization, motivation towards so called "lifelong learning" and finally the capacity to think critically and synthetically, much like the clever students alluded to above. The reality is that such a model of education is just another road to pathway and algorithm, albeit from a different starting point. The student starts with clinical problem and the pathways to diagnose and treat it, reaches back into conceptual space to teach themselves the basic medical sciences (albeit never deeply) before returning again to the problem, this time with a greater understanding of what the clinical problem "means".

Several points arise from the above. The first is that medicine and what it is to be a doctor becomes almost mechanized, even cybernetic in a sense, and notions of intuition, individuality and such become antiquated and silly, if not reproached as dangerous. Such a mechanized state of affairs becomes the case in virtue of the cognitive schemata of lists and pathway alone, without even approaching the influence of so called "evidence based medicine" dogma on the student's psyche, or even the reliance on standardized diagnostic and treatment approaches not so much for cognitively expedient reasons, yet rather as a group survival mechanism in a litigious world. That is to say, we do things so that the patient will recover.

This is granted. But often we do things more so as to avoid getting into trouble by instead locating ourselves in the centre of herd activity. Often these two goals and their outcomes only weakly overlap.

The second is that the medical student deals with the physical body as a kind of engineer of sorts. Despite the drive to abstractions they become in some sense at least grounded in something that has a material basis in reality. The more classically trained medical student will learn that there really is something called a heart. After all, they poured their concentration over it over a lengthy dissection process in some basement of an anatomy department where their olfactory apparatus was partially killed off by formalin, and their fingers became pickled like the cadavers if the gloves weren't up to the task. Parts of my thumbs remain hardened still. The same student will see under the microscope the cells that comprise it and what a heart looks like when necrotic (i.e. dead). They will learn about processes by which the heart muscle needed and utilized oxygen, and see the arterial and microvascular roads of supply for cellular demand. The same student will take the ECG, and quite rightly so, as the electrical representation of activity of the organ that's sustains them in its beating from the moment of birth (indeed from only weeks post conception) to the moment of death. After anatomy classes the medical student may never actually see a heart again as a material thing in the world, as opposed to an abstraction in a diagnostic or treatment pathway. All they might encounter is a patient in pain, what the blood investigations shows, what the physical examination finds etc. They will know what this probably "means" and be sure of the horizon of potentiality. No one would be foolish enough to question the existence of a heart attack qua dead or dying heart muscle as something concocted or confected by some vested interest group, a pharmaceutical company or as some "social construct". They know all too well that if push comes to shove (and it often does), the cardiologist will run a dye up the leg and demonstrate that there is a heart there just as they remember and that this heart is perfused with less than its fair share of blood. Beyond this the pathologist will have the final word in the pronouncement of the physical groundings to disease. In summary, the medical student becomes complacent in the justified confidence that in all that might be called disease, pathology or illness, they are working with the reality of a material, albeit biological, machine.

These symptoms, signs, investigations to be ordered, potential diagnoses and so on (all the many pathways and elements of pathways) amount to a formidable information overload to even the best and brightest of medical students, who are usually the best and brightest at school and college. The task is to survive,

remember, regurgitate, and apply correctly. Though all this requires a mind
of above average intellect in the sense of short term memory for "cramming"
exams and superior information processing capacity, there is nothing remotely
approaching authentic critical thinking of the philosophical kind, let alone to
recline in the garden of academe pondering the metaphysical questions that
might, nay should sometimes, be applied to the vocation of medicine. There is
neither the time nor the energy nor the compulsion, much less the inclination.
Long gone are the days of the appropriately famous medieval medical school of
Salerno, the Schola Medica Salernitana, which only accepted men and (just as
often) women who were first schooled in 3 years of philosophy as part of the
curriculum, having to prove themselves wise, willing and able to think clearly
and critically. Even contemporary medical school ethics becomes an uncritical
checklist balancing the so called 4 principles of Beauchamp and Childress (i.e.
autonomy, beneficence, non-maleficence and equity). The ethical calculus
usually excludes any superficial, never mind deep, analysis of one system of ethics
against another as philosophies within the "meta" question of the being and
value of ethics itself within the world. And never is it asked where ethics ends
and morality (let alone the rest of philosophy) begins. In summary, the game
is to uncritically accept what is, remember, answer correctly restricting critical
analysis to operations within the accepted system itself, and move on to the next
question or the next patient. That is what the mind of the medical student is
encultured to do. What hope do they have when confronted with the question
what maketh the man and what do I make of his apparent madness and misery?

With the all these wheels in motion, our medical student arrives at their term
in psychiatry. Unless they have a personal interest in the subject, they will never
have encountered the so called mind body problem (or mind brain problem).
Remember that they are accustomed to automatically assume everything they
encounter is grounded in physical reality. When their psychiatry lecturer voices
a piece of pseudo-scientific propaganda servicing the survival of psychiatry as
a profession (e.g. that schizophrenia or ADHD is a proven "neuropsychiatric"
or neuro-genetic" disorder, or claiming a delusion is fundamentally and
substantively different from non-psychotic beliefs, or that there is such a thing as
an "antidepressant" medication in the same manner and with the same nominal
justification that we have "anti"-biotic medication), the student will take all of it
as a given. Who can blame them? This isn't a product of a lack of intellectual
capacity or an uncritical temperament (though it might be). No it's a product of
pure philosophical inertia and an article of faith on the part of the student that the

psychiatric professor is telling them something about the world and the human condition as it is, as real as the broken bone (there is little doubt the psychiatry professor is a true believer in what they are preaching. Always a good quality in one who seeks to convince another is first having convinced oneself). I notice this especially in doctors who have been raised and educated in traditional societies not as historically touched by the Socratic method or the Protestant mood. When our medical student encounters another list of differential diagnoses in psychiatry they will automatically assume these to be as valid in themselves and vs each other as the existence of, and difference between, a myocardial infarct, a pericarditis, a gastroesophageal reflux, an osteochondritis, an aortic dissection etcetera as painful manifestations of the thoracic pathology. They won't hazard to question if these psychiatric constructs are even ontologically of different categories to each and every other field of medicine. What aids greatly in this will be the logical fallacy that any apparently salutary response to medication proves the existence of what some may call disease that in turn falls under the purview of the doctor. Though why not then make a doctor of a bartender escapes me, for alcohol also delivers a salutary response for many. And so the logic must be that millions around the world have a disease of excess of blood in their alcohol stream.

Along with all this will be the spectacle the medical student will first encounter with the first psychiatric patients they see. In the vast majority of cases, the medical student will first encounter "mental illness" as part of an attachment to large teaching hospitals with acutely and severely disturbed individuals, often the urban poor. They will accompany a consultant psychiatrist and their apprentice resident/registrar on their ward rounds. In one consult or corner of the room will be a girl curled up in a regressed state with more cuts and scars on her forearms than stripes on a zebra. She will say she surely wants to kill herself, and if so the blood will be on any others hands but her own. In the other corner will be the dishevelled and derelict man who mutters and occasionally giggles to himself as if in conversation with another whom he and the student cannot see, and yet whom he nonetheless "believes" is real. It will go unnoticed that in "reality" he probably has no one "real" to talk to, or at least no one caring who is worth listening to. The next might be the young adult liberated from an unenforced law against drug consumption by an overworked and nihilistic police force. He is high on methamphetamine, aggressive and speaking quickly and incoherently as he shifts in the chair and threatens to harm someone if he is not permitted to leave the locked ward to smoke. His aggression is 8 parts mania and 2 parts smokers craving? Or is it 2 parts mania and 8 parts smokers craving? Or is it a mix of the above with 8 parts deficiencies of character? Or is it 10 parts methamphetamine? Who can say? The next patient will be the straight faced person who tells you they are the God of Egypt and will order the CIA to execute the psychiatrist who does not release them from hospital now (they will of course not be able tell you what the acronym of the C.I.A stands for or why the God of Egypt does not use the Egyptian Secret Police, let alone be able to speak any ancient tongue).

For the medical student, this sort of thing can be quite confronting. For whomever has eyes to see can doubt these patients are disturbed and alien to normality, even vulnerable and unable to function in the world as it is unless aided by others who care. Who ought to care and how they ought to care is part of the subject of this book, for nigh on a couple centuries now care for these persons has uncritically accepted to be under the purview of medicine in general, and what has become known as psychiatry in particular. Even if our student vows to steer clear as much as is possible from psychiatry in their future career, I would submit to the reader that it is on the basis of this very confrontation with the greatly disturbed "other" that the medical student has cemented an uncritical acceptance of all they are told thereafter on the matter of madness and misery by their psychiatric masters. They never then will ask what makes the supposedly psychotic unfounded belief different from the supposedly non-psychotic unfounded belief vs a single spectrum with arbitrary differentiation of the normal from the pathological, or why from the meeting point between vulnerability and compassion towards another must flow compulsion towards involuntary hospitalization and treatment. They don't dare ask nor think to ask the extent to which the psychiatrists own psychological need to perceive themselves as a real doctor influences what they espouse to be true of the person and the world. The student might never ask if criteria for diagnoses is an exercise in carving nature at the joints (to quote Plato) as opposed to being a contrivance no better than a taxonomy of mythical creatures or the zodiac...and so on and so forth many more questions besides are never asked or asked rhetorically, for they have already accepted the answer psychiatry has readily available. A great number of non sequiturs that ought to be in view immediately vanish before they are even brought into focus in the presence of this great otherness of madness and misery. The uncritical turn towards faith is the same for the medical student (or junior doctor) who then decides to return to the same psychiatric ward later as a resident/registrar in the high church of psychiatry. Paradoxically it might be the inkling of the unsolved questions, the mystery that drives them inwards nonetheless. This want to sate the unconscious is a mistake, for psychiatry will constrain the horizon of acceptable answers before the questions are asked. It will invite the philosophically curious cat, and then proceed to kill it and proclaim it to be well all the same. But then of course the apprentice psychiatrist is too far from the shore of what they might have thought to question to swim back without drowning in the mistakes they have wrought on themselves and others in the diagnostic labels they too ascribe, the medications given to be imbibed and the deprivations of liberty prescribed. The junior apprentice has already detained people many a time against their will for treatment they do not want and who protest diagnoses they do not assent to. Who could then look back and call this deprivation of liberty monstrous, for to do so would be to risk calling oneself a monster. They have already put hours of study into "diseases" or "disorders" and "neurochemical circuits" that as explanandum of the psychological world exist more in the textbooks than in the world, or not in the world at all except so far as the textbooks project them outwards onto the person. Who could take this time invested and then easily admit it to have been futile to the cause of knowing what actually "is" in the world that is the person sitting across from them. Hubris and certitude are defence mechanisms one might say, though defence mechanisms are a mirror that cannot be ascribed to patient and physician both simultaneously. Often only the latter is educated enough to assiduously avoid self accusation, ironically without any conscious realization of their double standard. Freud after all would see a cigar as a phallic symbol, but sometimes a cigar is a cigar, especially when it was in his hand. Having mastered the psychiatric projection onto the world, the psychiatric trainee is too far from the great works of literature and the humanities they likely never read at all or at least not deeply, literature that might have provided a different more illuminating view of the human condition. They have given themselves over to the grace of a special kind of human indoctrination towards a special kind of secular priesthood. Welcome to seminary.

But I wish not to mix my metaphors too much here, and certainly not to the point of contradiction. To be sure I see the psychiatrist as a secular priest of a kind. To the end of convincing you of this fact I will provide evidence aplenty in the chapters to follow. Yet all the above talk of algorithm in medicine and psychiatry leads one to something perhaps more sinister, that being the mechanization of humanity. You see when the patient is situated upon the algorithm the patient ascends to the realm of abstraction and ceases to be as a human being. This is not to imply the malady in psychiatry is the misplaced primacy of the biological over the psychological, or a lack of kindness or apprehension of the pathos in the heart and mind of the psychiatrist. Heaven forbid I suggest anything so banal. What I am suggesting is that looking upon the patient as an object situated upon an algorithm or a bookmark to be placed in the appropriate page of the DSM is a red herring for the concerns of the humanities in psychiatry (or medicine in general for that matter). For what is assumed not to be lost, this assumption being entirely false, is that the psychiatrist has themselves retained their humanity. You see when the psychiatrist sees you as an object of a flow chart they must first have taken into themselves the being of "flowchartedness", of "differential diagnosis", of DSM and all that makes for the method. Having identified on too deep a level with their method, they are like Heidegger's carpenter where the hammer is ready at hand, and indeed the hammer is an extension of himself, and he of it. And the method of squashing humanity out of psychiatry is an essential part of psychiatry itself, for how can it be otherwise. The method being what it is, without it psychiatry would cease to be. Even the psychiatrist cannot escape the technocratic method of approaching the person, for the method sits "meta" to he (or she), in the body of knowledge and the bureaucratic imperative for how the patient is processed through their own mind just as their body is processed through the hospital. These metastructures, like Adam Smith's unseen hand of capitalism, take on a life of their own that in turn reflexively sets to mould both the psychiatrist and patient alike. The imperatives are efficiency, comprehensive "mental health assessment" and documentation, "risk assessment" and risk minimization, accurate diagnosis according to the accepted nosology and so on. Each one of these is a place upon which the patient is situated. And then the psychiatrist feeds the method and bureaucracy in its insatiable need to consolidate and expand itself, to sustain its own lifeless being. And in each and every psychiatric transaction there is nothing but method as far as the eye can see. Unless one is inoculated by a congenital hatred of it, one fails to see technocratic slavery save in such examples where the method approaches absurdity. Take for example the adolescent in state care. He is wilful and violent, this in some way related to adverse events of early childhood, chiefly being witness to violence from adult others. It does not take a genius to recognize the developmental connection which is its own explanation. And his supposedly psychologically trained residential care workers follow their method when he is violent, the method as directed by their own cognitive schemata and the directive of their hierarchy.

They call the police or paramedics, for he requires a mental health assessment, or so says their method. And the police or paramedics dutifully respond, bringing him against his will to the hospital with the powers invested in them by the state and its mental health legislation. Their motive and orders too are the same. And all look to the psychiatrist to "assess". What is the diagnosis, this is one question? What is the risk is another question? What might the treatment be for this condition is yet another question as the adolescent is placed upon the assessment machine? The answer, alien as it may seem to some readers, is no answer at all. The child is badly behaving. There is nothing to explain that has not been already. There might be corrective action in order, likely not to be successful in his march towards criminality yet not to be considered "treatment" in any sane world inhabited by those who have retained their humanity and good sense. Yet these simple answers simply do not compute. All involved, from the emergency physicians to the police to the care workers look doe eyed and baffled when I say there is nothing to be explained that is not known to any competent adult, and no recipe to a remedy that is medical and not the analogue of good parenting. But what is the "diagnosis" and how might we treat it? What psychological therapy will "change him"? Let's talk medication another says. Good sense falls on deaf ears. The child settles. Most hot heads do. And he returns back to their care. And later that week he returns again under similar circumstances, the action activated by the method, and returns twice more the following week, and three time more the next. The humans who behave like stupid robots act reflexively. The questions are the same. The assessment is demanded by the method. My (non) answers are the same, as I refuse answer as an agent of the psychiatric machine. The failure to compute is thoroughly recalcitrant to good sense, for the person has given themselves, their mind, their individuality, their good sense, all given over to method. And on goes the circus. Even to negate the method by appeal to personal psychiatric authority as opposed to good sense of an adult human being is itself to fall victim of the subtly of the technocratic machine. There is no escaping it save to escape psychiatry. So yes welcome to seminary. Yet welcome also to the machine of what a technocratic psychiatry has wrought on the world. Only the joke is on you, for if you enter into psychiatry the machine is you.

ONTOLOGY. THE KEEPER OF THE KEYS.

"When we cannot be delivered from ourselves, we delight in devouring ourselves. In vain we call upon the Lord of Shades, the bestower of a precise curse: we are invalids without disease, and reprobates without vices"
E. M. Cioran

What is a psychiatrist?

The UK Royal College of Psychiatrists website "What is psychiatry?" offers a rather laconic description, prompting the question of the boundary between what is a mental health condition and what isn't. Whatever they say it is I guess.

"Psychiatry is a branch of medicine dealing with people with a huge range of mental health conditions. As a psychiatrist you'll help people to manage, treat or recover from these."

The United States American Psychiatric Association, "What is psychiatry?" provides a longer, yet altogether equally prosaic definition. They say...

"Psychiatry is the branch of medicine focused on the diagnosis, treatment and prevention of mental, emotional and behavioural disorders. A psychiatrist is a medical doctor (an M.D. or D.O.) who specializes in mental health, including substance use disorders. Psychiatrists are qualified to assess both the mental and physical aspects of psychological problems. People seek psychiatric help for many reasons. The problems can be sudden, such as a panic attack, frightening hallucinations, thoughts of suicide, or hearing "voices." Or they may be more long-term, such as feelings of sadness, hopelessness, or anxiousness that never seem to lift or problems functioning, causing everyday life to feel distorted or out of control."

The US guilds definition is equally provocative of questions. An emotion is not a behaviour granted. Yet is an emotion not something "mental"? Are substance use disorders a matter of mental health, or the product of choice? And in what sense is substance use a "disorder"? Is disorder "a thing" in the sense that cancer is a thing? And when I was going to school "anxiousness" was not a real word. My how things change when psychiatry is the lexicographer.

In Oceania the Royal Australian and New Zealand College of Psychiatrists define the psychiatrist thus

"Psychiatrists are medical doctors who are experts in mental health. They specialise in diagnosing and treating people with mental illness. Psychiatrists have a deep understanding of physical and mental health – and how they affect each other. They help people with mental health conditions such as schizophrenia, depression, bipolar disorder, eating disorders and addiction."

The Royal Australian and New Zealand College of Psychiatrists at least makes an attempt at something more, succeeding at defining a psychiatrist in obviously narcissistic terms, explicitly confident in being internal medicine physicians ("deep understanding" of physical health), and having solved the mind body problem ("how they affect each other"). Most disturbing at all is the claim that psychiatrists are experts at mental health. Do they really know what health of mind is, and by extension what it is to be a healthy person? No. Even the great philosophers wrestled upon the question of what it is to be and the life well lived. Turns of phrase betray deeper meanings and motivations. In my experience it is said all the time, "the patient has no mental health history", which is to say they have no history until the present of being mentally unhealthy. Or put another way, they have no history of involvement with mental health, i.e. psychiatry. There is no paradox. Mental Health is semantically an antonym for mental illness. Mental health is practically speaking, a synonym for mental illness, or the institution of psychiatry.

All these definitions are, in petitio principii, assuming to know what mind is, the existence of what they say is mental illness and these illnesses (plural) being what they say they are (i.e. a question of construct validity), along with the psychiatrist's rightful place in the world as ministers to the mind (a political question). The Americans, though not as narcissistic as Oceania (on this occasion anyway), nonetheless metastasize out of the hospital in suggesting that the psychiatrist is even the specialist over problems that impact upon "everyday life", without at least speculating on the possibility that problems of everyday life are sometimes the problems causing (not impacting, but causing) the symptoms themselves. This is to say the so called mental illness is, at least sometimes, American everyday life itself, and what passes for the symptoms of the illness are epiphenomenon. Is this not self-evidently obvious in an Anglo speaking world of relative morality, undermining of personal responsibility, destruction of family and community, wage slavery and a popular psychology that for decades has been all about the "me", myself and "looking after number 1"? And what totalitarian havoc can be made from taking that tiny step from declaring oneself master over the impact from the problem of daily life to declaring it the business of psychiatry to be master over the problem of daily life causing the impact. The Americans are at least honest in using the word "qualified", for to be qualified is what psychiatry is all about. True enough they are correct definitions in the sense that a psychiatrist must be a medical doctor first, or at least to have completed medical school before they embark on a radically fast unlearning of all medicine inferior to the neck and outside of what is between the ears (and forget much of what is between the ears also, i.e. neurology). What all these definitions lack is the real sine qua non of the psychiatrist, what actually sets them apart from other doctors, and by extension with every other individual within their jurisdiction (and I use the word jurisdiction deliberately as we shall see). Any common or garden variety doctor can take a special interest in the mind and what passes for "mental illness", or mental health for that matter. Not every advanced western country even requires a single exam be sat in order to be annointed as a psychiatrist, though all of the examples in the Anglo speaking world do. Historically not requiring exams outside of medical school was even more universal, and not too long ago at that. After all, a psychiatrist was historically simply the doctor who was the warden of the asylum, otherwise known as an alienist. And so specialization is a term wanting of elaboration of the necessary and the sufficient factors and historical context. What it means in the case of 21st century psychiatry, whether in free market USA or in the semi socialist health systems of Australia, Canada and the UK, what really sets psychiatry apart, is simply this; the psychiatrist is a doctor who, in virtue of a the tripartite collusion between the state (i.e. government, particularly the legislature who in part defers to a registration body), a registration body (who defers to the guild), and a professional guild (who defers to themselves as a law onto themselves) is given a qualification that invests them with the legal right to practice independently (i.e. unsupervised) in the community and the legal right to authorize involuntary detention and forced drugging of the person who they assert requires it for reasons of "mental illness". And the terms of the argument the psychiatrist offers in favour of the deprivation of liberty viz a viz mental illness are set by the very profession and guild who exercises power. To have this authority is to be a psychiatrist. To be a psychiatrist is to have this authority. Other doctors can treat without consent the delirious, elderly with dementia and younger children without any involvement of psychiatry, this hardly being controversial. And other doctors may be able detain and treat a patient thought to be "mentally ill". Yet this is only for very limited periods of time, usually as an interim measure awaiting psychiatric evaluation. As such these other doctors' authority to detain is psychiatry res extensa. Some jurisdictions even have it instantiated into law that the garden variety doctor can only exercise powers to detain for mental health reasons under the promise that psychiatric evaluation will be available and forthcoming. The final say is always had by the psychiatrist or necessarily involves a psychiatrist as the key informant in whatever legal panels where a member of the judiciary notionally decides the person's fate. So you see that no one has the power to detain another for reasons of mental illness if the profession of psychiatry were to cease to be. The necessary criteria towards psychiatry is medical school. The necessary criteria in being a psychiatrist is to the authority to wield a kind of power which is underwritten by the philosophy and advice of the very guild of practitioners that wield it, and anoint the apprentice to be granted the power of the master. This is not to say, or not yet even to ask, how a psychiatrist morally ought to wield such power and if they are doing so correctly. Nor is this to channel (a reading of) Foucault and imply that power politics rule the world to the exclusion of all else. It is to simply say that it is power that defines the limit of the boundary between psychiatrists and all others who might consider themselves practitioners of, or in the case of the patient, objects within, the so called mental health system or medicine. Why is this profession specific capacity to exercise such a powerful authority over person's liberties not explicitly mentioned in any definition from any of the guilds themselves? Not a single one! I can only conclude from this either unconscious or deliberate desire to dissimulate the truth under cover of talk of helping and treating, or care and cure, of expertise and illogical talk of health when they mean illness. What do they fear by declaring their power? Personal embarrassment or public reaction at the implication?

Writing of psychiatrists as specialist doctors who practice mental health is like speaking of priests as being specialist choir boys with an interest in theology who also like to "help" people. The word help is used in each of the three above mentioned definitions, contra the fact that many patients do not wish to be helped and run across jurisdictional borders to avoid it. Is help not at least potentially something subjective and defined by the one who is being helped? Just as a priest is better defined as the one ordained by a select guild to have the sole power to administer the sacraments, the secular priest could also be defined on the basis of the power he/she wields, and much more so given there is no transcendent authority above the psychiatric guild as there may well be above the priesthood, this transcendence being something that redefines the priest in turn. Would it not be more honest for these professional guilds to state something such as....

"Psychiatrists are that species of medical doctors, who, in virtue of a collusion between the professional guild and the state, have the sole authority to bill certain items to the tax payer and/or insurance companies, work unsupervised in the so called free market, and lock you up +/- administer medication against your will when they believe it is suitable on the basis of a criteria designed by the very same bodies who create the psychiatrist in the first place. Psychiatrists have the additional authority to make themselves immune from challenge in the court of science and argument as guild members control the journals, the narrative and the standard of practice against which both malpractice and the notion of mental illness are measured"

All the above being granted, one might say that psychiatrists are defined by not merely what they are as agents of power, yet also by what they do in practice as specialists of their craft. This would be problematic. Allow me to explain.

Give one hundred orthopaedists the same fracture and one will get one hundred doctors diagnosing the same pathology, doing more or less and with varying surgical skill much the same thing. Being surgeons, they will even all agree that they personally (i.e. individually) did the superior job. Part of the challenge in providing the answer of what a psychiatrist is in being and in praxis lay in the fact that psychiatry is by far and away the most internally heterogeneous of the specialities in which a doctor may find his/her vocation. (note I do not call it a medical speciality per se, for such would be counter to the thesis that psychiatry is historically and conceptually something of a secular priesthood masquerading as medicine, science and art). The psychiatrist is well aware of this heterogeneity. When challenged, rather than feel anxious they will psycho-defensively reframe their castles built on shifting sand as a badge of honour, saying if one is too "linear and "black and white" one ought to become a surgeon. To properly do justice to just how internally heterogeneous would easily occupy several hundred pages. Herein will be two examples, with a preface to the first.

Unlike every other speciality there is a vast gulf between how public and private psychiatric practitioners diagnose and treat. This is even if the same practitioner works in both sectors, being public hospital one day and private practitioner the other. The differences within psychiatry dwarfs the closest other point of comparison, that of obstetrics wherein private (i.e. small business or large business private hospital) practitioners will often see a dire need for caesarean section more than their public hospital counterparts were they to see the same patient at the same time, and certainly more so than their nemesis nurse midwives would think necessary. Notwithstanding patient preference, the cynic would say this is in virtue of the Caesarean section being more lucrative in private land than that of an old fashioned vaginal birth. In the public system the obstetrician is paid the same regardless of how the newborn enters into the world, so why risk anything under the scalpel?

Returning to psychiatry, take for example this hypothetical case; the young woman named Amburr attends the psychiatrist (funky names and spelling are almost diagnostic). She is emotionally troubled and feels herself to be out of control, causing distortion in her everyday life as the American guild would say. That is to say she is open to abdicating personal responsibility from her actions in the word play of being "out of control" and requiring a locus of control to be placed with the psychiatrist. The psychiatrist asks questions. Do you have a family history of mental illness? Yes, Aunty Bertha was manic depressive (the psychiatrist immediately considers her genetically at risk of the same, and it will be difficult to escape this diagnosis sooner or later given such genetic "loading"). Do they have mood swings, sometimes this lasting days of highs and days of lows? Yes. Do they sometimes have abundant energy and drive, sometimes lacking the same? Yes. Do they spend too much money or engage in promiscuous sex that is out of character, i.e. that they later regret when the chickens come home to roost or behaviours they want you to believe they regret? Yes. Do they sometimes have difficulty focusing and others tell them they flit from one subject to another, sometimes even thinking at an accelerated rate? Yes. Do they sometimes feel like they are on top of the world and can do anything, not literally anything as in leaping over tall buildings with a single bound, not to the point of taking leave of their senses and reality (whatever reality is, please tell me if you find out). No. Just enough of a high mood to have been significantly elated and long to be back there? Yes. And so more than enough of the boxes are ticked. It does not take much more for the psychiatrist to diagnose the patient with type II bipolar disorder, or what might have otherwise been called mild manic depression had the DSM decided to invent a new construct whilst keeping the Kraepelian name "manic depression". Mild mania, which is pathognomonic of type II bipolar disorder, is called "hypomania", a kind of state of being almost yet not quite insane of an elevated mood. What causes it? The psychiatrist will say it's a brain disease of course, albeit a poorly understood one. This is code for there being no evidence of it being a brain disease whatsoever. They will say it's genetic within an environmental context of events "triggering" of episodes, invoking automatically within the unconscious the vision of victimhood, for who pulled the trigger? "Surely not I". Consequently, in one stroke and though not explicitly stated, the secular priest will absolve them of the sins of excessive spending and excessive sexing, of impatience and verbal abusiveness and many more besides. This is a pastiche of priesthood; confession and absolution, passing through a muddled dualism. For the sinner is the disordered brain and its fallen nature, perhaps even the "sin" is in, though not of, the father (or mother) and their genes of mental illness. "I cannot be responsible can I, having been dealt the genetic hand" they might say. And so the absolver is not only the priest psychiatrist, yet also the patient themselves. This is to say in the absence of God, the ultimate source of absolution is the ritual between the psychiatrist (qua priest object) and the patient as collectively one agent, the other object being the brain without responsibility as the sinner who never need suffer pain of conscience. In point of fact, no one need suffer pain of conscience. Even substance use will not be seen as co-causative of the problem or heaven forbid a personal choice to befuddle one's mind. Instead substance use will be framed as a result of the mental illness itself driving them to use. Their only act of penance will be to take valproate, lithium or quetiapine or some other powerful psychotropic medication that is touted by the pharma representatives (we must not be too harsh with pharmaceutical representatives, see elsewhere). Inevitably all these drugs will have a partial effect, insomuch as they all have non-specific sedative and emotionally blunting actions, leaving alone for now the actor that stands on every pharmacological stage, i.e. placebo. But these drugs will not effect any cure. Whatever it is, the basic fault will still be working its way within the psyche, likely created in childhood and cultivated by choices each day of what one wishes to be and become. There will be regular reviews and tinkering with the medication, as the psychiatrist leans over the caldron and adds a sprinkle of this, a pinch of that. There will be further confessions and absolutions under the heading of "psychoeducation", and "relapse prevention" or exploration of "early warning signs". And there will be a steady stream of income for the practitioner. Psychotherapy, the so called talking cure, will only ever be suggested as a method to manage the psychological consequences of the burden of the illness itself, not as a remedy suited for addressing the illness directly as a psychological thing in and of itself.

Likely the psychiatrist will outsource the therapy to a psychologist. The vast majority of psychiatrists do the ever decreasing bare minimum of psychotherapy during their training, and do as little as possible afterwards.

Now let's look at the same young lady from a different angle. Perhaps since her teens and perhaps before she had difficulty keeping a reign on her emotions. Like a cork bobbing up and down in a sea of (usually relational) events without any internal ballast, she is "out of control". When things go well her mood sits high upon the crest of a wave. When things go poorly her mood falls below the horizon, and cannot see the sun afar. Sometimes paradoxically when things go well her mood is low, perhaps out of fear the good times won't last, which of course in life they never.....ever....do! In virtue of her dissatisfaction with herself and her lot there may always be a tendency for the mood to drift down, and likely she will have been diagnosed with a 'major depression" before. Often this "depression" is stated to be a harbinger of the hypomania to come in cases of alleged bipolar disorder, with bipolar disorder a justification for why the antidepressants did not work (no doubt is cast upon the antidepressants themselves, or the veracity of the diagnosis). She may or may not have been sexually or physically abused or neglected as a child, this being arguably more likely than not, yet far from being universal as is often assumed. Often somewhere in her upbringing there was at least some loss or lack of even what Winnicott would call "good enough parenting", for perfect perfecting never exists and were it to exist would be paradoxically bad parenting in ill preparing the perfectly coddled child for a fallen imperfect world. This basic psycho-developmental fault can come in infinite forms; The parents broke up or were never together, ergo the perceived rejection from one or both (though this being at odds with the politically correct notion that broken homes and single parent homes are necessarily equivalent, my extensive experience would suggest exactly the opposite and the solo parent to face an uphill battle, often to their credit against the odds crafting the well-adjusted child), the perceived rejection of peers might have occurred, there is the parent who hovered too much or hovered at the wrong time and for the parents own reasons, the parent too busy nestling the cannabis bong in their arms as opposed to the child to their bosom. Perhaps the child did not see mirrored in the parents face and heart how and when to be emotionally calm, and when to delay gratification and how and when to delay it. And so on and so forth. The possibilities are as endless as the list of twentieth century theorists and experimental psychologists who did the work giving us all the hypotheses we might map onto this particular person who is Amburr. Yet we mustn't take up torches and pitchforks and go on the witch hunt for bad parents. Sometimes the parents were perfectly adequate, did their best and the child simply had the misfortune to be born with an insecure temperament or was not insulated enough from media that makes a mockery of parental authority, basic morality and dismantles any message promoting self-control. Life neither guarantees perfect parents or perfect children. In any case, there is something to be lacking in the psyche of the young lady of our example (or young man also), some emptiness looking to be filled. And sometimes it will be filled in its turn. Perhaps a new love or hope or love will enter the scene, as the patient reaches out in irresponsible and often dangerous ways. There is no medication as powerful as infatuation. This will be a time of "high". Perhaps the "high" follows from simply boredom with being down in the dumps and loathing of the self, the psyche finding time in prison served and time now to throw off the shackles of the superego enough for a little happiness and gay abandon (there's the "hypomania"). Yet the good times do not last long before doubts and self sabotage creep in. Then back we are in a morass of unhappiness and angst. Or she meets the love interest, soon feels comfortable, then just as soon doubts creep in, acting dramatically as if to hurt the other and force them to prove their love is unconditional, a comfort left wanting from the absent bosom that was her childhood. The object of her affections might weather the storm and his/her apparent reciprocation of love (or lust) might persist long enough for our insecure patient to feel comfortable again. Yet this sense of comfort is not to endure for long. And so the sadomasochistic like cycle repeats, often with some quasi sadomasochism from the love interest, for they often have their own psychological issues. When things go well there might be promiscuity and intemperance of all kind, including mood altering substances, the use of which may or may not be confessed and which certainly causatively upsets the psychological apple cart all the more. When things go poorly the mood will be lower, with or without thoughts of self harm. The reader will note this is the same patient as the first, with identical boxes checked. Only in the latter case with a different psychiatrist she is diagnosed instead with borderline personality disorder (DSM), otherwise known as emotionally unstable personality disorder (ICD).

Both diagnoses, i.e. type II bipolar disorder vs borderline personality cannot be simultaneously correct, for they rest upon entirely different theoretical substructures of aetiology and "pathogenesis", though there is a growing vanguard of psychiatrists incoherently attempting to meld them as one "bipolar spectrum". Regarding my own experience, I'd be on safer rhetorical ground to say something like "most patients I have seen fit much better the latter formulation", i.e. borderline personality disorder, in so doing appearing to be a little more conciliatory, a little less extreme. Yet the truth is that after having seen literally hundreds of (usually female) patients diagnosed as type II bipolar by (usually private practicing) psychiatrists, I have yet to see a single one who is not personality disordered as a crystal clear complete explanation of the case. Not a single one!

I have even seen many dozens of patients falsely diagnosed by many a psychiatrist with the full enchilada of type I bipolar disorder, i.e. that subtype of bipolar disorder (manic depression), where the upward swing of mood renders the person insane and needing hospital admission or urgent intervention, i.e. a full mania. Or so the diagnostic criteria in the bible (sorry DSM 5) would require of me to make the diagnosis. One recent case of many comes to mind where it was uncanny how the mania always occurred when the husband was cheating on his wife, sexting his mistress dozens of times a night and driving recklessly enough to attract the ire of the police. It was truly remarkable how his mania, or depression, would switch off the moment his wife forgave him or the psychiatrist arranged a letter of support for his crime of reckless driving, absolving him of his sins. I guess one could marvel at the power of love and compassion or advocacy or "stress" have been taken off his shoulders. I would marvel at the mendacity on the part of the patient, and fraud (or stupidity) on the part of the psychiatrist.

Or there are the cases where, as a trainee, the patient would sit across from both myself and the supervising psychiatrist, the patient narrating with modulated (non manic) speech and tempo of thought how their "bipolar was acting up". And so there lay the attribution for the hefty bill received by the credit card company when they spent too much. The psychiatrist would agree their bipolar made them do it. If push came to shove the debt would climb and the psychiatrist would write a support letter in an attempt to absolve the person of their debt, or an application for state (i.e. tax payer funded) assistance with an invalid pension. Some would call this compassion and patient advocacy. Some might also call this fraud.

I ask the reader to forestall from concluding that I don't believe bipolar disorder exists at all. Putting aside for now the far more interesting question of what it is for any psychiatric diagnosis to "exist", I've been convinced of about a few dozen cases of type I bipolar disorder over the years, where to be "convinced" means a certain level of comfort with applying the construct of type I bipolar disorder to the patient, not to be convinced of any greater ontological truths about the construct itself as a brain disease. These few dozen patients are extremely low numbers as a proportion of population, far below the rate at which a sizable fraction of contemporary psychiatrists diagnose bipolar disorder and far below what the guild intelligentsia state is its prevalence (i.e. its commonality in the community).

But enough of digressions from the point, for these examples are mere illustrations. The point for now is not what "exists" of bipolarity in the world (for this is but an example), but what "exists" in psychiatry in the world, what psychiatry can claim to know, and what psychiatry does. Plenty of my colleagues are uncritical true believers in type II bipolar disorder and see hypomania (if not mania) and mixed mood episodes everywhere they look. And plenty of my colleagues conversely also cast a jaundiced eye on the construct that is type II bipolar disorder and the supposed commonality of type I bipolar disorder. In conversations with colleagues, some of those disbelievers privately admit to using the diagnosis as something to work with, as a pragmatic metaphor to offer the patient who is looking for the comfort of a label, without disclosing to the patient that they lack the faith in the diagnosis themselves. It follows that the patients are not always fully complicit with this benevolent little white lie (actually another fraud), whilst the practitioner is wantonly ignorant of the fact that diagnoses have consequences, these rippling far and wide beyond the immediate comfort of the label to the patient. When I have been bold enough to challenge patients on what they call their "bipolar acting up" when it is obviously their characterological deficiencies acting out, I often get more of an inkling they know the truth beyond the lie, and so their previous psychiatrists (if they are not the more common true believer) have been lying to them and vice versa.

Were the construct of type II bipolar disorder ever to be revealed or discovered to be the fiction that it is, I have no doubt mainstream psychiatry would dodge embarrassment by rewriting its own history, with unanimous claim that the expert class as a whole knew the truth all along, with a couple scapegoats thrown under the bus along the way and only ever if absolutely necessary. Overdiagnosis by psychologists and family/general practitioners will do as a nice scapegoat. The guilds of psychiatric story-tellers are as skilled at managing historiography as they are lacking skill at managing what was once called hysteria. Yet from a patient's perspective, never will you see a jaundiced eyed psychiatrist tell a patient the colleague who previously made the diagnosis was just plain wrong or likely lying. A diplomatic psychiatrist seeking to revise a diagnosis might go so far as to say something akin to diagnoses being a work in progress evolving over time, which is actually to say the truth can be x yesterday, y today, and z tomorrow, a convenient timelessness where there is no "now" in which to capture and indict the psychiatrist as being wrong or mendacious. This is like Parmenides by the river into which he can never step twice. Nothing ever is the case and everything always is the case in such a state of flux where a diagnosis is never allowed solidify. Conflicts over diagnostic constructs or applications of these to individuals never ever see our secular priests defrocked or schisms within our secular church, unless the church is absolutely forced to. Internal dissent within the guilds is castrated of any real gravitas in the first instance, and smooth on the surface to all outside observers. As several psychiatrists have said to me, the greatest imperative is "we must not bring the profession into disrepute". Why not? This is a question they never ask never ask and the answer is never provided, for protecting the profession is axiomatic. It is canon.

So far in our journey I might have succeeded in taking the reader into a state of scepticism with type II bipolar disorder as the appropriate diagnosis, or a diagnosis that exists at all as opposed to borderline personality disorder being the authentic diagnosis that "exists". But let's take things further, for we haven't escaped the DSM and psychiatry just yet, as opposed to simply flipping pages. Let us speculate on what the core of borderline psychopathology might be, or type II bipolar disorder if we choose to check its boxes (the patient may also check the boxes for ADHD and dysthymia, or cyclothymia and a dozen other diagnoses very easily). Without elaboration, nor me being fixed on this speculation to follow as anything more than speculation through and through (which is to say not a fixedness to what we might call attachment theory, and explicitly I say not to devalue the role of what we might call "trauma", for many of these patients have had horrible upbringings), let us imagine the core problem in borderline personality or emotional instability is something we might simply call unfinished business of childhood. The infant is most certainly and justifiably insecure. And as any parent well knows, the child can behave in a dramatic way to attract and sustain love, connection, reassurance and nurturance. Now let us imagine this insecurity scaled up to one in whom it can be said has reached the legal age of majority, i.e. an alleged adult. When faced with threats to perceived security, loss of love, a painful memory or a million other speculative "triggers", there may be a drive to drama within the psyche. In the sense of which certain hot headed shallow males might act out their insecurities with bullying others, lusting after things they must steal to "own", and wanting to acquire security by dominance, they might add to the suicidal ideation some intimidation and beating upon others. And like an infant, their capacity for authentic empathy may be fragmentary or absent. Ergo with the same basic fault, the same insecurity and immaturity, this young man may be diagnosed as having an antisocial personality disorder when what he really has is a borderline character. On the other hand the young woman who usually introjects (that is inwardly directs and quasi identifies with) her insecurity is taken to acts of self cutting and self loathing, relational manipulations and marshalling around her others anxious to help and anxious to save, these others made all the more anxious by her distress (curiously often the two sit in inverse proportion to one another over the course of the psychotherapeutic transaction, as if to imply a transfer of neurosis from patient to the therapist or parent. The unsaid exchange is "when I have given you my problem, it is no longer my own"). We tacitly ignore the fact that she may have harassed and repeatedly texted the love interest, and stated to the clinician that if he/she does not save her from herself the suicidal blood would be on the psychiatrists hands. Can this be thought of as anything other than antisocial behaviour of a kind? The reader should see where I am heading, towards the question if what we usually diagnose as borderline in females and antisocial in males is but a product of sexism, with the core often, yet not always, the same. Yet the approach normally taken, the meaning in practice when drawings the boundaries between these "disorders", is vastly different.

Now we have diffused outwards, from a justified insecurity of a different kind, i.e. a diagnostic and conceptual blurring between bipolar disorder and between and within two discrete kinds of personality disorder. Let's not stop there, for there are many other personality disorders besides. The lay reader may not be acquainted with the idea of "clusters" of personality disorders, as is still dominant in the DSM. Borderline and antisocial personalities fall within the so called "cluster B" personality disorders, along with narcissistic and histrionic personality (the other clusters are cluster A; paranoid, schizoid and schizotypal personality, and cluster C, dependent, avoidant and obsessional personality). Let's imagine a different core problem, one that exists within the person just as strongly as undefined insecurity or a tendency to being a hybrid adult-infant emotional soup with unfinished business of childhood. Let's imagine that all cluster B personality disorders are different manifestations of the same core, i.e. narcissism itself. In the case of the pure narcissistic personality disorder, the narcissism is directed to the ego or self as self, which is to say "I am superior and I'd like you to accept this fact". In the case of the histrionic personality the narcissism is directed towards a specific kind of outward behaviour, one of shallow embellishment and being the centre of attention, which is to say "be I better or worse, it is all about me. Look at me". In the case of the borderline personality the narcissism is directed towards one's immediate emotional perceived needs and one's own emotional pain at the expense of everyone else "it's 2am in the morning but you all be damned I'll kill myself if you don't admit me to hospital, the blood is on your hands. No one's pain is as important as mine. My pain is my world. My pain is the world". Then there is the antisocial personality, whose narcissism is directed towards having and doing whatever they want, and damn the rules and social harmony "I do what I want, when I want, to whoever I want". I have not even considered how other times and cultures may formulate peoples behaviours, all of which are as plausible as that offered by the best of psychiatrists. In any case, is a person's character the business of medicine? This is very strange.

One final example, moving from infantile adults to child and adolescent psychiatry per se. Into the consulting rooms comes the 10 year old boy Jaxxson, his concerned mother and his latest off several stepfathers. He has been irritable lately and stating in various ways and forms that he is unhappy. Perhaps by the side table upon which sits his enticing smartphone is the bed where he has a troubled sleep. Perhaps his appetite is reduced. Never excellent, his grades have slipped and his teachers are noticing some conflict with peers and the teachers themselves (always the royal road to mental illness is being a nuisance to others and embarrassed parents searching for an excuse). He might have even become anxious at the prospect of going to school, the last few weeks playing video games instead of attending to studies. Things may have come to a head when he started talking about death and drawing himself in the stick figure way a 10 year old draws himself as hanging from a tree. Various shades and permutations of cases such as this are typical and we need not dissect this hypothetical example, missing the forest for the trees. It does not matter really whether the child is 8, 10 or 12, boy or girl, white or black, rich or poor.

Let us imagine a multiverse. Exactly the same child presents on exactly the same day and says exactly the same thing to exactly the same questions to 5 different child psychiatrists, only in each of 5 different universes. The psychiatrist observes the interactions with the family, speaks to the mother/stepfather alone also and consequently takes the history and examines the mental state.

Child psychiatrist number 1 might formulate the case thus; the child is weighed down by a major depressive episode. At the hands of a sufficiently skilled sophist psychiatrist, major depression in everyone is quite a protean construct when attached to a person to whom we might say is "unhappy". But it's malleability is especially the case in that of children and the aged. As one can see in that enormously successful best seller of fiction that is the DSM, a child need not be depressed in mood to be depressed for reasons of diagnosis. They can merely be irritable, for somehow it is thought depression only then appears as depression. His lack of recent success in school is seen to be a product of the cognitive deficits that are part and parcel of the depressive illness. Similarly, his recent lack of hearty eating and the difficulty falling asleep are "neuro-vegetative dysfunctions" of the illness. These add to the diagnostic criteria in our checking of the boxes, and given the "neuro" prefix by extension taken automatically (though it is a non sequitur and semantic play) that the depression is a biological disease. Suicidal thoughts check another box. Psychiatrist number 1 may explain to parent and child alike that there is some brain mechanism for the depression and the remedy is, principally and in principle, an "antidepressant". There are no shortages of first and second degree relatives also having been diagnosed with a mental illness. Up to a third or more of the females on both sides of the biological tree had been diagnosed with depression and/or bipolar disorder. This lubricates the mind of the psychiatrist into immediately assuming genetic vulnerability, and each generation the likelihood of diagnosis is made greater from the labels applied to those of the past. Like a pebble against the gravitational power of the sun, I have seen thousands of patients drawn into an almost inescapable orbit of attracting some diagnosis or another simply on the basis of what their parents, grandparents and Aunts and Uncles have been diagnosed (or diagnosed themselves) with. I guess in Salem witches had family too, and God help the family of the alleged witch if the diagnosis is made more probable by the idea of it being "genetic". And so the script is written, the money exchanged and the subsequent appointment booked. And the show goes on.

Child psychiatrist 2 formulates the case thus; the child has developed an anxiety disorder. Anxiety is the kissing cousin of fear. When we are afraid we take flight or fight, i.e. in fight mode we manifest aggression under a range of behavioural and affective modes which includes irritability, if not frank violence. In flight mode we may simply withdraw. Anxiety explains the recent truancy, the inattention, the neuro-vegetative dysfunction and, given the unpleasantness of the anxious child's inner world, can lead to thoughts of suicide. Anxiety isn't fun and can lead to feeling depressed under the weight of fear. In any case, all roads lead to Rome. Another script of antidepressant is written, for as luck would have it, so called antidepressants are also anxiolytics. Or so they say. This psychiatrist might also refer to a psychologist skilled in the childrens version of CBT, depending on age and maturity.

Psychiatrist number 3 will diagnoses little Jaxxson with ADHD, attention deficit hyperactivity disorder (which is actually an umbrella term which should read attention deficit and/or hyperactivity disorder). How will our psychiatrist manage to accomplish this diagnosis? Actually it's a simple affair, for if you read the literature of academic and clinical fans of the diagnoses, ADHD can be had in those who are high achievers or low, in those who are dreamy absent minded introverts or rambunctious spinning toys of boys tearing around the classroom like a whirlwind. With a pinch of imagination and an ounce of inclination (the latter of which I lack), I could easily formulate about half of my child and adult patients with ADHD, including of course most drug addicts. With Jaxxson, we could say his recent lack of attentiveness and drop in academic achievement is merely an unmasking of the so called "neurodevelopmental" disorder that has always been there. Perhaps they will justify the diagnosis on the basis of being "unmasked" in virtue of the growing mismatch as schooling progresses between expectation and capacity vs his peers. Perhaps things will be explained in terms of the current teacher being less entertaining, for ADHD kids respond better to novelty and wither on the vine of routine unless domesticated with medication. On a similar vein, we can explain how the child can sustain attention for prolonged periods on videogames and other devices, and not on schoolwork. These little machines are enjoyable. Small victories along the way of the game provides the little squirts of dopamine that the childs brain lacks in virtue of the chemical imbalance they are thought to have (though the savvy clinician won't use the term "chemical imbalance" now the critical psychiatric community has run it out of town.......for now). Why the apparent depressive symptoms? Being hyperactive or inattentive leads to conflict that can lead to a challenge in ego strengths, a sense of knowing one lacks academic competence or comparative social successes. The child is irritable (or downright depressed looking) on account of these frustrations and failures. Psychiatrist number 3 will prescribe a powerful stimulant that is illegal in recreational use, plus/minus the antidepressant for the mood symptoms. As a footnote, I might add that the criteria from which ADHD is formulated in the child can also be seen as a reflection of immaturity per se. There is abundant evidence that the diagnosis is overrepresented and can be predicted by the child simply being the youngest in the class. The diagnosis can also be explained by a certain mix of what psychologists call the "big 5" personality traits and, in boys at least, a "pathological" mismatch between the child's needs for stimulation and rough and tumble activity of village or tribal life and the schools demands for moulding the cog in the machine as he is told to sit for 6 hours. It is worth noting in closing that ADHD is the example par excellence of the fallacy of the response to medication proving the existence of a diagnosis. Amphetamines (and methylphenidate) have psychotropic effects on persons taking them, be they diagnosed with ADHD or not. And these effects can be notionally salutary to both in similar domains of behaviour and function. This has been known since the time of Smith, Kline and Frenchs early marketing of benzedrine and Bradleys early experiments with stimulants on the grab bag of traumatized, rejected, intellectually delayed, delinquent or basal gangliopathic children he treated. Amphetamine aids the concentration of all up to the mind it renders them only thinking they have improved cognition, this being the mind they are half way to drug induced madness. Finally, it is worth noting that the evidence does not support the conclusion of long term benefit to children of taking stimulants. Over the long term they are either useless or harmful.

Psychiatrist 4 faces an uphill task vs the first three, though let's see if he/ she can manage it anyway. To the proverbial hammer, everything is the nail. Just as there are the psychiatrists and paediatricians who are known to diagnose many, if not most, of whom they see with ADHD or depression or bipolar disorder, there are also the psychiatrists on the lookout for autistic spectrum disorder (ASD), or what might in little Jaxxsons case been called "Aspergers" or "high functioning Autism". You see if there is the slightest sense in which he can be said to be alienated from his peers, by which we mean a subjective sense or behaviours where he is awkward, lacking in social acumen, misreading or not reading body language, response cues, irony etcetera, Jaxxson is on the radar of such a psychiatrist or paediatrician as the free spirited girl dancing in the forest was on the radar of a Salem witch hunter. This is also the case if the psychiatrist is unable to click with the child, the countertransference of alienation being projected outward from clinician to patient (or in other words, "if I don't connect with you, the fault is not my own or tough luck. It is a diagnosis"). Our childs interest in videogames is not a bad habit or the outcome of bad parenting. It is interpreted a symbol of his autistic alienation from flesh and blood people and towards their digital counterparts. And just as the social and self-evaluative sequelae of ADHD can result in mood disturbance, the high functioning autistic child may also feel frustrated and be irritable, down in mood and even threatening suicide. He may even want to connect with others, yet cannot. The more he and his family are educated as to what ASD is and the funding support packages available driven by the diagnosis, the more they will come to take on the part of what they have been diagnosed to be (I say "they" as the childs behaviour and the parents interpretation of it are in toto one phenomenological reflective system of meaning and becoming in the family unit). In addition to opening the door to various supports, Jaxxson will likely be prescribed some medications, including an SSRI antidepressant and perhaps some medication usually given for high blood pressure to calm his irritability. If he is especially irritable and misbehaving it will be difficult for him to avoid powerful tranquilizers usually reserved for those patients with "psychosis". These are powerful medications often difficult to wean off, and often ironically pharmacodynamically completely at odds with the ADHD medications co-prescribed. It makes as much sense as rubbing faeces in a wound of ones making and then washing it out.

In our fifth and final universe, our child encounters the final psychiatrist (though there might be many more examples). He or she might eschew over-diagnosis and be more "family" and "systems orientated". True enough the low mood or anxiety and the various other signs and symptoms won't be ignored. Yet this psychiatrist will look for other explanations such as the child's symptoms being a reaction to the disconnect between parents and child, e.g. in virtue of the parents cannabis use and being too stoned to parent. The parent/s of course won't realise this themselves and not be inclined to continue paying the psychiatrists bills if told something they do not wish to hear. After all, they will say they are only "self medicating" their own mental illness. (the term self medicate is predicated on there being a medical illness, which as I will argue does not exist in those who make the claim their illness is mental. Psychiatric diagnoses are not medical illnesses, and every drug user can be said to self medicate something within their mental selves they wish were not the case). Or perhaps the child being bullied? Or they are reacting to the parents separation? Or there may be any number of other reactions and reasons in the child's world of relationships and groaning towards and through maturation. Usually psychiatrist number 5 will prescribe an SSRI also, if for no other reason than "pragmatism" and its use as a therapeutic object they can hold in their hand, though usually the parents want something prescribed anyway and medication is the purview of the psychiatrist. To prescribe it is a ritual of protecting the interests of the profession against the psychologists and social workers who need compete with inferior products (psychologists for example will fight back and market the utility of certain trademarked psychometric tests that only the psychologist is authorized to administer). It's a very rare psychiatrist who won't offer the family the symbolic power of a diagnosis at all, along with the medication the family and/or the psychiatrist crave. Why? Drugging the child and providing an easy answer is, well, easy. Effecting cure by treating the child alone is difficult. Effecting cure in the child by having to "treat" the parents also is extremely difficult. Effecting cure in the child by treating the child, parent, school and society is nigh on impossible. Sooner, rather than later there is something or someone out of the psychiatrist's hands. How does the child get well then? By the psychiatrist's gentle hand of course. Or so they will say, though I'm reminded of the old adage that medicine is the art of amusing the patient whilst nature (or time) effects the cure.

The above examples of Amburr and Jaxxson are but tiny drops in the ocean of the same heterogenous muddle of snake oil. My point is not to say that there won't also be vast chunks of homogenous agreement within psychiatry. There certainly will be in cases of what passes under the banner of chronic schizophrenia for example, and the DSM is intended to be an aid towards increased interrater reliability (i.e. enabling different psychiatrists to diagnose the same person with the same thing, though the empirical evidence and my experience has failed to show it increases reliability, and this says nothing on the subject of construct validity, i.e. if the disorder exists as they say it exists in the first place). Nor is my point that any of the above psychiatrists are more correct than any other. Though I could argue that those who believe in type II bipolar disorder are delusional, and though I have some sympathies with psychiatrist number 5 above in Jaxxsons case, I have seen some patients lives turned around for the better under the care of the ADHD guru who prescribes them legally sanctioned and otherwise illegal amphetamines (or a life turned around for a while anyway). No. My point is saying that psychiatry is a church so broad as to be stretched beyond the breaking strain of its own credibility, inhabited by persons blindly fumbling around in the dark with a Rumi's elephant of person in the midst of the human condition in a fallen world. The same deconstructive critique could be levelled at any of the diagnoses, and future chapters will cover some of these. My point is that psychiatry does not have any epistemological foundation for any of psychiatrists one through five to lay claim to being correct. We might as well include in the example above a psychiatrist number 6 who formulates the case as a boy with Sagittarius disorder. A star sign is also a physical referent as much as a gene, and as equally convincing as a determinant to those who do not approach the topic of genes (or celestial bodies) critically so far as determining the psychology of the individual patient who sits across from us. With regard to the first patient example (i.e. the young emotionally unstable woman), my point is not simply to argue the non existence of type II bipolar disorder as to argue the non-existence of it and the cluster B personality disorders as anything more than convenient descriptors that all fail to adequately capture the person. And so they do more harm than good, or at least no better than the obvious fact of emotional dysregulation, a fact for all to see who have eyes to see. If the core problem can be almost whatever I argue it to be, then what really do we grasp in our intellectual hands? And if, as narcissism implies, the real "pathology" is, at least in our example, a "me, myself and I"-ism, might we have sailed so far from the shore of science and medicine that we are more in the misty lands of the humanities, of moral philosophy and even theology as ultimate formulations as to what maketh the man (or woman) in good cheer and bad? Yet another example might drive home the point. Following the suicide of the nu-metal rocker Chester Bennington of Linkin Park, I overheard some learned psychiatrists talking of his "depressive disorder" killing him via suicide, as if he succumbed to recurrent infections with some foreign agent. This was certainly the theme of all the many articles written in the wake of his passing, the infection of depression that he caught, the disease of depression he carried. I never once read or heard it pondered if the lyrics were not entirely the outward reflection of some mental illness as claimed. Deeper still were these lyrics to hold oneself in a constant choice of becoming not simply depressed, but were the lyrics within the world the beingness of depression itself, a constant meditation uttered over countless concerts, the aural dark cloud spreading out into the world again and again and reflecting back upon him. To quote only one of the songs,

"I tried so hard and got so far. But in the end It doesn't even matter I had to fall, to lose it all. But in the end It doesn't even matter".

If so, where is depression? In some simple causal medical model? In the voiced expression of depression? That is to say, the tautology of one suffering from depression because one says they are depressed. How banal. Is it in some deranged neurochemical system? I can assure you no such "chemical imbalance" or serotonin or bio-amine deficiency has been found, and I doubt it ever will. Is the depression in the lyrics themselves? No. These can be interpreted as depressive nihilism or a beautiful poetic and liberating retelling of the book of Ecclesiastes. Rather I think that in the appetite for the potential nihilistic interpretation of the lyrics, is attached the mood that speaks to a sickness in mood of the world, an ever present proclivity in man to something destructive that the collective mind of psychiatry is hopelessly ill equipped to apprehend.

Psychiatrists are neither scientists and God forbid they be considered philosophers with the will to truth. They are narrators, story tellers, salespeople, engineers with medical degrees and medicinal tools and, to the degree they are bound together at all, a kind of secular clergy of a materialist faith. I'm amazed at how some patients wait months for an appointment with an in demand psychiatrist and walk away actually believing they were just diagnosed with something as solid and true as lung cancer or the Rock of Gibraltar, when the psychiatrist is more like an epistemological Wizard of Oz, all puffed up beyond the optics of the real image. Psychiatric stories are like the proverbial turtles, it's convenient pragmatic stories all the way down. We are back to where we started. The ties that bind the definition of what a psychiatrist is, is the power itself to tie and bind, and the fallacy of authority makes the bondage stay tight.

Now the reader may wonder how such potential for (and often real) heterogeneity of opinion does not implode into infighting, psychiatrists cannibalizing each other's credibility to mutual death. How do they stay strong and appear so coherent for so long? Guilds have evolved several mechanisms to counter this, and perfected these practices over decades. Some examples are included or implied within the text above. I will give three additional examples here...

Firstly, the Guilds control the publications and the conferences. True science and true philosophy are intellectually brutal endeavours, something akin to Spartan midwifery. The strong infant lives. The weak infant is cast out to die. In a similar vein, one knows in advance that an idea or hypothesis will be tested against either a dialectical process or an experiment. And that idea might too have to be cast out and die. The very statistical methods employed in data analysis in what passes for scientific method nowadays place the cherished idea as guilty until proven innocent. By way of a different analogy, the scientist must adjust their thinking and take on the role of an attorney for the prosecution against their own cherished hypothesis. Only in attempting to prosecute against their idea and failing does the idea have the right to walk out free into the sun. In philosophy the idea placed in peril might be philosophy itself. Several philosophers have laid claiming to ending the whole philosophical enterprise and been given their chance to do so. Some might argue otherwise, yet I would historically connect the scientific method as above described as in turn connected to that Christian drive to dying to oneself so that theosis, like scientific verisimilitude towards the truth, might take the place of self instead. One will never find the same glorious attitude in psychiatry. In the church or corporate body of psychiatry, what passes for robust debate always passes first through a filtration or screening process of guild and professional self interest. If critique is presented in a way that threatens the psychiatric church doctrine and its power, it will not even be declared anathema. It will simply not be published and will disappear in silence. They will probably allow the DSM to die in time and mock it in generations to come, but only when they safely have something else.

Secondly, renegade psychiatrists are like heretic priests, only worse in a sense. For if one studies the true history of the early church from which I make my numerous analogies, the patristic fathers who advanced what was called heresy were by and large left to their own devices. Even Galileo was not imprisoned in a tower as opposed to the family vineyard, and story of him being tortured was a myth. Renegade psychiatrists who criticize psychiatry in a substantial sense will not be tortured of course. They will be alienated and find it impossible to gain employment except in private practice or where they have the already secured the firmest tenure. They will find it almost impossible to publish in mainstream journals. I have even seen up close a case of a patently perfectly sane heretic psychiatrist (not myself) reported to a medical licensure board to be mentally ill themselves, this an act of bad faith in an attempt to slow the agitator down. And this was by more than one anonymous complainant psychiatrist, on more than one occasion!

Finally, bear in mind that the psychiatric trainee / resident (in the UK, Australia and some other Commonwealth countries a trainee is called a "registrar") is a member of an underclass, though an underclass of a special kind, one which has ample chance of upward mobility. And so mine is far from being a pro Marxist argument of class warfare. This upward mobility depends upon capitulation as opposed to entrepreneurship. On the road to freedom, prestige and a doubling or tripling of income overnight upon completion of training, the proverbial boat shall not be rocked. For if the heretic priest is vulnerable, how much more vulnerable is the heretic deacon or acolyte? After all, unlike Luther, the heretic cannot just uproot and create his own church. The system simply won't allow it. The state underwrites the power of the psychiatric guilds. In each nation there is but one single guild, one road to the top, with an absolute prohibition to what might otherwise have been a free market. Or put another way, specialist medical guilds are the best example I know of a state sanctioned monopoly of power, this being another proof of psychiatry working hand in glove with the state, as state. To the extent psychiatry has supplanted the church as the minister to mens (and womens) souls in the secular state, there most certainly is no separation of powers, not even in the United States. Despite its vain ramblings as to the holy constitution, freedom ends where psychiatry begins. Returning to the life of the trainee; I have seen a curious thing happen many times. If one psychiatrist does not agree on some matter with another, there might be a debate between the two, usually behind closed doors. Usually there isn't conflict at all, a kind of ecumenical pluralism within the fraternity. If a trainee were to have the same opinion of one of the consultant psychiatrists and come into conflict with the other, the two psychiatrists would close ranks and put the trainee in his or her place. The trainee would be told they are not considering the complexity of the case, need develop a more sophisticated or nuanced view of things, and so on. The truth be damned if what really matters is institutional power. Were one secular priest to weaken the authority of the other they would weaken the class as a whole, and by extension weaken themselves as individuals and the guilds to which they belong. This will not do! The trainee capitulates easily, for they wish to get a good report and eventually be anointed a priest with all the trappings of power themselves. And so the cycle will continue into the next generation, and the next. Such is the blessing and curse of upwards mobility in providing a disincentive to needed change, a class divide that exists without class struggle. Should some time the trainee be fortunate enough to encounter an honest iconoclastic priest in the church of psychiatry, they will almost always find only a partial, and rarely public, ally. The advice will be "you cannot change it, I cannot change it and I do not wish to. Play the game. Be pragmatic. Pretend if you must. Give them what they want and you shall have your freedom". But the church of psychiatry itself cannot be raised to the ground, and no iconoclast will leave it. Play it or not, the game must go on.

None of this gives a window into psychiatric praxis itself, a day in the life of a garden variety psychiatrist. In this closing half of the chapter I'll tell you all you need to know.

Apart from the ontological question of a psychiatrist qua authority with legal power, there is the matter of what they do. And what a psychiatrist does in praxis is nothing more complicated than the praxis itself, and being confident and practiced in the role. This may be summarized in four terms; history, mental state exam, diagnosis, formulation and treatment (I say four terms as formulation is often done poorly or omitted entirely).

History; So you visit a psychiatrist in their private rooms, or find yourself sitting across from one in a state hospital, plus/minus a security guard or two standing by lest you commit a crime from which you will rarely be charged or prosecuted (you are mentally ill after all and what's the point staff pursuing a charge that will receive little to no sentence). After the pleasantries are hopefully exchanged, psychiatrists begin by asking basic questions of demography. How old are you? Where do you live? etc. This is how I would start, for one achieves a basic skeleton of knowledge of who the person is by where they reside, with whom they reside, what they do for work (if they work), if they have children etc. This gives one an idea of the ties that bind along with functional capacities, if these are being utilized at this point in time or if there has been a drop in function. Then what is approached is the question of why you came for help, your own subjective complaints, i.e. your symptoms and the surrounding narrative. Are you sad or anxious, confused, obsessed, having strange experiences such as hearing voices or has life become mundane and not strange enough? Do you think of killing yourself? Are you here because someone else wants you "to get help". Have you tried to take your life in the past? What is the impact of the symptoms in terms of work, relationships, sleep, appetite and the like? How have you been coping, i.e. self-managing symptoms? (this can be a guide about how you can generate your own recovery and participate in the process. This can also be an opener to asking about drug use as "self medicating"). Many more questions are asked besides. What ought to be explored in depth is the childhood experience. More often than not a developmental history is not explored in anywhere near the depth that is it's due, if at all. Psychiatrists Instead often make a big deal about family history of mental illness. They do this under the assumption of looking for bad genes. I ask about family history with a view to looking for experiences of other alleged mental illness in the family and the impact of this upon the patient. As suggested elsewhere, genes (in my humble opinion and having evaluated the evidence) are overrated where they are highly rated (risk of bipolar disorder, depression and schizophrenia for example), and under rated where they are over looked (personality and genetic propensity to anxiety for example). In any case, nothing can be done about them. If you can ask questions of a typical comprehensive history and cognitively apply them to the next three steps to follow, you are on your way to being in practical terms interchangeable with the psychiatrist (though of course without the power invested by the state).

Mental State Examination; Genuine doctors perform a physical examination where they bump you knee (or just south of it) with a tendon hammer, listen to your chest with a stethoscope, and many things more steps besides. Anankastic physicians of internal medicine who take themselves too seriously (and most do) will kick up much of a fuss in favour of following conventional steps of physical examination to the letter, even castigating the physician trainee who approaches the patient from the wrong side of the bed or dares do anything out of order. The psychiatric equivalent is the mental status examination, or MSE. On one hand the MSE is an unconsciously desperate attempt on the part of the psychiatrist to consciously realize themselves to be a real doctor, and so they obviously adopt (or dissimulate) the parlance of the real doctor, having a conversation masquerading as an "examination". On the other hand, the MSE is simply a list of variables from what you tell the alleged doctor and what they themselves observe. History could easily have dispensed with the MSE and its elements be incorporated in one paragraph of synthesis written about the therapeutic encounter. In any case, the MSE is here and here to stay, for no psychiatrist is critical of why it need be there in the first place. An example of the elements is provided below. The MSE ought to flow from the history and be congruent with the diagnosis and formulation. If not, something is amiss.

A brief and simple example of an MSE might be this, in a homeless schizophrenic IV drug user. For the most part I've omitted the specific terminology employed by the psychiatrist, though this is easy to learn

"Patient presents as older than stated, dishevelled malodorous and not attending to self cares of hygiene and grooming. Rapport was poor and he had an irritable attitude to interview, with poor eye contact and stigmata of IV drug use. Occasionally he paced, though was not aggressive. Speech was monotone. Appeared to be responding to non apparent auditory stimuli (i.e. talking to himself) and reported voices telling him to kill himself. Affect (usually taken to mean facial emotional expression) was lacking reactivity and restricted to a mask of seriousness. Mood was subjectively euthymic (i.e. says his mood is fine). Significant thought disorder with tangential responses (i.e. the response might make sense yet do not relate at all to the question asked) and thought content included persecutory delusions of being followed by the CIA, leading in turn to thoughts of suicide. Lacks insight into his psychosis and non-compliant with treatment (i.e. denies having a mental illness and does not take his medication). Fully conscious"

Diagnoses; It is not at all uncommon to find psychiatrists with genuine disdain for the DSM or the ICD 11, these being the diagnostic nosology in use throughout most of the world. Often they might parrot the usual party line that such diagnostic manuals or criteria are "just guidelines" and be critical of some diagnoses, choosing to value the criteria as enunciated in the DSM for research purposes and consensus of what makes for a name for purposes of inter-practitioner (and often international) communication. Occasionally one might encounter a psychiatrist who would rather the DSM go away. But what is extremely rare is the psychiatrist who attempts, in practice, to do away with the DSM entirely and explain the patient as a formulation alone, or a narrative akin to that one might read in literature. However much a psychiatrist might pretend to be "anti DSM", when taking the history their mind is invariably ticking over as to what DSM and/or ICD 11 checklist criteria are included and which are excluded. All psychiatrists almost always implicitly use it and almost always are explicitly required to. To not do so and not do so well for many years would render it impossible to complete training and enter the priesthood. If we could conceive of a modified Turing test where the robot was to take the history and record the mental state exam, each congruent with the resultant being diagnoses as per DSM or ICD 11, then this robot would be indistinguishable from almost every psychiatrist I've ever known (the exception being the one I am not permitted to be).

Formulation; Formulations are explanatory little statements of a few paragraphs, linking the patient's presentation with the symptoms and some speculative link to a "theory" of mental illness most applicable to the case. Formulations are a game for true believers of the theorist and sophists alike. The five different explanations of the child's case (vide supra) are crude approximations of formulations, to which one might add a comment on what may foreseeably make the patients mental state worse in future, and what strengths and resources the patient can draw upon. A tongue in cheek example of a crude formulation for now might be this fiction...

"Sigmund presents with suicidal ideation symptoms and the full suite of symptoms consistent with a diagnosis of major depression. The current episode seems to have been precipitated the revelation his brother likely had sex with his stepmother, Sigmund being angry he himself did not succeed in the conquest, this anger introjected (i.e. turned inwards) and transmuting itself into the depressive symptom complex itself. An additional contributor to his depression may well be the ambivalence Sigmund has towards his father, enjoying the fact his father qua Laius object has been slain, this satisfaction not sufficient to overcome the punitive superego against his psyche in response to the enjoyment itself. Thankfully Sigmund is functionally quite strong, has an excellent capacity for insight and is agreeable to taking the therapies prescribed (principally opium, along with, of course, analysis), though there may be countertransference issues with the therapist whom Sigmund believes is of inferior mind."

Developing a robot to construct a formulation would not be as easy as developing one which could take a history, document a mental state exam and narrow to the point of choice from the smorgasbord of diagnoses in the DSM or ICD 11. Nonetheless there are now artificial intelligences that are amply up to the task. A program has now been developed to replace journalists, beginning with the first paragraph it can mine the internet and complete the article from there. Psychiatric formulations are the same, fake news that might be real, and real to the trainee to the extent they might dialectically defend its use as applied to the patient (as opposed to it being the truth of the patient), and real to the patient to the extent it is convincing. No one really cares how or what the formulation is. Providing it is done well, you could complete two or more disjunctive formulations and choose your favourite. One can formulate according to a biopsychosocial, or object relation orientated or Freudian or systems minded or Jungian or existentialist or Eriksonian or anywhere up to another dozen other theorists/theories I can think of. Psychologists often do formulations which are almost entirely bound up in numerical scores of psychometric testing, and appear more like summaries of finance reports rather than something about a human being living amongst other human beings.

Many formulations nowadays are banal statements composed of the "5 P's", i.e. the presenting complaint, the precipitating factor, the predisposing factors, the perpetuating factors and finally the protective factors. A fictional example that may match many patients

"Krystyll, a 20 year old mother of three (all children are at all times in their grandmothers care and the fathers are nowhere to be found) arrived in the ED via ambulance after over dose whilst having an argument with her boyfriend, this within the context of intoxication with alcohol and cannabis, and on background of multiple past overdoses. Krystyll has a genetic diathesis (i.e. family history) of manic depression. Thankfully Krystyll is help seeking and well supported by her grandmother, though has limited other supports having become estranged from her parents and the fathers of her children due to drug use for which she is pre-contemplative to change. I'd speculate that much revolves around her early attachment, this being anxious avoidant."

Notice how I cover the "5 P's" without actually using the "P" words. When I was training and this method of formulation was coming into vogue, explicitly stating the 5 P's was considered insipid and lacking sophistication, I can only conclude for reasons of a drive to dissimulation, appearing to be something literary, something greater and tailored to the individual, while being something systematized and technocratic.

Insomuch as formulations are a choice of theories, they are the art of the sophist and a pretence to sophistication, and nothing more than pastiche. The greatest authentic formulators were Dostoevsky and Shakespeare. Read their works, their descriptions of people. Neither of these were psychiatrists. Psychiatric formulations are, in comparison, quite embarrassing really. They are, like the symbolism in the cover of this book, a taking apart of a beautiful thing, subsequently unable to put it together again whilst horrifyingly thinking they have all the same.

Treatment; This last step is rather easy, and I could teach any junior doctor the basics in a few weeks of on the job training. Start with the guidelines into the disorders as published by the local guild machine APA (USA), CPA (Canada), NICE (UK), RANZCP (Australia, New Zealand) etcetera, and apply this to the patient. For all of the many pages and for all the appeal to expert judgment, these guidelines are just glorified flowcharts. Actually it is simpler still for the psychiatrist, as most will have their favourite few drugs or drug combinations for each of the disorders, be it the so-called antidepressants/anxiolytics, mood stabilizers or antipsychotics. For example, take the depressed patient. If the depression is mild start with CBT. If it is moderate add CBT to the SSRI. If unsuccessful move to a tricyclic, if unsuccessful still augment with lithium or antipsychotic. The end of the line if all else fails is ECT or an MAOI, or both

Granted the doctor need be aware of dosing considerations, if and when to test serum drug levels, exclusion of organic causes of depression (i.e. medical causes of depression such as underactive thyroid), when and how to switch medications and so on. Yet this is not too daunting, also just a memorization or reference to flowcharts. The psychiatrist might be able appear more erudite by justifying specific medication choice on the basis of what receptor systems they act upon and which they do not. These are by and large convenient stories, mirages of oasis that vanish when one looks closer at the literature. The psychotherapy is more often than not outsourced to psychologists as psychiatrists take upon themselves a managerial mantle, this being convenient for psychiatrist is by and large as neither competent at, or interested in, the "talking cure". If they are, they will have their pet little approach that is also easy to learn in practice. Surely this fact is not controversial.

My example is a deliberate one, for it is worth digressing at this juncture to hurl grenade at the myth of the power of so called antidepressants, these also often marketed as first line for anxiety. Once again my little spiel will be unreferenced. Suffice it to say for now that these agents correct no chemical imbalance in the brain, for no chemical imbalance has ever reliably been found, nor any other biological pathogenesis accounting for any but a tiny subset of depressed (or anxious) patients. It is the same also for schizophrenia. What these medications do is run the risk of creating a chemical imbalance, for the brain reacts to an excess of neurotransmitter with altering its neurochemistry such that it then becomes imbalanced, as the brain "fights" what the drug is 'attempting" to do. Oft times the consequences of imbalance is not recognised until one attempts withdraw from the SSRI or SNRI (or any psychotropic really), and whatever attendant symptoms emerge is reinterpreted by the psychiatrist as a relapse of the imaginary biological illness, not a withdrawal phenomenon pure and simple, i.e. a side effect of the drug. And so they wind up on the medication yet again, and the circus continues. But you might say that you, or your patients, have an undeniable salutatory effect. Irving Kirsch, the Harvard psychologist and doyen of the placebo effect, has provided us the best evidence yet that the vast majority of what might be considered the drug effect is actually placebo, what beneficial effect there might be being below what a psychiatrist will subjectively judge as the minimum possible discernible improvement. This is the best evidence that evidence based medicine has given us, and Kirsch's deflationary findings have ben replicated at every turn to date over now more than two decades. As it happens I am disposed to the view that SSRI's and SNRI's have a function that extends beyond the placebo, though this hardly offers any consolation. I have lost count of the number of patients whose anxiety is substantially reduced in correlation with the takings of these drugs, and who claim to not be as depressed as they were. Indeed the anxiety may be so reduced as to be negated altogether. Where once they were crushed by anxiety over public speaking or an exam, now when the train is late and they walk into the exam an hour late they take it in their stride. They can sometimes tell me, when one is so bold to explore, that they wonder if they would react with even a tint of worry if a bomb were to explode in the quad. And the patient who might have been labelled depressive no longer feels as depressed, their mood has moved from 2/10 to 6/10. Bravo. Yet they are not moved by anything. No longer depressed, they no longer feel the suspense of a thriller and the tears no longer well at the reading of melodrama or the attendance at the opera. And if they were anxious about their job, their battering husband or whatever the mood is now is more "Hmm cest la vie", untouched they are from the passions that are a signal to change, and the driving force behind change itself. The battering husband no longer feels the pangs of conscience on mind altering drugs, and so on goes the circus. Were I to be a dictator of a docile minimally functioning people, the first thing I would do is commence the populace on an SSRI, plus minus some cannabis. The children I would give low dose stimulants. Some adults, or children also, I would administer so called antipsychotics. And no revolution would ever disturb my sleep.

Having returned from digression, let us return to what defines the psychiatrist, as an adjunct to the police with powers to deprive persons of their liberty. To the reader who is a non-patient, there but by the grace of God (or good fortune) go you.

EPISTEMOLOGY. COGITO, ERGO COGITO.

"Human beings are complex biological systems, with mind as an emergent property. For this reason there are inherent uncertainties regarding diagnostic formulation and optimal care. It is anticipated that this guideline will assist clinicians to better navigate complex and challenging clinical scenarios. Tailoring care to the individual in the context of an effective working relationship is the foundation upon which the proper application of this guideline relies."

The above quote was taken from the elsewhere mentioned Guidelines into the management of mood disorders published by the Australian and New Zealand guild of psychiatrists. The amphibology is almost impenetrable, as the text gives us no clue to the relation of the parts. Are the "inherent uncertainties" in the process of minds alleged emergence from matter (matter as material and efficient cause?) or in there being the mind per se after having emerged? Or is the challenge in the human being a complex biological system, where being can otherwise imply an experience of being as noun or as verb, as much as denoting this or that member of the species homo sapiens? Or is the complexity in the irreconcilable combination of the two elements of mind and matter as I will claim, or the human qua a human person and not a scientistically formulated "biological system"? And what on Earth has this ontology have to do with profane issues of psychiatric diagnoses? I will argue it matters greatly, this being the subject of the present chapter. Such is the matter of mind.

There is no inherent uncertainty in diagnosing a heart attack when this diagnosis is properly made, this despite the heart attack being in the minutia of its pathophysiology a complex biological event in a complex biological system, with the attack certainly emergent in the sense that it had not occurred a day before, yet not emergent as anything outside its own physicality and temporality. And so we have to ask, as later we will, what is meant by the word "emergence"? In any case this guild, as do others, nail their colours to the wall in acknowledging that to know the maladies of mind requires a knowledge of the mind itself, this being the solid ground upon which they need stand when diagnosing and treating. This is not a controversial expectation. How can pathological anatomy be possibly understood without a knowledge of the normal? What is mental illness without a knowledge of mind in general, either as noun or verb? This being so, the mind nonetheless renders psychiatry "inherently" different to other specialties which might make a claim to be medical. And so with that acknowledgement made, let us not dishonour what they have seen to be the case and state the matter simply; psychiatry cannot know itself or the patient either, unless it first knows the mind. I would argue its predicament is direr still, as the psychiatrist cannot know either itself or the patient without looking itself square in the eye as a participant in a social and political transaction, this also in part defining the patient to whom they might relate and who in turn relates to others. What was missing in the bio (complex biological), psycho (mind) formulation was the greater collective (socio) component of this greater complexity, which has also been called, in toto, a biopsychosocial model. And yet whether bipartite or tripartite, the latter so called biopsychosocial model is nothing more than a collection of considerations that can be placed under three differentially listed columns and so is not any model of the person at all, where model implies an explanation of where and why the boundaries between the categories and what are the interactions between these and their elements so as to produce the final product. A model is an explanation of precisely how components statically and dynamically fit together, not merely a three columned list of spare parts sitting on the shop floor.

To all this the reader may counter, with a pragmatic refrain, that the psychiatrist does not need to know or even conjecture on what the mind is in order for its praxis to be meaningful. All that matters is if treatment and diagnostic formulation "works" (I have included diagnosis as something that "works", as diagnosis has as much utility as treatment in the psychiatric ritual, it is a shared fantasy that "treats" the psychiatrists and the patients anxiety not knowing what illness they "have"). The psychiatric pragmatist may state that in times past all physicians may have administered a perfectly suitable remedy without any knowledge at the time of what it chemically was and how it physiologically worked, and the patient none the worse for it. They might cite the example in our own day of general anaesthesia, where it remains only dimly known of how it works (where dim is a charitable overestimate). And fair enough. If one wishes to be rendered unconscious and insensate to avoid what would otherwise be agony at the surgeon's blade, then who cares how this is to be achieved, and who cares how the sevoflurane or propofol interrupts the mystery of consciousness. This theoretical question is only of interest to the philosopher, and not at all when the philosopher is prepped for surgery. Such an analogy between general anaesthesia and psychiatry would be misplaced however, as general anaesthesia has no claim or calling to be anything other than a wholly self contained pragmatic exercise. It entirely explains itself by its success to bring the patient to deaths door and back again, and does not attempt couch itself in any greater narrative of the human condition.

Psychiatry on the other hand necessarily asks grander questions and pretends to have grander answers into mind and its maladies. In its pretences it tells people who they are in their symptoms and the relation between normal and abnormal, and in its omissions cannot avoid the charge of assuming what the patient is not (as spiritual beings for instance, the cohort of believers run roughshod over in the above quoted guideline elsewhere purporting to have sought and respected submissions from a broad audience with broad values and beliefs). It really does matter if the patient asks what mood is, and is told mood relies upon a harmony of certain neurotransmitters and that indeed good mood is an epiphenomena of the operations of these neurotransmitters. Or alternatively is depression inwardly directed anger or the outcome of laziness or not living up to expectations? It really does matter if the patient is told their addiction is a "highjacked" reward pathway or alternatively more a moral matter or distraction against life's meaninglessness with neuroscience having little of substance to offer to the question. It really does matter if we posit the unconscious to exist at all, let alone it being the warzone from which bursts forth our anxieties. It is only in begging the question towards a philosophical pragmatism (see chapter to follow) that these and countless other questions do not matter.

The current chapter, perhaps to be the shortest in the book, hardly addresses a survey of what the mind is or is not. Nor is it a survey of C.D, Broads taxonomy of mind as consciousness or an answer to Chalmers "hard question" of the same (i.e. the explanation for consciousness itself as the ground upon which all mental operations must stand and be experienced as mind in either noun or verb). Nonetheless I'll take a stab at a defence of a radical agnosticism with respect to mind. Should I be correct, it will make of psychiatry forever a speculation longing to become the place it can never arrive. And if that is the case, psychiatry sits upon a level playing field with the pastor or wise grandmother as to what maketh the man (or woman).

Brain and Mind

Take a garden variety neuron. One neuron is first excited into activity by another, and so do we begin with the second or the first? But the first is also excited by another, and so on ad infinitum back to some embryological point where somewhere some first neuronal pair was excited to act. Thus our entry point into the brain is arbitrary. And so we are back to the garden variety neuron at an arbitrary space and time in the adult brain. A starting point of excitation for neuron 2 might be, in the simple case, a neurotransmitter floating around in the fluid space between neuron 1 and neuron 2. And the neurotransmitter might form a loose chemical bond with a protein in the seething semi fluid membranous coating that wraps around the neuron and is its cellular "skin", this membrane being the place within which this protein "receptor" is to be located. This loose chemical bond results in a changing of the receptors structure, the change in structure being entirely explained on first principles to be a physical event, much as a door is explained by where the hinges are located and from where the force is applied when the wind slams it shut or swings it open. For the moment we are imagining neither a mind forcing its will upon the neuron or a hand forcing a will upon the door. This is a change in receptor structure that might, once again in the simple case, result in the receptor becoming a channel or loch through which flows positively charged sodium ions. Why do they flow in and not out? Actually they flow both ways, yet the nett flow is in one direction, this the result of random movement of a physical thing and an initial imbalance in concentration either side of the membrane. The original state of separation of charge and concentration imbalance across the membrane of various ions is driven in large part by other subcellular machinery whose operations can also be explained on the basis of one chemical bobbing up against another, changing the shape of it and so on, the principle chemical unit in this case being a little molecular machine that pumps sodium out and potassium in, in a ratio the resultant of which is more electrical negativity on the inside of the membrane at rest. The events of neuronal activation are similarly entirely explained by basic physical and statistical principles at play. The fact that the positively charged sodium ion is not at a temperature of absolute zero permits motion. The differential concentration either side of the membrane predicts the statistics of bulk nett flow (from high to low concentration). The second law of thermodynamics explains the same (the increase in disorder if energy is not applied to increase order, in dissipating a concentration gradient) and so on. The state of affairs can collectively be readily explained by calculations of both the Nernst and Goldman Hodgkin Katz constant field equations. Should enough sodium enter into the cell to alter the electrical state of the neuron to the requisite threshold, there will be another species of sodium channels responsive to changes in the electrical milieu whose shape will also change, so called voltage gated channels. These will conform into an open state and more sodium will float on in, this sodium diffusing sideways within the neuron, the resultant being more electrical change and more sodium influx propagated along with length of the nerve (so called depolarization and propagation). At the terminus of the nerve the voltage change will activate yet another species of little intramembranous proteins bobbing around like icebergs in the semi fluid sea that is the cellular membrane. These admit calcium ions which in turn come to activate a chain of events that allow for a change in shape of an internal scaffolding within the neurons terminus such that vesicles (little bubble like structures) containing neurotransmitter fuse with the membrane of the neuron itself, releasing the transmitter into the space between neurons to float on over to interact with neuron 3. To imagine vesicular release, imagine a lava lamp where the bubble within the tube is hollow, contains a chemical transmitter substance, and releases it to the outside world if allowed to partially fuse with the glass of the tube, in this case with the outside of the tube composed of the same substance of the bubble and not the glass of the tube in our analogy. The released transmitter will float around between neuron 2 and neuron 3, perhaps resulting in activating the latter when enough quanta of transmitter arrives at its destination. There also will be subsequent processes returning the neurons 1 and 2 to the state of rest and excitability, returning initial charge separation and vesicular separation from the membrane, and refilling the vesicle with transmitter.

The above is the most basic model, explained in the most basic terms faithful to the physicality of the system. Nowhere in all these happenings is anything like that which we know to be the case in our being aware, in feeling and thinking and in directing our intentionality inwards and outwards. Where in all this is the spontaneous emergence of the language of consciousness and mind and persons, let alone the raw beingness of consciousness and mind?

The reader may make the obvious objection. They might say that two or three neurons does not a brain make, and that consciousness and mind is the "emergent" product of complexity.

And yet how can this be the case? There are no convincing analogies of emergence the likes of which we are asked to believe happens in the relationship between brain and mind. One could say that the wetness of water is an emergent property from the combination of billions of water molecules. Yet this is a nonsense. Wetness is the subjective sense of a person with a mind who "feels" water. Wetness needs mind. The fluidity of water on the other hand results from the properties of the water molecules themselves and their arrangement at a given temperature and pressure. Fluidity can be understood with a language already contained within a semantics of physical chemistry. Are we to propose that from placing the straws on the camels back, that somehow emerges this alien state of crushing the camel, like a giant phantom hand has appeared in the midst of the straw or come down from on high. And yet the potentiality of the crushing was contained within the mass of each straw, this pitted against the physical carrying capacity of the camel. Something happened for sure yet nothing alien emerged. Or it is like a revolutionary society, which in its emergence is more than the conversation. And yet what is so alien here? Is not the revolution of the same properties of the conversation in the café or the first call to arms? But where in the brain can we find mind, even in its proto or partial emergence?

That having been said, let's entertain the nonsense anyway, and pit it against our intuitions. Let's scale up the complexity. Where there were three neurons and two synapses, we now have billions. And so what? From heaping lead upon lead upon lead do we see emerge an ounce of gold? Billions of more of the same is greater mass without effecting an alchemical transmutation of what that mass is composed of. Now it's in the arrangement they might say, the spatial complexity is the wellspring of emergence. Fair enough. Let us put one train upon a track, then multiply the tracks into an elaborate system of a national railway, with thousands of miles of tracks and hundreds of trains coming and going in extension and recursive loops. And yet we still have nothing more than trains and tracks. Nowhere in all this does the great train God emerge to know itself as something beyond its material and efficient self. Or at least the train God has not acquired a communicative apparatus to communicate its existence to us, and so we have exercised the option to hypothesize its non-existence. Those of a pan-psychic persuasion think every material thing is conscious. Even a grain of rice has a tiny packet of proto consciousness. How a consciousness not conscious of itself can be a meaningful consciousness is for them to say before the proof in the rice is found. Digressions aside, we might say it is not in the spatial complexity so much as the complexity of elements that mind emerges, of there being a potpourri of different neurotransmitters and different types of neurons and glia, along with a bewildering complexity of intracellular machinery. Yet once again so what? In an age when we have many who literally believe that oxytocin is love, that dopamine is hedonism and reward, that serotonin or GABA is calm, that anandamide is bliss, in even dismissing these scientistic horrors, how does the immaterial property "emerge" from the complex co-existence and operations of all these neurotransmitters in the same brain. Does consciousness emerge in there being a half dozen herbs in the chemical soup, or is it less, or is it more? How does the complexity in neurotransmitters interact with that of glia and neuronal shape and size to create mind? And where might the threshold be found between zombie and person? And once again we are appealing to an alchemical argument in the emergence of one from the other. Now they might say it is not in the complexity of the spatial properties, or the number of arrangements, but in the temporal complexity. Once again so what? And once again we can return to the train analogy. How might we conceive it to be possible for the train God to emerge from the fact of some trains always running in perpetuity down the tracks, others released at a given frequency from their stations, some traveling under contingent modal schedules of supply and demand of special occasion etcetera. Music also depends greatly upon temporality of physical events and yet the instruments and sound waves can neither compose the music nor listen to themselves. Or we might imagine it possible for us to build a computer in the imago of the brain, building up the elements of the circuits within circuits one by one, testing dynamic frequencies of substructural components until somehow what emerges is the conscious computer that we have taken as an article of faith to have passed the test to convince us has a mind like our own (and contra Turing, this will always necessarily involve an article of faith). After all, what is so special about proteins, fats and fluids when these might simply be material realizations of on/off functions and spatial arrangements which might be achieved by other non-biological material means, or even the abstractions of a model that, like mind in mind, be the idea of a model. One day they might say "aha, a circuitry of a billion neuronal switches arranged like a spiral within a spiral here running at 70Hz, and a 5 billion unit helix shaped circuit there running at 10 Hz, with each node in the helix connected to fixed points in the spiral, this is the basic model from which consciousness emerges and a mind comes to say 'cogito ergo sum' when we attach up to some communicative output". If the spiral is to appear similar to that of the galaxy or if the helices to resemble DNA there would be those to ponder the spatial correspondences. The esoterica in the shared symbology would be the stuff of many new age books. Is the universe then conscious they would ask? Is DNA? As above, so below. But regardless of what spatio-temporal correlate to consciousness is the threshold of its apparent emergence, what would they have really found if they think they found it? What have they explained, except to open the door to mystery all over again.

The fact that the above is a gross simplification of the brain is acknowledged. Yet I would submit to the reader that when one takes a partial Cartesian turn and comes to dwell within their own mind for a reflective moment and seeing it as the you who you are, and then takes an honest look at brain as the material thing it is, that they can only be left with the conclusion that words such as property and substance dualism and emergence are stand ins for others better fitting the occasion, those being supra-material alchemy or, better yet, a miracle. Now an alchemy implies an alchemist I'll grant you, just as a miracle implies a miracle worker. And so what? Let us not yet launch into that question or recoil from the implications of the same, foreclosing on what ought to be the moment of being caught suspended in confrontation with the miraculous. My contention is that mind and brain are metaphysical categories so radically different as to be radically irreconcilable. Just to restate, I am not proposing this to be a devilish problem for which we have yet to arrive at a solution, like an understanding of what caused the plague in the days before microbiology in its current form. I am proposing that the metaphysical gulf between brain and mind is so great as to not allow for the possibility of a solution. The horizon of an answer in the distance that the neuroscientist sees is simply a projection of their own wish, a faith in their own scientistic eschatology. And I am willing to wager in particular that what Chalmers calls the hard problem, i.e. the explanation for consciousness as the ground upon which all mental operations must stand, can and will never be solved to the satisfaction of an honest neuroscientist. Any awaiting of a new science or paradigm shift is as much an article of faith as the belief in a miracle.

Part of the problem lay in the language. Neuroscientists speak of the "reward circuitry" of the brain without there being a silicon chip or electrical wire in sight, and in full knowledge that so many loops of connection are found in the brain as to make the analogy of "circuit" trivial. And computer scientists program what they call "neural networks" without a single neuron to be found anywhere outside of their heads and on the desktop in front of them. Psychologists increasingly talk of the nature/nurture problem as being a hardware/software problem (in so doing an insidious move from nature and family towards computer science), and cognitive scientists talk of the mind of a person as a processing unit of packages of information, and of the on/off state of neurons in terms of the binary "language" of the computer. Military engineers develop "smart" bombs and we talk of computers "solving a problem", the smart phone app "suggesting" we buy something or the satnav in the car "telling" us the way. We live in an age when the computer is described in terms of mind and mind (and brain) in terms of computer, just as every age has chosen the apex technology of the day as an analogue for both mind and brain. And so with the lubricant applied to this psycholinguistic crime, we might be incredulous to hearing the fact that no computer, even an "artificial intelligence" (which dare I add has no consciousness), has ever calculated anything at all, any more than it would be true to say an umbrella protects us from the rain. We protect ourselves from the rain using the umbrella as a prosthetic. We build clocks that have a mechanism, the output of which is what we call the time. Yet a clock does not "work out" the time. It does not "tell us" the time. And an artificial intelligence might propagate and elaborate an output that might be fruitful, even unto novel fruit and better than we can imagine with our feeble minds. Yet so does a tree yield its own fruit. An artificial intelligence does not invent, innovate, compete or win at anything as there is no winner there within it, no internal witness to innovation. Likewise, there is no binary language, no ones and zeroes within the computer, and in its complexity we do not have calculation qua mental activity. We do not have intentionality between self and objects both internal and external with preferences driven by emotion, desire and telos. We simply have statics and dynamics of matter and energy, complex machines that we anthropomorphise into being like us. Similarly, no book communicates things to us. We read meaning into it or extract meaning from it that the authors mind is communicating to us through words on the page. But without two minds this is just ink and paper. As a test of the degree to which we have allowed these semantic conflations between man and machine cloud our judgment, try and explain the operations of any complex technology or machine used by a human without use of any terms that might be more properly descriptive of a person with a mind, of feeling and thought, of intentionality and teleology. And try and explain the operations of the mind without recourse to the language of technology. It is harder than you think, and more difficult than I wager would have been the case were we not indoctrinated in a philosophically malignant overreach of analogy and metaphor.

Returning to emergence

One way out of these troubles is to imagine that the "emergence" is not some kind of immaterial ghost from the brain (a substance dualism). Rather there is no immaterial mind at all and emergence is some kind of stand in term for a focus on a heretofore unacknowledged physical property no more special than any other (property or semantic dualism). And so the second dimension of a drawing emerges from the first and the third emerges from the second. If the 3 dimensional object is materialistic then heat emerges from it, mass and gravity emerges in interaction with other masses and mind emerges in a way consubstantial with its own materiality. Or it could be said that a brain qua supercomputer is doing its super mechanical thing and the mechanism has certain functions that require a partitioned "language", functions of "modelling" itself in relation to other computers or modelling future outcomes so as to optimize future outputs in accord with a programmed equilibrium state and so on. This language being distinct from others in the machine includes terms like as "I", "me", "you", "feeling" and so on. And that is what mind is, semantically emergent yet materially (and metaphysically) non-existent. Or so some might say.

I have sometimes been tempted to walk some way down this line in an objection to Descarte. When Descarte thinks he can step outside of the perceptions given him that he doubts the authenticity of, and instead rationalizes his own existence as a mental actor, he is using language that is not his own, language he acquired from a source that he has already considered suspect and unknown. He remembers once having been a child and learning a language. But was he and did he? His is a conversation that he has been thrown into with a game which is not his own. It is impossible for him to extricate himself and start anew, even if he imagines himself as come into being a second ago with false memories given him by the demon. Every way he might know himself, in its language dependency, is suspect. And so he cannot say "cogito ergo sum" (I think therefore I am), yet rather "cogito ergo cogito" (there are thoughts, therefore there are thoughts), or "sum ergo sum" (or I am therefore I am), both statements empty of meaning. What is left of the person when void of language used to communicate self to self? There would be raw consciousness and qualia, with little else besides. In a primitive sense there would be mind without the one with the mind, this leading to contradiction.

And yet here we are confronted with a reality of our own consciousness that is neither rationally a priori or axiomatically true, yet simply proven a phenomenological fact in our being. And thank heavens we have our own personal consciousness as it is our only strong proof we exist at all as mental beings. Clearly our mind is not a material thing. Contra hard materialism, to argue anything successfully is partly an analytical exercise and partly an identification with the argument. A mind/brain material monism with emergence as merely property or operation of a biological computer (to not, in a stronger sense, exist), demands an almost mystical nihilism to successfully argue, let alone identify with it as an idea that is comfortable like hand in glove. In its radical self-denial, it is more Zen than science and yet neither at the same time. I am not proposing that mind brain monism is not true. I am arguing simply that to my mind it has not been adequately argued and I doubt it ever can be. It denies the undeniable. It is a hypothesis with which I cannot (as opposed to choose not) to identify, where non-identification is not trivial.

The brain won't go away

One might say that we can philosophize until the cows come home, yet the mind is undeniably dependent on the brain. In its rather severe dependency we might have the proof of emergence at of least a ghost contingent on the brain for its ethereal existence (a substance dualism contingent on the brain), or the proof that mind is the workings of the brain (in which we return to a property dualism). I'm so frequently encountering people who argue these positions to have been the recent findings of post enlightenment neuroscience, though we can be reminded that Hippocrates (or someone claiming to be Hippocrates) stated over two millennia ago

"Men ought to know that from the brain, and from the brain only, arise our pleasures, joys, laughter and jests, as well as our sorrows, pains, griefs and tears. Through it, in particular, we think, see, hear, and distinguish the ugly from the beautiful, the bad from the good, the pleasant from the unpleasant, in some cases using custom as a test, in others perceiving them from their utility. It is the same thing which makes us mad or delirious, inspires us with dread or fear, whether by night or by day, brings sleeplessness, inopportune mistakes, aimless anxieties, absent-mindedness, and acts that are contrary to habit. These things that we suffer all come from the brain, when it is not healthy, but becomes abnormally hot, cold, moist, or dry, or suffers any other unnatural affection to which it was not accustomed. Madness comes from its moistness."

Now Hippocrates was perhaps, nay was, working on false premises. He would have seen the changes in perfusion and colour to the body and face in various states of disease and might have made inferences as to corresponding humoral imbalances in the brain. In all likelihood he never even witnessed a brain dissection, if for no other reason that the brain turns to mush unless pickled. Not until the age of Thomas Willis was this problem overcome. But what I think would have been driving the mind equals brain hypothesis in ancient Greece might have been a common knowledge of many in antiquity. When, for example, a Greek strikes a Persian with a weapon or a Persian strikes a Greek, there are different outcomes following a central chest injury vs a blow to the shoulder or the leg. And all these might result in different outcomes, very different outcomes, to that of an acquired brain injury from a blow to the head. Most preliterate persons might well have well known that a knock on the head can profoundly change a person, if not kill them. And so it is not only the premise of Hippocrates observation, yet his place in the intelligentsia also as the one with licence to discover, both as further questioning the scientific metanarrative we have made for ourselves. In any case, the Greeks did not deny the embodied lifeforce that is the psyche or soul.

Now we can say that we have moved beyond Hippocrates and Neuroscience texts such a Kandel and Schwartz "Principles of Neural Science" include the above quote as a throwback to the time when natural philosophers (i.e. scientists) were interested and conversant in history and the liberal arts, a projecting of persona to being the gentleman scientist. It's quaint isn't it. In any case we have moved beyond Hippocrates. We now know the parts of the brain correlating with vision, olfaction, muscle movement and so on. If a part of the brain dies, there can be a more or less predictable range of outcomes such as loss of speech, vision, smooth sequential movement and so on. With respect to vision for example, we can even locate the place in the brain correlating with the perception of objects with certain orientation and movement. The teasing out of these modular brain regions and also more distributed so called circuits are what Chalmers calls the easy problems. Nevertheless, like shining a light in a furnished room containing an infinitely deep well at its centre, all we have simultaneously done is to resolve the even greater darkness of the hard problem, consciousness itself. Its edges are illuminated, this leading the neuroscientist to think they are closer to the solution when they are further away than ever. And so what have we gained from saying, for example, that vision is dependent on the unexplored whole brain to now say it depends on this particular part of the brain into which we have journeyed? Neither tells us what seeing is, let alone what it is when "I see". And have we answered the question if mind drives brain as a necessary instrument, or brain drives mind, the latter as its secretion?

An answer in favour of materialism might be in the fact of just how profound the changes to mind can be in disease or in states of drug intoxication. A congenitally blind person is likely never to describe a visually vivid dream and never say "I see with my mind's eye, yet lack the apparatus to see in the world".

Helen Keller "saw" and held memory in her fingers. A demure introvert might experiment with phencyclidine and become a raving homicidal lunatic. The older person with dementia might not simply lose their memory, but their memory of having lost memory, and indeed their whole connectedness with themselves and the world goes with it. These are prima facie devastating blows to a non-materialist account of mind or accounts which place mind on a pedestal as anything more than epi-phenomenon, though their claim to being fatal blow is more a neuro-scientistic mode de jure, than a fact beyond other interpretations.

One such non materialistic objection, and one which has been played out in religion and popular culture (cross culturally) from antiquity, is the notion that the person is primarily a non-physical substance that becomes attached to a material structure into which it grows and comes to identify. To a behaviourist the phenomena is actually a supernatural Pavlovian experiment without extinction being easily achieved. Just imagine it to be possible that there is something which is better described as spirit that comes to be shackled to a brain and grows with it. With time it would forget what it is in the greater sense, and contra Plato might never have known to begin with what it was then to forget. It might only know itself in the phenomena of its conscious awareness and in its intentionality, particularly its intentionality of moral faculties and the like. But this is the bitter joke, for the mind never achieves an emancipation from the attachment to the material brain, and neither ignorance of neuroscience nor a knowledge of its limitations is to any avail. When the brain bleeds the mind reflexively bleeds in its own way, even unto the end of the person as they knew themselves and were known to others. I am not proposing this ontology to be true, much less expecting it to convince the diehard materialist. Yet it is a fair opening gambit to an ontology that could be developed and indeed has been developed by better minds than mine. In its accommodation of both the facts of neuroscience and the miracle of consciousness as per outlined above, it is far from being the least parsimonious formulation either. The fact that it lay partly outside the bounds of what is ordinarily considered science provides no a priori's to abandon it as a possible (nay plausible) way to see self in world.

The glimpses we have into this supra-material self may be within aesthetics, morality, peak experiences and the givenness of consciousness, along with certain aspects thereof. One of many places to which I was taken to marvel when I was younger was the spatial location and extension of consciousness. And this was a sense of marvel only to be amplified by a knowledge of neuroscience, as its answer to the mystery was as unfulfilling as an answer could possibly be. Take something sharp and jab it into your finger tip. The pain you feel is of course in your finger, not somewhere behind the eyes. Now I could tell you that there is a sensory representation of that same finger in the brain, this homunculus having been resolved with clarity by Wilder Penfield and others nigh on a century ago. Stimulate that finger part of the brain and you may have the very same sensation in your finger as if you dug into the fingertip itself. Ablate that same area in the brain and you might prick your finger a thousand times and feel nothing. We could also do, as nature sometimes does, cross wiring experiments where one physical stimulus leads to a different physical sensation, or where removing a limb results in the sensation that your limb still exists out there where it was and yet now only empty air has come to fill the space (see in the use of the word "wiring" the ease with which the technological metaphor creeps in). Now I, as well as anyone else cognizant of neuroscience, can dismiss the mystery here. I can say that the feeling of the finger as being spatially outside the brain and in the finger is simply the brain performing some strange ventriloquy, like the performer who projects the voice as if coming from the doll in their lap. But this neuro-ventriloquy, if true, is much more profound and cannot be simply believed without pause. For neuroscience would say, and say rightly, that the only the brain itself has the requisite complexity to effect the emergence of the finger consciousness. Certainly the "wiring" in the finger is just the ramifications of a simple nerve. There is no little brain in one's fingertip sufficient for the complexity argument to hold, and so I am not in my finger they will say. And yet I do not experience things within the head as if to say "I the one behind the eyes feel a pain and know that it is associated with a noxious stimulus to the finger". If I take upon myself the cap of the materialist neuroscientist I cannot liberate myself from the experience as being in a place (and time) which, so says the dogma, lacks the neurological complexity to be experienced. That is to say I cannot convert the beingness of the finger from spatially within the finger to within the head and somewhere behind the eyes simply in virtue of knowing about the sensory homunculus. Even an assiduous change in language to prohibit "in finger" consciousness cannot alter the basic fact of being out there. And so back we are to dismissing things as a trick of our ventriloquist brain, and the case is closed. The mystery does not go away however, nor does an evolutionary explanation which might pretend to answer the "why" or "how". How am I, qua nothing but an emergent product of the brains complexity, consciously existing res extensa in the finger, a place of neurological austerity? I would suggest to the materialist that if they admit to the possibility of any ventriloquist act as they apparently must, then why not countenance one of a different kind, i.e. not one where matter automatically in the act of emergence thinks that it is mind (for lack of a better turn of phrase), and not one where the brain qua mind thinks it is spatially located "out there". If the concept of ventriloquism exists in the world at all and it admitted into argument, then why not allow for the hypothesis that an immaterial mind confuses itself with the walls of its jail and automatically thinks that it is matter?

Another possibility, terribly unpopular nowadays more for falling out of fashion than plausibility and more a result of the sycophantic want for philosophers to cling on as scientistic appendages as opposed to the philosopher telling the neuroscientist how to think and where they have failed to think, is another kind of mind brain monism. Only in this case the monism is not material but mental and usually, though not necessarily, religiously informed. In such a world view what we think of as brains and rocks and the orbits of planets are thoughts within a greater mind. In their regularity and radical separation from our own little minds, certain of these thoughts are experienced as something solid, separate and "objective". Our perceptions of this solid world out there are internally valid of course. Yet the solidity of the external world is a category error. For in the greater mind all in creation is weakly consubstantial, with thoughts merely crystalized in various forms in time and over time. Our own mind is a thought made free from the greater mind, with some limited agency to change itself and effect change. And what we cannot easily change is the brute facts of the material world. To disavow the existence of this greater mind is a projection of our own narcissism in defending the limits of what our own can know and do. We might think that if we cannot be more of ourselves, then this greater mind cannot be at all.

As Ronald Knox wrote, when thinking of the immaterial monist Berkley

There was a young man who said "God

Must find it exceedingly odd

To think that the tree

Should continue to be

When there's no one about in the quad."

Reply:

"Dear Sir: Your astonishment's odd;

I am always about in the quad.

And that's why the tree

Will continue to be

Since observed by, Yours faithfully, God."

All of the above is not offered as proof of what is, this being impossible. Rather it is a briefly reasoned defence of what might be. When multiple hypotheses explain the phenomena, we must in dint of reason be agnostic and know what we believe as an article of faith.

My own inclination is that things are of one of three possibilities. The first would be a mind brain material monism which denies the givenness of personal consciousness. This is so profoundly nihilistic as to require something of a paradoxical transcendent or mystical turn to explain mind away. And so for this and other incoherence in the argument besides, it lacks appeal both logically and intuitively. Then there is the (substance dualistic) notion that God has a sense of humour, making mind emergent each moment as a miracle of upmost immanence to us, with the brain being both the tool upon which mind works and the manifold upon which it stands to know itself. And yet in us being half mind and half matter we are not fully anything of either except a reminding of our own mortality, perhaps the one miracle which really can die and stay dead when its time is up. The final possibility is something akin to Berkley, where there is certainly only a monism, but it isn't matter and any transcendence can only be found in placing a faith in a mind greater than our own to either not forget us or remember us in some hyper-time.

Now what has all this to do with psychiatry? Well we are back to where we started. There is nothing lost to the renal physician thinking the kidney is a glorified filter or the heart a glorified pump (yes they are both endocrine organs too of course). Both subspecies of physician may play about happily in metaphysically smaller ponds. But psychiatry has thrown itself into something deeper without being able to swim, and the village has invested it with the power to be our lifeguard.

RELATIVITY. THE TRUTH MAKERS.

Alice laughed. "There's no use trying," she said: "one can't believe impossible things.""I daresay you haven't had much practice," said the Queen. "When I was your age, I always did it for half-an-hour a day. Why, sometimes I've believed as many as six impossible things before breakfast."

Alice and the White Queen (Lewis Carroll)

"Only in psychiatry is the existence of physical disease determined by APA presidential proclamations, by committee decisions, and even, by a vote of the members of APA, not to mention the courts"

Peter Breggin (maverick psychiatrist)

As I write this chapter a current best seller is a certain "12 Rules for Life" by professor of psychology Jordan Peterson, who is also the hottest ticket on the speaking circuit, commanding upwards of fifty to seventy-five thousand dollars per appearance. Now part of the good professor's shtick is the thesis that our current relativism with respect to truth, the attack on so called "Western" or "Judeo-Christian" values and even the tyranny of political correctness all flow from the postmodernist school, this being the scourge of the current age. And the postmodernist school in turn, whether we are talking Lyotard, Derrida or Foucault et al consisted of disillusioned Marxists who could no longer sustain their former allegiances in light of certain revelations as to the failure of the communist utopian project. The failures to which one might refer are the evidences in the 1950's and 1960's as to the brutality of the soviet regime and a material standard of living within the USSR that could not come within a country mile of rivalling that of an middle class white America surfing the wave of post war prosperity, something easily achieved for a nation whose mainland was not invaded to the tune of 20 million dead. Then there was Khrushchev's 1956 revelations to the international communist world that all was not rosy under the regime. And there were the writings of Solzhenitsyn as another of just two examples.

And so, goes the conspiracy story, the maleficent forces infecting these brilliant young French minds against Western and Judeo-Christian values morphed Marxism into this thing called postmodernism, the latter being equally hostile to the west, yet simply using different dialectical weapons of "deconstruction", identity politics (read class struggle) and the like. And then the infection spread to the Anglo western world as it had done already by the method of Gramsci, also in a disguised form. By extension what is implied is that certain political forces today to which Peterson is opposed are covert or at least rebranded Marxist Communist, a call to suspicion that in a sense is a recasting of the Mccarthyist upturning of the mattresses to find the reds under the bed. These are the views held by most of the so called "intellectual dark web", self-styled classical liberals and many neoconservatives alike. And all without exception vie for preening themselves a product of the enlightenment.

Never mind that Marxism itself was a product of the west, a secular Jew situated in a German dialectic in a most enlightenment atheism. Never mind that the youth and academia of a post war France were struggling to find a grip on any moral and ideological firmament after a reign of terror, a mistake of Napoleonic proportions, the fin de siecle and two wars to end all wars, both of which were valiantly fought by the French with the latter war also contaminated by Vichy shame. And so why not at least try on for size the official ideology of those who won the Eastern front and the war in toto. Any port in a storm in a country where perhaps a quarter of all the post war populace had socialist leanings anyway, this proclivity evidenced from a time long before Marx was a glint in his father's eye. Never mind that Peterson is a deconstructionist and reconstructionist himself in seeing Christ as a Jungian archetype of Christ, as opposed to Christ as the Christ, a definite article, one without a second. Never mind that to the nuanced eye there are considerable differences between those to whom might be given the descriptor postmodern. Never mind that that there many different formulations and expressions of Marxism to whom the postmodernists are supposedly too intimately connected, as "the new skin" of Marxism. And just as Marx was influenced by, and a response to, Hegel, there emerged and continue to emerge different Hegelians. Are leftist, right and contemporary branches of Hegelianism the same given the common root, and despite otherwise having considerable differences between them? And never mind that postmodernity could not have existed in thought much less in name were there not the modernity to which the current crop of "classical liberals" find themselves purporting to be a part of, an enlightenment project that also included the French revolution and the reign of terror. And was not modernity part of the slow creep away from Christian values towards the worship of the individual "me" and the coming to terms with being the happy orphans of a dead God, the victim of our own patricide. And never mind that "Western" in the "classical liberal" sense is not at all synonymous with "Judeo-Christian" either, and there is as great a degree of similarity between the "Judeo.." and the "Islamo.." as there is between the "Judeo..." and the "...Christian". And one final never mind is the never mindedness to the fact that the so called Judeo-Christian values as having become part of the modern western politics has also been influenced by the Romans and Greeks, and further east besides. Are we to say Pagan Christian values? Or Socialist Christian values after the book of Acts? You see we can build the cladistics of our own ideology as being parented however we wish. All these words are just slogans towards a political end, an attempt to pick the best and prettiest of histories, draw a wiggly line between them and say this is me too.

Now this book is far from being either a defence or critique of Marx, Marxism or Marxoid thought here. Specifically, I cannot engage with the strength of any putative connection between what Marx thought and said, the horrors that might be said to have been committed in his name and the avant-garde continental philosophers of the latter half of the twentieth century. It is beyond the scope of this book, my experience and my learning, though my intuition suggests to me such an association is at least somewhat misplaced and frankly silly. But I will say I'm bemused at the ignorance of others to notice what I think is a far stronger and pernicious assault on the traditional Christian values and presents a stronger push to relativize truth. But this is not from continental philosophy. It goes instead by the name of pragmatism and its evils hide in plain sight, even hidden from those who think it to be benign and live out the philosophy daily. Peterson, incidentally, despite all his virtues which I duly acknowledge, is a pragmatist.

You see the story begins with Charles Sanders Peirce (from whom we get the term pragmatism, and later pragmaticism. When he thought the former term was being misused he invented yet another "ism"). Peirce, an American philosopher and chemist, once wrote in 1878 an article on epistemology titled "How to Make Ideas Clear". Well I must confess his article was not always clear to me, and I dare guess many others who may read it. And I wish to make clear myself that Peirce held a belief in truth existing beyond the particular bearer of the truth. He held faith to a positivist eschatology that someday somehow science will irresistibly approach a point where belief (as a truth assertion) will be held without the possibility of an argument that would prevail against it.

That said, this eschatology was obviously an article of faith without empirical evidence. It also in no way could be interpreted as a correspondence theory of truth, where truth exists "out there" as something to be discovered and our beliefs must accord to it in order to be "true". He saw belief (qua an assertion of truth) as having a psychological utility in discharging doubt, the resultant being a sense of peace for a time, a comfort with the thought held, this comfort being the affective side of belief. Doubtless this is all carrying a survival value and could be argued to be part of the Darwinian project, another pan explanatory "ism" extremely pervasive at the time and one that remains so to this day.

He (Peirce) also makes a number of other statements that point towards a concept of truth in the here and now that is our daily life, even the life of the scientist. And that is that belief or truth is a function of the utility of the belief. It is true if it works for the singular or collective "you". The repeatability of science points towards a truth which is utilitarian, not a communing with an ontological truth "out there". X is true because it works, not because it is true.

e.g. "Consider what effects, which might conceivably have practical bearings, we conceive the object of our conception to have. Then, our conception of these effects is the whole of our conception of the object"

In other words, if it is practical to believe in x and ascribe to X the word "true", then believe in x.

Someone who was greatly influenced by Peirce and had both the intellect and the clarity as a wordsmith to take pragmatism to the masses was William James. James meta-philosophical project was to save those who carried what he called the "tender minded" philosophic temperament from the "tough minded" ones. That is to say he wished to save the humanities and spiritually minded philosopher from the corrosive effects of materialism, scientism and the excessive austerities of pure logic, much as Kant and Wittgenstein tried to do the same in their own and far better ways. Pragmatism was James answer as a happy mediation towards both the tender and the tough. James pragmatism can also be encapsulated beautifully into his story of the squirrel in the published account of James second lecture.

"Some years ago, being with a camping party in the mountains, I returned from a solitary ramble to find everyone engaged in a ferocious metaphysical dispute. The corpus of the dispute was a squirrel — a live squirrel supposed to be clinging to one side of a tree-trunk; while over against the tree's opposite side a human being was imagined to stand. This human witness tries to get sight of the squirrel by moving rapidly round the tree, but no matter how fast he goes, the squirrel moves as fast in the opposite direction, and always keeps the tree between himself and the man, so that never a glimpse of him is caught. The resultant metaphysical problem now is this: DOES THE MAN GO ROUND THE SQUIRREL OR NOT? He goes round the tree, sure enough, and the squirrel is on the tree; but does he go round the squirrel? In the unlimited leisure of the wilderness, discussion had been worn threadbare. Everyone had taken sides, and was obstinate; and the numbers on both sides were even. Each side, when I appeared, therefore appealed to me to make it a majority. Mindful of the scholastic adage that whenever you meet a contradiction you must make a distinction, I immediately sought and found one, as follows: "Which party is right," I said, "depends on what you PRACTICALLY MEAN by 'going round' the squirrel. If you mean passing from the north of him to the east, then to the south, then to the west, and then to the north of him again, obviously the man does go round him, for he occupies these successive positions. But if on the contrary you mean being first in front of him, then on the right of him, then behind him, then on his left, and finally in front again, it is quite as obvious that the man fails to go round him, for by the compensating movements the squirrel makes, he keeps his belly turned towards the man all the time, and his back turned away. Make the distinction, and there is no occasion for any farther dispute. You are both right and both wrong according as you conceive the verb 'to go round' in one practical fashion or the other."

In the above excerpt from James, his claim to truth and belief rest upon a clarity with which the problem is stated, and is a better illustration of what Peirce wished clearly to say. In what sense is the question asked, that the man goes around the squirrel? It hinges upon a definition of "going around". There's a third option also. After Einstein and without any aether or universal reference frame it might be as true to say that the man's legs move yet he does not go anywhere, as the squirrel, tree and indeed the whole universe orbit around him. Perhaps in the 22nd century there can be additional formulations of man, squirrel and tree, bounded only by our imagination and the new scientific paradigms that may come...or may not as the case will be. But as is clear in the example and in further of James lectures, truth is not arrived at by a clear sense in which terms of the proposition are made. Neither does truth find it's ground in clear grammar providing a correspondence between words about the world and the world as it is. No, for James truth is entirely instrumental. It is as true to say that man revolves around squirrel as squirrel revolves around man depending on the ends to which the question is asked and what one wants. James, in the land of the free marketeer capitalist and contra the Marxist temperament, even accords to truth the descriptor "cash value" and also additionally writes....

"Any idea upon which we can ride, so to speak; any idea that will carry us prosperously from any one part of our experience to any other part, linking things satisfactorily, working securely, simplifying, saving labor; is true for just so much, true in so far forth, true instrumentally. This is the 'instrumental' view of truth."

And where the anti-communist conspiracy might have it (and probably has it correctly) that certain Marxist infiltrations entered into the universities, media and the like by Gramsci 's inspired "march through the institutions", pragmatism also had its inroads into the same institutions in the United States by John Dewey and his disciples, even leading to the foundation of American public school education and social work.

Dewey, a democratic socialist with friends in high places and philosopher of many areas, was the last of the trio of classical pragmatists, classical pragmatism having taken root and flourishing as the first home grown American philosophy. Not surprising for an atheist, Dewey also rejected truth as an ontological, dare I say transcendent, state of affairs, that knowledge is or ought to be a correspondence between the reality out there and how it might be represented in the mind or the collective "sciences". Instead truth was for Dewey, as it was for James and Peirce before him, that that is the case when we reliably get the outcome we are wanting. Truth is teleological where the architect of telos is mortal man.

Now I'm not stating that Pierce and James' pragmatism was entirely as it could be cynically interpreted. On a deeper reading it was actually quite nuanced and I confess not to have read the entire corpus of their works. It's entirely possible, though this is very much to be doubted, that somewhere they might have inserted a caveat not to be taken too seriously. That having been said, we are at least discussing the effects of their pragmatism, a reading of their pragmatism which by their own lights is the "cash value" of their philosophy on truth.

Now what on Earth has this to do with psychiatry I hear you ask.

Firstly, I take it as a given from my own experience that psychiatry has no faith or sincere interest in objective transcendent truth, never mind the good or the beautiful.

Secondly, I take it as a given that contemporary psychiatry is dominated by North America, its publication machine and the DSM. To the extent to which it exports its ideology beyond its borders and to the extent psychiatry is bio-political (as is certainly the case), American psychiatry colonizes other nations. It does this under the guise of caring words just as it does using propaganda words such as democracy, rights etc. And these other nations welcome becoming colonies.

Thirdly, when the effects of a various philosophies are found to be existing in an Anglo nation and can be attributed either to being manufactured locally or to have been imported from the European continent, it is the more parsimonious conclusion that the effects are from the local philosophy (i.e. pragmatism), though this of course is not to imply other influences are impossible (Marxism, postmodernism, other isms).

Fourth, Pragmatism qua truth being what is useful was an invitation to a power hungry hedonistic epistemology that was too much for modern (and post-modern) Americans to resist. It seeped into all areas of its culture and indeed even into psychiatry. It is evidenced by the words psychiatrists use. It placed a perverted epistemology in an unholy marriage with an ethics that would be unable to resist becoming perverted in kind. It is a question of human drives and motivations as to what people wish the truth to be in being directed to a desired end, ends often impacting upon other persons. In this sense pragmatism is necessarily a political philosophy. And the will towards a desired truth is the manifold upon which psychiatry can slide incoherently and effortlessly between appeals to reified truth as a science of the objective world (an appeal to scientific legitimacy), and also an appeal that the truth can be whatever is according to some other self serving end that it wishes (the continuance of power cloaked in the language of care, patient values etcetera). The truth is my truth. And who am I? I am the psychiatric guild. And the truth I trade in derives its "cash value" from verification. And who verifies? It is the guilds of psychiatry that verifies. If psychiatry verifies its own truths, it creates its own capital. And who owns the capital? The guilds do. Domestically they are monopolies. Internationally they are oligarchies. And then the public take these false "truths" as fact, via a focus on what the guilds call science at the time in a game when the doublethink makes opportune to invoke the word "science". Surely this is an economy that can only survive as long as the metaphorical mint keeps printing the metaphorical cash, always borrowing on a future that never arrives, a society where the will to real truth has lost the "cash value" of a former age. This is the age where Oprah can speak of "my truth" and "your truth" with nary anyone taken aback at the horror of three hundred million truths, and few wishing to champion even the notion of "the truth". This is the age where psychotherapies are more concerned with what "works for you", as opposed to a confrontation with "what you are" or "who you should be".

Fifth; Take a critical look at all the uses for the words pragmatic and pragmatism and their variants or subtexts in the psychiatric literature. It is everywhere. What follows is but one particularly egregious example from the Australian literature, a country where I once worked for a time, citing American psychiatric intelligentsia of course, this being consonant with my thesis.

The 2013 Royal Australian & New Zealand College of Psychiatrists (RANZCP) Mood Disorder Guidelines is the specimen to be studied, at its time the most up to date international guidelines in print. It remains perhaps the largest undertaking into mood and its disorders, so long in the planning that the previous guidelines were published a full decade prior. Weighing in at greater than one hundred pages, with more than a thousand references and a few dozen committee expert authors and advisors, it includes the claim to have consulted widely with many stakeholders including the laity.

The first section titled "Classification of mood disorders" opens with subtitle "A pragmatic approach to mood disorder classification."

It continues; "There is growing consensus that psychiatric diagnoses are akin to social constructs (Insel, 2014; Zachar and Kendler, 2007). It is nonetheless appropriate for the structure of this guideline to adopt an accepted mood disorder taxonomy because, (i) there is broad agreement about definitions, and (ii) diagnostic terms have accrued valuable meaning through scientific (e.g. clinical trials) and social processes (e.g. advocacy). (See: Figure 1). Using the terms as pragmatic organising constructs should not translate into their reification – the optimal classification of disorders must await a quantum leap in our understanding of the aetiology and pathophysiology of abnormal behaviour."

The references are these.

Insel TR (2014) The NIMH Research Domain Criteria (RDoC) Project: Precision medicine for psychiatry. American Journal of Psychiatry 171: 395–397.

Zachar P and Kendler KS (2007) Psychiatric disorders: A conceptual taxonomy. American Journal of Psychiatry 164: 557–565.

We will dispense at the outset with the words "akin to". This is written I suspect to allow one to evade critique by denying having made a definite statement, only something akin to the statement. The same is the case with the word "consensus", as I suspect were I to say the consensus is the RANZCP they would say "no not us", and have me running down labyrinthine alleys searching for the target.

The RANZCP guidelines are a lesson into the dangers of secondary reading and that bloating an article with references (or a book, hence my refrain) neither adds to the weight of scholarship or the strength of argument. You see neither the Insel or the Zachar and Kendlar articles state anything like approaching that diagnoses are akin to social constructs. Insel speaks of the DSM, "like other medical disease classifications". His article is thoroughly wedded to the so called medical model and it would dishonour the man to suggest a social constructivist subtext that clearly is not present. It simply posits that medical science (under the RDoC framework) will grant the tools to reorganize a taxonomy of mental illness that would be an improvement on the existing one. There is not one single mention of any psychiatric disorder being etiologically either a psychological or social phenomena, much less specifically a "social construct" designed by a consensus group of powerful stakeholders.

And what of Zachar and Kendlers paper? Having been published pre DSM 5 in 2007, it's a curious choice, with both authors publishing widely since. For Zachar this has reached its peak as a contributor in a multi-perspective wonderful series of articles in 2012 in Philosophy and Ethics in Humanities and Medicine. Suffice to say for now, Zachar sides with the American psychiatric guild and its colonies (Australia included) on the side of philosophical pragmatism. To use Allen Frances baseball metaphor of truth, he thinks the reality of an umpire's call lay in how he uses it (Frances was chair of the various DSM IV committees). Or to speak of psychiatry, he considers models and explanations as more or less as a means to an end. For Kendler, he was a task force member of DSM IV and a member of the psychotic disorder working group, the group in which one hundred percent of its membership were in receipt of monies from the pharmaceutical industry. He also was part of the DSM 5 mood disorder working group 2007-2010. His views on the DSM are sympathetic at the very least, even whilst paying lip service to their imperfection. The cited 2007 article speaks of a need to revise the DSM for sure, though posterity has shown this revision to the DSM 5 be modest, to capture more people under diagnostic umbrellas than in earlier editions, and the DSM has continued to underwrite psychiatric diagnoses as bona fide medical illnesses. The article takes us on a journey not of consensus to social constructs but of many ways in which psychiatric classification may be considered. The authors do this by comparing 6 sets of dipoles as dimensions of categorization. (Causalism vs descriptivism, Essentialism vs nominalism, Objectivism vs evaluativism, Internalism vs externalism, Entities vs Agents and Categories vs Continua). Nonetheless at the end of the day and of the article the use of the word "construct" is endorsed as being synonymous with that of a scientific hypothesis that can be empirically tested within a scientific framework. The authors make no statement as to their diagnoses being a consensus held (presumably by a powerful interest group) and thus a "social" construct.

Returning to the RANZCP guidelines and the quoted text above; we need be clear that social constructivism is essentially antithetical to metaphysical naturalism. Water as being two parts hydrogen to one part oxygen is not socially constructed. It is a fact of the world, as is its boiling point at a given pressure. As is the location of brain in the skull and not the chest and the fact that it contains certain component parts that if ablated will result in blindness etcetera. The list of these natural facts are endless. They are not established by opinion of an individual or a consensus group or contingent in any way on the same. Compare this with social construction in the ordinary language use of the term. Though both made art and placed paint upon the canvas, the distinction between the baroque and rococo periods is a matter of social construction, as are endless lists of human belief and behaviour in fashions and politics. A bone is either broken or it is not. The sport played in which the bone was broken is a social construction, as is its rules. Whether unhappiness is to be seen as part of the human condition, a challenge to change one's life or to be medicalised as if it were disease (though it is not), this too is a social construction.

Now the psychiatric guilds wish to have their cake and eat it too. They are forced to acknowledge that they can no longer claim all psychiatric diagnoses to be naturalistic medical facts of the world of a broken body or brain. The evidence simply is not there. Yet they hold onto pretences to scientific legitimacy and an appeal to the status quo whilst holding out a faith that "the optimal classification" would involve greater knowledge of the "pathophysiology" i.e. they are nailing their colours to the wall that mood and its disorders are naturalistic phenomena whose pathological mechanism is yet to be discovered, whilst acknowledging it isn't at this time. The acting "as if" to a pragmatist is all that matters, as we have discussed above. Why? Because to act "as if" if directed to a given end of prosperity to the guild is the end of the journey to truth. The rest is just persuasion and propaganda, again to a desired end. It's pragmatism through and through, where pragmatism is what one does when one has abandoned all principles. Pragmatism is the philosophy of choice for the merchant. It is a trading of the staff of Aesculapius for the caduceus of Hermes.

Perhaps I could make my point clearer by an analogy with religion. Imagine that some grand ecumenical council were to convene and issue the following edict;

"There is growing consensus that our faith in anything transcendent is akin to social constructivism and by extension God or Gods probably don't exist as such. It is nonetheless appropriate for the way of life of humankind to continue practicing, living in hope and dying for faiths following the status quo mix of religious doctrines because, (i) there is broad agreement about the operational notion of the God or Gods as defined, and (ii) religious ways of life have accrued valuable meaning through sacraments and observed "miracles" (e.g. prayer, fasting, confession, healings and resurrections etc) and social processes (e.g. churches, monasteries, martyrdom, faith based wars, charities, alliances of church and state, orphanages etcetera). Using the notion of God or Gods or anything supernatural as a pragmatic organising construct should not be reified and translate into their genuine faith or belief in them as existing beyond their identity as akin to a social construct – the optimal determination of theological truth must await a quantum leap in our understanding, a miracle never before experienced".

Surely we would be aghast to read such a thing and question the seriousness, logical and moral coherence of those who would say such nonsense. A move towards a view of religion as socially constructed by a mortal consensus group must surely be followed in lockstep by an immediate move towards apostasy and an overnight dismantling of the church. The want to avoid a vacuum would offer no excuse to fill the void with the ghost of what came before that moment of terrible consensus, when the substance of the ghost is found to be meaningfully lacking. Similarly, from the revelation that psychiatric diagnoses are social constructions must follow a dissolution of all the pretences of psychiatry to science and to medicine. And the mad, bad and sad would need return to the community from whence they came as persons amongst people. Any doctor reaching for the prescription pad would need admit that s/he is practicing at best cosmetic psychopharmacology, at worst placebo medicine. An expert class of professional liars would be superfluous. Naturally with the death of psychiatry what would follow wold be the death of the link between it and the state. Society would need find other ways of managing misery and deviancy. Whether or not society is successful in this endeavour is immaterial to the fact that what is socially constructed must properly return to its home in society.

Why Psychiatry is a Secularised Exorcism?

The state and the church never separated. The church was simply replaced by psychiatry. The transaction between an enquiring patient and their doctor might go something like this.

Patient "I feel poorly and have a cough"

Doctor (having auscultated the chest, viewed the X ray and other investigations) "you have pneumonia"

Patient "and what is pneumonia?"

Doctor "in this case it is an occupation of certain parts of your lungs with bacteria and the outcome of the war between the bacteria and the immune system, that being pus and such".

The reader will note the linearity in the explanation, and the appeal to something real. Yet take what might be a dialogue between patient and psychiatrist

Patient "I have a low mood, poor sleep, poor appetite and life has lost its lustre"

Psychiatrist "You have major depressive disorder"

Patient "and what is major depressive disorder"

Psychiatrist "major depressive disorder is when you have low mood, poor sleep, poor appetite and life has lost its lustre"

The reader will note the circularity here, that the diagnosis fails to point through, as it were, to something beyond the symptoms and signs. Rather the symptoms and signs point only to themselves, they are denotatively void. Now the reader may object and suggest the symptoms and signs of depression point towards some truly causal and explanatory event or thing in the world. Yet the thing in the body does not exist, there being for example no chemical imbalance causal to the depressed mind, no neuroplastic change in the brain causally related to an addicts drug use, no dopamine deficiency in the ADHD brain unmolested by drugs. And events in the sense of providing explanatory power are empty or at best partially formed explanations. Am I coughing and sick because I am old, or because someone similarly sick coughed upon me? This transfer of coughing does not define bacterial pneumonia. Does it really say anything to say I am depressed because I was raped or because of unrequited love, having been fired from my job or the bank to have foreclosed on my mortgage? These may play their causal roles in their way to the mood that I feel, though this is not to say depression is these events, certainly not in the way it is presented by the psychiatrist and accepted by the patient with the ontological force as pneumonia is pronounced upon the patient. Usually the antecedent events and speculations as to their causal significance are an afterthought or in any case secondary to the symptoms and signs as defining the diagnosis. And yet the shared experience between psychiatrist and patient alike, the belief, the affect, is as if none of these deep intractable problems existed. The psychiatric diagnosis is pronounced as a recognition of a "this" that is "there", as real as a bacteria and the purulent expectoration from one's lungs. It is as real as the invisible demon for those who believe in possession, that malevolent other that is in the patient yet not a part of them. To be sure I'm not proposing anything supernatural is going on in psychiatry. Yet to speak of persuasion and suggestion, of placebo, faith and empty belief is too banal. It does not capture the magic here when the non-existent other is invoked and given an ontological status far beyond its due. The psychiatric pronouncement makes something real that remains unreal. The magic is in the ritual and its impact upon the world. And psychiatrists, those most unholy of demonologists, create the demon whose exorcism they seek credit. This sort of bewitching can only be done be master pragmatists

DEMONOLOGY. I, FATHER KARRIS

"At first art imitates life. Then life will imitate art. Then life will find its very existence from the arts"
Fyodor Dostoevsky

"Television has done much for psychiatry by spreading information about it, as well as contributing to the need for it"
Alfred Hitchcock

"Is the accuser always holy now? Were they born this morning as clean as God's fingers? I'll tell you what's walking Salem—vengeance is walking Salem"
John Proctor to Hale (Arthur Miller's "The Crucible")

Act I; Multiplicity

From time to time the psychiatric guilds lament at how their profession is portrayed in cinema and popular culture. I say "lament" as these philosopher kings and queens do not like being portrayed as cruel and stupid, or just plain weird, and film never seems to administer ECT humanely under general anaesthesia. Lamentations aside, never is the question turned on its head. Never is it posed if psychiatry itself is the virtual image, that is to say if psychiatry is a portrayal of film and imitator of popular culture, if life imitates art.

This chapter will attempt a study of just that very question, and explore a couple of occasions when psychiatry, if not the product of the screen and novel, was at least in an uncritical symbiosis with it. The problem is in the realization that both the film crew and film goer can discern the difference between fantasy and reality when the curtain falls. But can psychiatry do the same? And what might these historical episodes reveal as to the personality of psychiatry and its guilds?

Our journey begins with the psychological concept of dissociation, which is to say by way of rough definition a certain degree of consciousness and behaviour persists in the person which is split off from normal perception, memory consolidation or even a loss of continuance of personal identity. And so in war or rape one may dissociate from the body or surrounds so as to feel a sense of separation from the horror of the moment. In a limited sense this stepping back from, or outside of, the self can be said to mimic the cruder less sublime elements of so called put of body or near death experiences. These near death experiences tend to be hyperreal and often life changing, in this sense entirely different to dissociation. The quasi out of body experience is one kind of dissociation. We might also have dissociative fugue and dissociative amnesia, wherein the person claims to have "lost time" after having been otherwise potentially observed going about this or that activity in their own identity or in a trance like state of automatic activity. And finally we have dissociative identity, in the latter twenty years of the twentieth century known as multiple personality, in which the person as we know them is replaced by another identity with a different name, personality and stream of consciousness. It is optional if these second, third or nth personalities/identities can sit aside and observe the behaviour of the primary personality at the times when they do not hold the reigns to the body and their voice remains unheard by the outside world. In this sense dissociative identity is a parallel topography of consciousness with different identities sitting side by side, rather than the layered up down of traditional formulations of seeing consciousness as unitary and conceptually placed above the primitive and alien unconscious or subconscious.

Behaviour for which we might be inclined to use the descriptor "dissociation" has probably always been with us. Historically we might imagine the first therapist of multiple personality disorder to be the Christ, who cast the multiple identities of the demonic "legion" out of the Gerasene. Yours truly offers such a formulation only with tongue in cheek, without the hubris other authors have had when talking of the allegedly possessed of antiquity as obviously epileptic, obviously schizophrenic, obviously "x" or obviously "y". To the extent Christ might have been an early psycho-therapist of a kind, it is to be noted that remission was achieved in a single session and in record time. Insomuch as the patient was male, neither was it blatantly chauvinist, the medicalization of female "hysteria" that has otherwise been the case in the current century and a half of psychiatry. Hence even the secular progressivist must bow their head whilst simultaneously groping to medicalize.

Peri and post enlightenment, dissociation was of interest to European occultists and magnetists, such as the German Franz Anton Mesmer in his Dissertatio physico-medica de planetarum influxu of 1766. The connection between the communing with the inner selves and others and the netherworld of the dead and familiar spirits never really went away. However, as a psychological theory with treatments, allegedly serious study only comes into its own in the post enlightenment.

Despite there being many of a German or English interest in dissociation, in many ways post reign of terror France was the centre of it all. One early case of extreme dissociation was that of Antoine Despine (1777–1852) who employed "magnetic therapy" (what James Braid would later call hypnosis admixed with mineral waters, forced rest etc) on a young 11 yr old girl Estelle L'Hardy in 1836, published two years later in monograph form. Estelle did not quite manifest what we might call MPD, though had a severe dissociation with conversion disorder (she was paralysed without any organic explanation in an age when one had limited ability to organically explain anyway). Despines case is emblematic of what would be the attitude of the physician with respect to dissociative disorders in general, i.e. the want to believe there was not the slightest conscious design on the part of the patient, the want to believe they (the physician) could not be fooled. Much to the chagrin of Despines wife, he took Estelle into their home as an honorary member of the family, and described her thus

"because of her age and youthful frankness, she cannot be suspected of emotionality, conceit, or the wish to cause a sensation. Finally, her extreme innocence made her incapable of deliberate deception"

Ergo, children cannot lie, the corollary of which is that the wise physician cannot be deceived.

There were other French physicians who took an interest in dissociation. There was Moreau de Tours, who a decade after Despine and a century before the experimental work in the 1960's studied drug induced dissociation, his drug of choice being hashish. There was also Étienne Eugène Azam, who in the 1958 case of Felida described the "doublement de la vie" of multiple personality, perhaps the earliest case.

But the master of dissociation was to be the alienist, neurologist extraordinaire Jean Martin Charcot at the Hospital de la Salpêtriere. Much has been written about Charcot, who by his own narcissism and others accounts likewise was considered the greatest physician of his age. Most would fawn over Charcot. Few if any would defy him in his own lifetime. One who was not backward in coming forward was the Swedish physician Axel Munthe. Munthe, though compassionate to the poor was independently wealthy and aristocratic in nature. He was a polyglot and at home pretty much anywhere in Europe, whether in Capri where he often resided or his native Sweden where he was at one point the physician to the royal house. In short he didn't need Charcot and his sideshow where young women would swoon or convulse and perform under the guise of medical science and its hypnotic discoveries of the deeper parts of the psyche. And so in his memoires "The Story of San Michele" Munthe writes of Charcots presentation of dissociated patients at his theatre of medical hypnosis

".....these performances of the Salpêtriere before the public tout of Paris are nothing but an absurd farce, a hopeless muddle of truth and cheating. Some of these subjects were no doubt real somnambulists faithfully carrying out in a waking state the various suggestions made to them during sleep-post hypnotic suggestions. Many of them were frauds, knowing quite well what they were expected to do, delighted to perform their various tricks in public, cheating both doctors and audiences with the amazing cunning of their of their hysteriques....."

Munthe knows this as he partook in the hypnotism itself, even on one occasion fighting fire with fire in hypnotizing a girl to attempt escape Charcot's clutches and return her to the nobler path of assisting her ailing and aging parents back on the farm in Normandy. What Munthe did not reckon on was that Charcot was the greater hypnotist, and more importantly the girl did not wish to relinquish her place as Tuesdays main event at the Hospital de la Salpêtriere. Munthes bitter lesson was to discover that a patient can like their mental illness and benefit from it, hence his conclusion as quoted above. Insomuch as some pathetic hypnotized young french hysterique nursing a top hat in her bosom like it is a baby or walking around on all fours thinking she is a dog, are both a step beyond mere multiple personality, it would be a bold step for psychiatrists of today to dare claim they are less gullible than the gentlemen scientists and physicians who fathered their profession before it even had a name.

Neurologist and Sorbonne professor Pierre Janet was one disciple of Charcots, as was Blueler, Gilles de la Tourette, Babinski, an early Freud and most of the other founding fathers of neurology from which we have eponymous diseases, signs and syndromes today. Freud we will mention only in passing. For all his many faults he never embraced the notion of multiple personality, and also swung on the pendulum from believing in neurosis and dissociation into multiplicity as a manifestation of bona fide childhood trauma only to later abandon it as a symptom of the fantasy incest within the unconscious. Notwithstanding the sceptical Freud probably believed in his own shift in view, it was a politically shewed move. Both the neurological intelligentsia and his Bourgeoisie clientele would not wish to be told the daughters of their social class were neurotic messes on account of childhood sexual abuse. The truth is likely somewhere in between.

And so it was in France and not Vienna that MPD continued its nascent advance with Pierre Janet. Janets prize case was that of "Lucie", a young woman who could be brought to dissociate by way of hypnosis, behaving in ways inexplicable to herself when not hypnotized. One day whilst hypnotized and dissociated, Lucie qua Lucie was engaged in conversation completely undistracted from what she was suggested to do, i.e. write on a piece of paper. This is the automatic writing that fascinated neurologists and occultists alike. For if the message was from another part of the self, might it not be channelling a message from the other side of the life/death divide? Janets own 1889 thesis "L'Automatisme psychologique" includes mention of possession, Spiritism etc

As the French philologist Taine writes

"two thoughts, two wills, two distinct actions, the one of which he is aware, the other of which he is not aware and which he ascribes to invisible beings."

Digressions to the spirit world aside, under Janet's watchful eye Lucie was conversing and split off from "her" hand which was busily writing. Only on this occasion the letter shockingly came to be signed "Adrienne". Just who, or what, was Adrienne? Adrienne, as would soon be discovered, was the woman who inhabited Lucies body when Lucie was not, so to speak, as a stream of consciousness and identity, "at home". Janet hypothesised that Lucie had developed this proclivity to dissociate into Adrienne after the small 't" traumatic experience of being frightened by two pranksters when she was a small child, a far cry from childhood sexual abuse which many contemporary trauma theorists would assume occurred. Indeed, many contemporary therapists assume the sexual abuse must have occurred in all hysteriques, and so are forever suspicious against family members who may very well be innocent. In any case, Janet developed a complicated though coherent system of topography of consciousness and subconscious as static and dynamic layers of component parts in flux and where traumatic events could result in the perturbation we call dissociation, even onto multiple personality disorder. His was a contribution that printed deeper on the map of what would become psychiatry the connection between trauma and dissociation, of unity and multiplicity.

Outside of the society set that attended Charcots human carnival of hysteria and some of the scholarly work that trickled down from those hypnotists and occultists of the fin de siecle interested in that sort of thing, arguably the next major seed into multiplicity was sown with R.L. Stevensons medically titled 1886 novel. "The Strange Case of Dr Jekyll and Mr Hyde". Many cinematic renditions have been made since, commencing almost as early as film in 1908 and ongoing to this day.

On the silver screen this was soon followed up by less science fiction fare, including the overtly MPD themed "The Case of Becky" which first played the stage in 1912 and adapted to film in 1915 and 1921. Hypnosis and childhood trauma were motifs of this and other films since, with Becky flipping between herself and the evil Dorothy. Elmer Clifton directed a variant of the Becky plot with "The Two Souled Woman" in 1918, with Priscilla Dean playing both Joy and her alter ego Edna.

It also not be lost on the reader that following Janet and Jekyll/Hyde and before the first eruption of early films, MPD was imported into the USA by Morton Prince, himself a neurologist/early psychiatrist who once was a visiting scholar at the Carnival of Charcot. Later he would adopt the same Parisian showmanship in Boston, and with the same ideology after rejecting the rival cult of Freud. Prince realized what is still practiced today, i.e. that in order to retain the prestige and scientific legitimacy one needs publish in scholarly journals. And so to tailor the peer review to his liking he started his own journal, the Journal of Abnormal Psychology in 1906, this soon followed by the Harvard Dept of Psychology, also his creation. Both continue to this day.

Prince wrote the case of Christine Beauchamp written 1906 in "The Dissociation of a Personality". Beauchamps real name was Clara Norton Fowler. She was a garden variety neurotic whose first manifestations of multiple personality emerged, not surprisingly, after hypnosis. Like the case of Eve (vide infra), Clara also had three distinct personalities, Clara being the first, Sally being born of hypnosis and later the saintly "B.I".

In the 1907 review of "The Dissociation of a Personality" in the Journal of Nervous and Mental Diseases, Beauchamp/Fowler was described thus "an actual case of Stevensons Jekyll and Hyde". This descriptor is perhaps a trivial flight into literary licence, though perhaps not. It is consonant with the thesis of the present chapter. It matters not that Hyde was not entirely the alternate personality of Jekyll so much as Jekyll deliberately wanting to exercise his moral vices behind the disguise of Hyde's face and brute strength. What Jekyll/Hyde and Beauchamp/Fowler speak of is a confusion in motive and fact, that being to create multiplicity and then argue the creation to be a discovery. The narcissism and moral deflection is preserved with creator or discoverer alike. The discoverer can say they did not create the evil alter. The patient can say it is not I, but "she" or "he" or "they" who does wrong.

Later McDougall would write in the 1926 An Outline of Abnormal Psychology

"It has been suggested by many critics that, in the course of Prince's long and intimate dealings with the case, involving as it did the frequent use of hypnosis, both for exploratory and therapeutic purposes, he may have moulded the course of its development to a degree that cannot be determined. This possibility cannot be denied"

In the end Clara was unified and married one of Princes assistants who was involved in her care.

Popular cultures next best exposure to MPD was to be the 1954 novel "The Birds Nest" by Shirley Jackson and the 1957 Richard Boone film adaptation "Lizzie", about the boring Elizabeth sharing the same body with the evil Lizzie. The plot was typical. Both were successful enough to further the idea of multiplicity trickling down into the American psyche. They were to beat "The Three Faces of Eve" to the market, yet not in becoming a household name. What is ominous in the tale of Lizzie is the treatment, which was to be seen as a success. In the end Elizabeth, Lizzie and whatever else indigenous to her psyche was killed off leaving only "Victoria", the new creation of therapy. Like Adam naming the products of creation before the fall, the doctor has become the original perfect man, and stands aside God in their own private garden.

The Three Faces of Eve

Eve White (aka Christine Costner Sizemore) was a troubled young woman, separated in a 6 year marriage and forced to live apart from her ostensibly dearly beloved 4 year old daughter. She lived with the maternal grandparents as Eve worked. According to some sources Eve had been diagnosed with "atypical schizophrenia" and fled from the psychiatrists who wished to give her electro-convulsive shock therapy. And who could blame her. There was never any evidence of psychosis.

She soon after attended the primary psychiatrist (Corbett Thigpen) with blinding headaches, dissociative fugue (day walking without memory) and a grab bag of aches and pains. One day a letter arrived at the psychiatrist's rooms, seemingly started by Eve White and ended with a different emotional tone and a different micrographic handwriting. Soon after during a subsequent psychotherapy session Eves body language and whole demeanour underwent a sudden and temporary metamorphosis. The demure submissive Eve White, with all her restrained repressed anger, vanished. The tacitly seductive devil may care Eve Black emerged. Though Thigpen and Cleckley did not formulate the case thus, the two Eves were a beautiful playing out of the Madonna whore complex, not in the mind of her husband or men in general but in the life of the Eves themselves. That said, one can always speculate on what was projected out from the therapists from their own libido into their suggestive patient. Freud would have preferred analyse them than Eve I'd venture to guess. The therapeutic journey as documented by Corbett Thigpen and Hervey Cleckley seems to be little more than exploration and hypnosis, in time effecting a much easier calling out of the alters desired at the time, in this sense adding to the instability of her psyche. Actually, as the months progressed in some ways the two Eves deteriorated until one day when a new personality "Jane" emerged disorientated and bewildered into the light of the consultancy room, a birth of a newborn adult. Jane was neither Eve W or Eve B, nor a mixture of the two. By the authors own admission, Jane might well have been a partial iatrogenic product, though they consider themselves "more catalytic than causal". This is a most interesting metaphor given that in chemistry some reactions will realistically never occur without the presence of a catalyst. And so what is causal here is a matter of semantics, and the psychological wish to admit what is necessary whilst retaining an innocent distance.

It is worth pointing out at this juncture a deeply moral and ethical conundrum which I have almost never heard raised by any of those who believe in multiple personality disorder and its treatment. Eve White was the patient who first presented seeking help. She was the one who was married, had a child and was the embodied identity known to the community around her. Yet Eve Black claimed to have always been there, with a continuity of historical narrative going back to childhood. Additionally, Eve White qua a stream of conscious identity, vanished into amnestic blackness when Eve Black ascended to take control of the body, whilst Eve Black retained a stream of consciousness at all times, even when just observing from the Cartesian depths what Eve White was doing with her body that they shared. Eve Black was often in control, and could even be the architect of Eve Whites amnesia when the latter held the reigns of consciousness. As the outsourced psychologist noted in his report, Eve Black was the maiden name of Eve White, and so could be formulated to being a regression of the same Eve, at an earlier time in her adult development. Yet why might the psychologist whom Thigpen and Cleckley consulted call Eve Black the secondary personality? This is all the more the case as Eve Black's consciousness and memory was an alternate personality that by all accounts emerged at a young age.

Accordingly, one can ask themselves who was the real Eve? Who was the bona fide owner over the body whose passport, if she had a passport, might have read "Eve Black" before marriage and "Eve White" after? But that devilish question we will dispense with, for the simple reason is that it is trivial compared to the next. The deeper, darker and much more disturbing question is this? If the deceptively named therapeutic goal of "integration" is successful, this is the annihilation of all alternate identities but one. For the true believer in multiple personality disorder, these identities have all the phenomenological components that the therapist themselves enjoys. They are living, breathing, embodied persons with emotions, thoughts and memories. These are not identities termed according to a priori qualifiers of subservience or supervenience. No, in MPD circles these are overwhelmingly termed alternate personalities or identities, even if the primary is called a host, a misplaced metaphor from the world or infectious diseases and demonology. For the true believer, nominalism does not save us from the essentialism revealed by the encounter with these identities, each who are other persons. And psychologists and psychiatrists are terribly confused on the basic metaphysical distinctions that the terms personality and identity provoke. One can have a fragmented personality and a unified identity. All over the land one might find the lady of the women's church group and the whore of the bedroom, the extrovert amongst friends and the introvert amongst strangers, the man of impeccable character to the town and the vicious wife beater at home whilst all the while maintaining the same unbroken stream of waking consciousness and awareness of who "I" am. But Eve W, Eve B and Jane were three different persons sharing the same body. And so in their bid to integrate via annihilation one or more alters, there is but one logical conclusion and I mean this in utmost seriousness. Every psychiatrist who believes in MPD is, in the court of their own metaphysics, a cold blooded serial killer. Even Thigpen and Cleckley, the only authors I have ever known to have scanned the outskirts of such a moral problem as this in understated utilitarian style, were to skirt it only shallowly and to have taken on themselves the assumed mantle of the philosopher kings who might decide the answer and the authority of judge, jury and executioner.

In the end their answer that Eve Black would be the better one to die in the gallows of psychotherapy, and like the fictional doctor in "The Birds Nest" they favoured the survival of their own "catalyzed" creation Jane as she had greater capacity to parent and flourish despite Jane being a 4 month old adult (if that makes any sense as she was born from hypnosis 4 month prior). Jane herself pondered making the self-sacrifice after bearing witness to Eve White one day saving a child from being struck by a car. But the two psychiatrists who were judge and jury became shy and cowardly at the prospect of playing executioner and working towards the annihilation of Eve Black, at the least. They speculated that another ought to do that. Their deference was that they knew her as a significant other in their own lives. This is of course to imply a moral logic that Judas can wash his hands in Pilates bowl as he did not personally drive in the nails. The psychiatrists were able to achieve this distancing from the gravitas of their own conspiracy by concluding also that these were not three separate people, this being incoherent to what they otherwise claimed. Death would not be death. And why? The eyes would stay open they said, the heart would still beat and whatever is unified come the end of the day is the person, with Eve Black merely a personality with the person. Would they not be terrified at their own interior world dying if another's were to replace it as owner of their own bodies? In this terribly obvious missing of the point, were they merely taking leave of their intellectual faculties? I'd speculate not as their two men write and think as those capable of writing and thinking with quality and adequate self-reflection, a throw-back to times when physicians did not abdicate their intellect to be mere vessels of what a guild or guideline or precooked "evidence" may tell them. No I'd do them the honour at least of speculating that Thigpen and Cleckley were grappling with something unfamiliar and caught in the moment of being bewitched, and perhaps their unconscious at least knew it was all a charade. Even Christ in casting out the multiples that were the "legion" did not annihilate them, perhaps leaving them to roam the world until that furthest eschatological horizon when even the demon will be reconciled with God. Does not even Eve Black deserve the same right to life is she exists as Eve White and Jane exists?

Thankfully for myself I never been placed upon the horns of the same moral dilemma, for I have only ever encountered two patients who came close to being as convincing as Eve arguably was. On both occasions it was clear that on some level of their consciousness the primary personality gave themselves over the secondary. In the sense that they are giving themselves over to a creation that is their own, the alter is a part of themselves. In the sense to which they choose to give themselves over, they retain responsibility in the same way that a drug user is culpable for crimes committed after they give themselves over to the drug.

Like the latter Munthe, I consider the whole MPD idea a farce. The therapist must treat the hysteric as an adult and refuse to talk to alters. That's the only acceptable contract and move towards recovery.

To Thigpen and Cleckleys credit, after Eve they kept their wits and did not make of their career ever expansive discoveries of multiples in other women. In their 1984 retrospective they look back to having only ever had the one case that fitted the multiple personality disorder diagnosis apart from the index case that was Eve. This is quite an admission as one would expect the two psychiatrists to have become the mecca for multiples. Indeed, this was precisely what occurred in being referred literally hundreds of patients. They lament at persons successfully using multiple personality disorder as an insanity defence for rape/murder charges and wisely advise thus

"The other cases manifested either pseudo- or quasi-dissociative symptoms related to dissatisfaction with self-identity or hysterical acting out for secondary gain. One particular form of secondary gain, namely, avoiding responsibility for certain actions, was evident in a recent legal case where the person was diagnosed as having the disorder and successfully pled not guilty by reason of insanity. We urge that a diagnosis of multiple personality not be used in such a manner and recommend that therapists consider the hysterical basis of the symptoms, as well as the adaptive dynamics of personality before diagnosing someone as having the disorder. If such factors are considered, the incidence of the disorder will be found to be far less than the "epidemic" recently claimed"

What Thigpen and Cleckley do not state in their brief retrospective was another factors that might have had occasion to given them a jaundiced eye, and that is what happened to Eve herself (i.e. Christine Costner Sizemore).

Soon after the 1954 paper was published in a scholarly journal, the case was adapted with a certain level of artistic licence and released in circulation the same year as a novel "The Three Faces of Eve", and soon after in 1957 a much celebrated film of the same name. Given the chronology of events, one need not be a cynic to see that things were happening with such apace that almost certainly from the beginning the plan was to convert curiosity into capital. The book sold handsomely (somewhere in excess of two million copies) and the film adaptation was likewise highly successful, earning Joanne Woodwood an Oscar for best actress. Christine was stung by signing a contract for $1 for each of the three personalities for the book and earned $7000 in total for the film when she soon realized she ought to have received a cut from the profits. And it is to be noted for a film in which the fictional ending was a complete cure, the contract was made out to Eve W, Eve B and Jane. She was also spurned in never having a chance to mix with Hollywood celebrities and MGM executive herself, as Thigpen and Cleckley did. The Three Face of Eve that was Christine were to have a major falling out with the two psychiatrists after mixing business with therapy, and she soon ceased contact with them. Christine's personalities only amplified though the next half dozen or so therapists, totalling somewhere in excess of 20 alters by the mid 1970's when, under the fourth year of care by Virginian psychiatrist Tony Tsitos, all the faces were finally and suddenly unified into Christine. By 1975 Christine announced to the New York Post her recovery and was unified sufficiently to tour the talk show and speaking circuit and launch her own 1977 book, with a follow up in 1989. Christine also needed be integrated to file suit against MGM and attempt negotiations to the rights over a remake of the film, though this did not come to pass.

The Eve Effect

According to some accounts, worldwide cases whose description approximated what we might call multiple personality disorder between 1816-1944 (128 years) number 72 persons. After the book and film, according to Thigpen and Cleckley alone, many hundreds were referred to them diagnosed by other psychiatrists and physicians, or those self diagnosed by the patients themselves. How many thousands more never reached the mail box or telephone of these two doyens of multiple personality? We can only speculate that the number is at least an order or two of magnitude greater than the preceding century or more. The expansion in diagnosis seems roughly to map onto those cultures and languages who had access and inclination to take in the fiction was "Three Faces of Eve". Naturally the vast majority of cases were in America, usually bourgeois neurotic white females, or males seeking an insanity defence for violent crimes. The third world had to live with good old fashioned demonology and stoicism.

Thigpen and Cleckley write in their 1984 retrospective

"some patients who ostensibly have the disorder there is a competition to see who can have the greatest number of alter personalities. (Unfortunately, there also appears to be a competition among some therapists to see who can have the greatest number of multiple personality cases.)"

Sybil and Shirley

In the somewhat punctuated retelling of the MPD story, for there were other films and novels, the next success of popular culture was to be Flora Rita Schreiber's "Sybil". The book was released in 1973 and the television miniseries three years later. On first release the book quickly sold out the 400,000 copies, with further printing topping out somewhere in excess of 6 million copies within a few short years. The two night miniseries (later heavily edited for VHS release), though a small screen affair, was arguably just as successful as "The Three Faces of Eve". By some accounts it was such a success in the ratings as only to be eclipsed in 1976 by the likes of the Superbowl. Sally Field earned an Emmy award and Schreiber, the author of this supposed true story, also had accolades heaped upon her, including eventually an academic chair in a university journalism department. Were there any doubt, after Sybil every American not living under a rock knew about MPD. Though Sybil was marketed as a true story, the real woman behind the pseudonym would not be widely known for many years. Not until 1996 (2 years before the death of the real Sybil) did Mark Pendergrast write the first critique of the case, and the public would wait a full 15 years later until Debbie Nathans excellent expose "Sybil Exposed" in 2011, a decade after access to Schreibers notes of the therapy sessions were unsealed. The plot of the film, brilliantly acted as it was by Field and Joanne Woodword (the latter who played Eve and now played Sybils psychiatrist), was uninspired and typical for MPD. Sybil has vague somatic symptoms and "blackouts" of amnesia, has a suicide attempt perpetrated by an alternate personality and comes under the care of Dr Cornelia Wilbur. Therapy follows, personalities emerge, Sybil remembers the trauma of childhood at the hands of a particularly sadistic mother whose character is assassinated in the makings of this "true story" and eventually re-integration is achieved to a happy ending and the delight of all. Sybil becomes the well adjusted academic she always aspired to be. The true story, complete with controversy, is much more interesting

The therapists were two, primarily Cornelia Wilbur whose name was curiously retained without change in the book/film adaptation, and sometimes Herbert Spiegel whose name was changed, for reasons that will soon be made clear. More on him anon.

Sybil Dorsett's real name was Shirley Mason (1923-1998), and by all accounts apart from living in an unusual particularly devout Seventh Day Adventist family who deprived her of the fun of a normal childhood, there is no evidence to suggest she was abused in any way from which to cast aspersions on her mother as worse than any other, and certainly not the monster the film would have us believe. Part of the film's success was the sordid details of sexual depravity metered out by her mother, such as ice cold colonic enemas and other sexual penetrative abuses, deprivations etcetera. The mother was also portrayed as being a closet psychotic, a lesbian, (something rather uncontroversial and passe in our day and age, though doubtlessly the notion also being an offensive accusation about a lady as religious as Mrs Dorsett (Martha Mason)

Shirley Mason first encountered therapy by Dr Cornelia Wilbur (1908-1992), an intellectually adventurous psychiatrist who embraced every new fangled therapeutic modality. Prefrontal lobotomy was not unknown to her, she regularly performed electroconvulsive therapy out of a suitcase and she was neither wedded to the esoterica of hypnosis or the so called biological paradigm, using mesmerism and sodium pentothal both and many more powerful drugs besides. Masons psychotherapy was extremely lengthy and protracted, somewhere in excess of two thousand sessions. This was conducted in two parts, the first in Minnesota and the latter in New York where Wilbur moved to open a successful uptown private practice and Shirley had also moved, ostensibly to attend Columbia University though one wonders if proximity to Wilbur was an additional motivating factor. In the latter New York phase, Cornelia initially rejected Mason, only for Mason to return manifesting for the first time an alternate personality. This latter therapeutic phase was, needless to say, following the release of "The Three Faces of Eve". Wilbur could not resist a multiple at her door, and therapy became so long as to essentially become a part time job for Wilbur, eventually Wilbur even setting up Mason with housing, rent and clothing so as to continue her career as a professional patient. Eventually there would be 16 personalities in total emergent from career therapy. True to the plot of the film, Masons mother was to be demonised and eventually Mason cut ties with all from her past. For the childless divorcee Wilbur who was 15 years Masons senior, she was just old enough to be a replacement mother figure, and the therapy can be formulated to be relational matricide committed under the language of cure. When Wilbur was given a professorial chair at the University of Kentucky, Mason was not far behind in relocating also, eventually moving in with Wilbur who died in 1992 of complications of Parkinson's disease.

Like Eve White, the fictional Sybil Dorsett enjoyed a happy ending. But like Christine Costner Sizemore, Shirley Mason was to remain with her multiples for many years to come until the book was to be released and their veracity might run the risk of being placed under the light of a more public examination. Then and only then did her alleged disorder remit. Strangely no one ever saw her multiple personalities outside therapy sessions, this despite the fact that some would have either been vulnerable children or infants prone to misadventure, or antisocial personalities provoking reprisals from others around her. Two were male and outside therapy seem never to have encountered the disappointing answer to what they thought was between their legs. Occasionally whilst Wilbur was away, Masons care was transferred to psychiatrist Herbert Spiegel. Spiegel wasn't taken in by Masons performance, describing her as a "brilliant hysteric". Records indicate that he refused to talk to the alters, and Shirley Masons response to a question asked from Spiegel ""do you want me to be Peggy or should I just tell you" speaks volumes. He refused to be part of the book deal unless the diagnosis be more honest and comprehensive of a wider view, and so his name and his character remains essentially unrepresented. We can ask why Spiegel did not cry from the rooftops his inside knowledge of what some might call a scam, this question all the more significant in seeing Sybil not an isolated case, as opposed to the stimulus for social contagion and further miscarriage of justice. He also would likely have been aware that Wilbur served as an expert witness for the defence, another being psychiatrist David Caul, in the case of William Milligan, the armed robber who raped three women yet who successfully obtained an insanity defence on account of the rapes perpetrated by his alleged alters. And how could poor Billy Milligan be incarcerated they plead, when Billy qua Billy wasn't the rapist? Milligan and his 14 personalities spent a decade in the mental health system before being released to unsuccessfully plan his own film. And on goes the circus.

The Sybil Effect

It is circumstantial evidence to be sure, as it was for observing the spike in MPD cases following the Three Faces of Eve. Yet we could be forgiven for drawing conclusions between the timing of Sybil (1973/76) and a certain inclusion in the best seller and bible of the American Psychiatric Association, the DSM III (1980). Certain members of the DSM working group on dissociative disorders considered Sybil a true story, emblematic of a rare yet very real psychiatric disorder. In turn we can speculate on the symbiosis between Sybil and the DSM III both, and the explosion of cases of MPD estimated to be at least 40,000 between Sybil and the mid 1990's. The casualties in terms of character assassinations are many more besides, given the assumption that childhood trauma begets MPD and that family members are not afforded due process in the court of the psychiatrists rooms. Every Shirley Mason has a Martha Mason who nursed her from when she was a babe, and who might not be the monster they are portrayed as being.

A Comment on MPD and Schizophrenia

From the above, it is hardly a subtle subtext of the plot of my own little drama that I view the construct of MPD with a healthy degree of scepticism, even mockery. In this sense, I may appear to stand together with the mainstream psychiatric opinion in 2020. The average psychiatrist seldom if ever encounters it and is similarly sceptical, many following with the herd believing "MPD/DID does not exist" even if they are unmoored, as they all too often are, from any knowledge of the history of the construct and even if this undermines the legitimacy of the entire DSM project. Rather they go along with the herd. However, yours truly might receive a conditional welcoming into the fold of MPD true believers in the following sense; I do not share the discriminative placing on a pedestal of any of the psychiatric diagnoses, and see schizophrenia or bipolar disorder as no more sacred than MPD. Ponder this for a moment. Schizophrenia, or psychosis generally, can be characterized in many (even disjunctive!) ways with multiple symptoms/signs from which to choose. Take classical non congruent affect. This is the case when the inner subjective emotional state or thematic nature of the conversation would predict one emotional expression, yet what the psychiatrist observes is another. So, for example, the schizophrenic may be grieving the loss of a loved one yet grinning like a Cheshire cat. Is this not congruent with the picture of a split personality locked in simultaneous inner emotional being of alter 1 and facial expression of alter 2, each without access to the other? And what of delusions, which could also be said to be the simultaneous expression of the alter in a regressed childlike state or dream state or the personality of the unconscious of alter/s manifesting within the adult living in the world? A similar argument can be had for hallucinations which are different personalities and neuroses of personalities talking amongst themselves or about themselves or dissociated across time, the voice of the other disavowed from the alter that has the reigns of the body in the now.

Finally, we come to thought disorder, which might be manifest as a breakdown in the architecture of thought, with clauses or even single words lacking articulation with one another towards a coherent response, let alone addressing the narrative or the question asked. If alters were rapidly cycling between one another without ever coming fully into the conversation, would we not expect fragments of dialogue or monologue from the first alter, followed by fragments from the second and so on? And so the architecture of thought and sentence as heard from the other appears to break down against the disunity of different personalities coming in and out. Schizophrenia has a rather weak correlation within monozygotic twins (8-30%) despite sharing an identical genome and an incredibly weak correlation with individual genes or combination of genes. Childhood trauma is orders of magnitude more predictive of developing schizophrenia in adulthood, though this too unreliable and most traumatized children grow up to be non psychotic, and certainly are not psychotic in childhood. So why not conceive of schizophrenia as just an incomplete or fused switching or rapid cycling between alters, with schizophrenia an MPD subtype? Though I'm as sceptical about this formulation as much as any other in psychiatry, it is easier to defend than the nonsense that schizophrenia is a neurodegenerative genetic disease. This latter formulation is more in keeping with the dementia praecox of Emil Kraepilin and Morel's pre fascist degeneration theory, whereas the Swiss born disciple of Charcot, Eugen Bleuler a decade later brought schizophrenia into the psychiatric lexicon with this description of the schiz (split) in the phrein (mind)

"(D)issociation of the personality is fundamentally nothing else than the splitting off of the unconscious; unconscious complexes can transform themselves into these secondary personalities by taking over so large a part of the original personality that they represent an entirely new personality."

Many other quote besides could be provided to indicate that Bleuler used splitting (Spaltung) in schizophrenia as an alternative to dissociation and similar to what later became known as MPD and DID. Bleurerian schizophrenia is very different to our current use of the term,

ACT II; The Devil and Psychiatry go to the Movies

The late 1960''s was a time of great foment and political upheaval. It was a time of communes and cults, of 1968 student riots and all manner of ideas and alternate religions filling the void from the slow death of Christianity and conservatism. This was a trend not to dissipate until the nihilistic grunge 1990's. And the late 1960's was the time Satan the dragon reintroduced himself on the silver screen as the grand conspirator interested in women and children, and willing to battle the white knights in psychiatric armour over the fates of souls.

The first entry to consider in this second act is the Rosemary's Baby, a 1967 horror novel by Ira Levin. After selling several million copies it was not surprisingly irresistible for other authors not to cash in on the theme, resulting in the devil and his possessed becoming one of several staples of pop culture. And not surprisingly the year after the novel was released it was made into a film adaptation written and directed by the now infamous Roman Polanski. The plot in the briefest of summaries involves the innocent Rosemary having a disturbing dream. In her dream she had been raped by the devil, something she does not realise consciously is true and that she is impregnated with his, and not her husbands, child. Several themes are important here, including yet not limited to a) Satan wanting to claim the child, and indeed the demonic nature being within the baby b) Satanic cults can be hiding in plain sight, even our neighbours might be witches and warlocks of the darkest of arts, c) the middle and upper class can be both victim and perpetrator, d) the satanically charged sexual assault can be repressed, save for the royal road of the dream and other unacknowledged clues and finally e) that the damsel in distress will be dismissed as a neurotic. "They" won't believe you, except of course whatever psychiatrists and psychotherapists might be watching the film and wishing to identify with their own hypothetical character, i.e. the wise and clever therapist who sees through the conspiracy and ostensive hysteria and knows the truth.

An enormous number of other (probably largely coincidental) tangled webs assemble themselves around Rosemary and her child of Satan. We have for example the same year of the film's release, Polanski's wife Sharron Tate brutally mutilated and murdered by the cultish Manson family in a manner suggestive of being a ritual killing towards apocalyptic ends, though it might have been nothing more than the manifest jealousy of a Charles Manson who would never have succeeded in earning his way to Cielo Drive. Manson was to fly like Icarus, close enough to visit the Hollywood Hills, but not rich or talented enough to stay there. Manson was allegedly motivated by the lyrics of the Beatles and John Lennon is gunned down in 1980 when exiting the very uptown Manhattan apartment block where Rosemary's baby was filmed. In 1977 Polanski took flight from the United States for sexual impropriety with a minor and has been dodging extradition since. And actress Mia Farrow (who played Rosemary) forms a relationship in 1979 with the worlds longest analysand Woody Allen, the marriage finally ending after revelations of Allen's affair with their adopted daughter. Presumably this began after the girl reached the age of consent, for in the court of public opinion it appears the scandal has not negatively affected Allens career any more than Polanski's scandal has affected his. Perhaps the connection most apt to provoke conspiracy was the gossip by Anton LaVey, the founder of the Church of Satan. LaVey spread the rumour that he cameoed as the devil in Rosemary's dreams, in so doing existing as a transitional object between the world of film and that of reality. It matters not that LaVey would be quick to say that he was, ipso facto, a materialist atheist who worshipped Lucifer as symbolic of the carnal nature of man and man's power to self-creation, making of himself a mixture between a third rate neo-Darwinian, Nietzsche and P.T. Barnum rolled into one hedonistic charismatic package. Perhaps he was an atheist, or perhaps his retreat to atheism was mockery to those who believed him, the "magic" being to both reveal oneself a believer whilst simultaneously remaining concealed behind a different mask.

Before and after Rosemary there were many other devil cult films. To name but a few Eyes of the Devil 1966, The Devil Rides Out 1966, Mephisto Waltz 1971, The Wicker Man 1973, Satans School for Girls 1973, Race with the devil 1975, The Devils Rain 1975, Suspiria 1977 and many others.

The next novel film duo to which we will our more considered attention is the highly successful "The Exorcist", these released in 1971 and 1973 respectively. Most will remember the film as the blockbuster in which the child actress Linda Blair was made up to look as the Hollywood depiction of a girl possessed, complete with projectile spitting, liberal use of vulgarity and spinning her head like more than a barn owl than a little girl. So shocking was the film that it provoked in at least five cases what was described in the psychiatric literature by Bozutto as a "cinematic neurosis" (symptoms included dissociation). And the viewer might remember the characters of the two priests who did battle with the arch-demon Pazuzu dwelling within the girl. Viewers might not recall that these priests were like traditional Jesuits of the Latin Church, priests for sure yet also men of academe. The elder, Father Lankester Merrin was the archaeologist who had previously partook in exorcism, and so was the veteran psychotherapist of a kind. The younger apprentice, father Damien Karras was, strange as it may seem, also a psychiatrist. The exorcist explores the journey of the child character and the priests alike, which includes within the plot of the film primitive diagnostic tests of the 1970's, this placing demon possession side by side with more conventional psychiatric and medical diagnoses. And the priest is the psychiatrist, the psychiatrist the priest, the younger to represent a scientific age integrating the spiritual world with science, a handing over of the baton from the elder archaeologist who is priest and classicist. I liken the two to Feud and Fenenczi/Jung, and the dynamic between the two priests to teach budding therapists much of what they need to know about psychotherapy and its ethics. The elder maintains his distance and pace, and more importantly does not allow his compassion and own inner conflict to be used against him. The younger rushes in where angels and wisdom would be more circumspect. Ultimately it is the younger priest, like Fenenczi or Jung, to ignorantly transgress the ethical boundaries. I am not about to place all my conspiratorial eggs in one basket, and don't suggest The Exorcist was the cause of the content of our enquiry to follow. What I will submit is that it was a reflection of the ingredients swirling around America. I will suggest that in its own small way, whether directly in the mind of the psychiatrist or indirectly in the psyche of the patients who are the psychiatrists market, The Exorcist made regular therapy with a regular patient trivial, even an MPD patient. A real psychiatrist was one who faced the real devil, and by extension a usurper of the church in making the priest redundant. Such is at the heart of the secular project. The real psychiatrist would be a philosopher sage and hero scientist bundled into one package. How irresistibly exciting.

And finally there is "The Omen", directed by Richard Donner and released to the screen in 1976. The Omen spawned two sequels to complete the trilogy, these being released in 1978 and 1980 respectively. The Omen furthered the themes that the devil can involve himself in the lives of child, in this case the innocent looking Damien being the antichrist himself. Once again there was conspiracy of Satanists amidst the pre-apocalyptic tension of the coming end to both century and millennium, and the idea that the Devil is a globalist corporation with international ambition.

The Stage was set for the Devil to call the audience up to join him on it.

ACT III. The Satanic Panic; Psychiatry, the Devil and MPD

Moral panics have always been with us. In AD 177 Lyon (then the Roman Empire) Christians were accused of

"holding meetings at which babies or small children were ritually slaughtered, and feasts at which the remains of these victims were ritually devoured; also of holding erotic orgies at which every form of intercourse, including incest between parents and children, was freely practiced; also of worshipping a strange divinity in the form of an animal."

Then there are the recurrent pogroms against the Jews with concocted allegations of Blood Libel, these but two of many examples.

Circa 1973, around the same year of Sybil the book and The Exorcist, Michelle Smith first attended therapy with psychiatrist Lawrence Pazder in his private rooms in Victoria British Columbia. Ostensibly the presenting complaint was depression after a miscarriage. Pazder was very well respected and well credentialed. Working at two of the cities hospitals along with running his own clinic, Pazder was a practicing Roman Catholic with a background in both psychiatry and tropical medicine, once living and working altruistically in Nigeria for at least two years. Sometime circa 1976 therapy was stagnating and Michelle felt she had something within her unconscious she could not quite recall, and yet was nonetheless vitally important (like a pregnancy she longed to deliver the psychoanalyst within me might speculate). One session in her struggle to remember she regressed to a screaming 5 year old. It was not long before Pazder resorted to hypnosis to bring to the surface what remained hidden. More adventures in psychotherapy followed and in the years 1976-1978 Michelle, with "benefit" of hypnosis, recalled the satanic ritual abuse she was forced to partake in as a child in otherwise boring mid-fifties Canada. The details became increasingly lurid, including many dark robed adults, the satanic black mass, infant sacrifice and even cannibalism. One of these rituals was said to last almost three months, this despite the fact her school records show attendance at the time. The sex within the rituals was salacious and fantastic, orgies, rape, paedophilia and even beastiality. Michelles alleged abuses extended beyond being a mere witness to all these devilish acts. She claimed to have been forced into a cage with snakes, buried in a coffin and placed in the trunk of a car with a corpse. The account stretched beyond medical credulity when Michelle also recalled having horns and a tail grafted to her body, something which would certainly fail either from immune rejection alone, if not failure to perfuse.

By 1980 Michelle had completed her therapy, this in part on account of remembering Jesus and Mary themselves intervening to save her and miraculously heal her of the physical scars of her abuses. This heavenly intervention failed to cure her of what eventually drove her to therapy, yet another implicit proof of psychiatry's narcissism to complete a healing that even the Christ and Theotokos could not. Along with Pazder she co-authored the successful book "Michelle Remembers", which quickly earned them approx. $350,000 in advance fees and sold well for several years. I say "them", as by this time each had brought their mutual affair out of the closet, had left their respective spouses (Pazder had 4 children also) and were set to marry.

Thankfully Michelles mother Virginia Proby, having passed away circa 1964, never lived to hear the allegation that she inducted her daughter into a satanic cult and subjected her to unspeakable torture. Her widowed husband Jack (Michelles father) is quoted to have taken 4 months to read the book and cried every day until the final page, thinking "Dear God. How could anyone say this against their dead mother". Michelle Smith and Lawrence Pazder were stymied from profiting from a film deal only after Jack Probys legal counsel issued a letter to the publisher with intent to file suit if they met with Hollywood. The publishers and Pazder/Smith were aiming high, fantasizing that Christopher Plummer would play the Satanist priest and Dustin Hoffman play Pazder.

The couple seem, on the surface at least, to have believed wholeheartedly in the reality of what Michelle remembered. In this battle with the devil and his vast network of covens they sought advice from Catholic Bishop Remi de Roo, who arranged for a meeting at the Vatican with Cardinal Sergio Pignedoli. The bishop was trusting enough to allow the couple the foot in the door of the Holy See, though would not give a naïve ringing endorsement. His quote in the preface of the book reads

"I do not question that for Michelle the experience was real. In time we will know how much of it can be validated. It will require prolonged and careful study. In such mysterious matters hasty conclusions could prove unwise."

What the good Italian bishop may not have realized is that North America any publicity is good publicity, and the couple had much more besides, be it People magazine, National Enquirer and several other well known publications. In the late 1980's Michelle appeared on the hugely successful talk show hosted by Oprah Winfrey, another guest being Laurel Rose Willson, author of her own bestselling memoir "Satan's Underground", which was published under the nom de plume Lauren Stratford. Willsons fraud was undone by, of all authorities, a Christian publication (Cornerstone) which explored her claims and found them untrue. This did not stop her adopting the name Laura Grabowski in the 1990's and writing award winning poetry pretending to be a survivor of the holocaust and Dr Mengles fiendish experiments. The Holocaust of course was real. Laura wasn't, and her final fraud was only uncovered when she allied herself with Binjamin Wilkomirski (aka Bruno Gosjean), when he too was exposed as a fake holocaust survivor (and so how could she have vivid memories of time in the camps with him). Both in their own small indirect way served to strengthen the false claims of holocaust denial. Winfrey would do her best to then forget her naivety in entertaining these fakes and many others such as James Frey, author of the fabricated memoir "A Million Little Pieces". But these revelations would take years to emerge and all manner of shenanigans were given carte blanche to wreak American havoc throughout the 1980's and into the early 1990's. Lawrence Pazder and Michelle Smith (now Michelle Pazder) were not resoundingly proven to be frauds, and Pazder the psychiatrist achieved much notoriety in the US speaking circuit educating psychiatrists, other mental health workers and law enforcement on the supposed reality and dangers of satanic ritual abuse. His "expertise" also informed the McMartin case (vide infra).

McMartin

Manhattan Beach is a laid back upmarket suburb of south Los Angeles, deriving its natural beauty from the Pacific Ocean and its money from the nearby aerospace industry. In 1983 the place to send your children for day care was the McMartin preschool, the oldest and most successful day care centre in South L.A. Run by matriarch Virginia McMartin, the school was a multi community award winning family business staffed also by her daughter Peggy McMartin Buckey and her son (Viriginias grandson) Ray Buckey, in addition to three unrelated teachers Betty Raidor, Mary Ann Jackson and Babette Spitler. Peggies husband Charles, an aerospace engineer, furnished the centre with his own creation of child size wooden animals, rocking horses and playhouses.

But before discussing their fate, the stage must be set with other players, first of these is professor of psychiatry Dr Roland Summit. Summit was effectively L.A. county's chief psychiatrist, and informed not merely the local understanding of incest and child abuse, yet also the wider American understanding of the same. Summits first formulation of incest in the early 1970's was the creepily named "family romance". He spoke of the semi traditional family, the fathers "horizons and dreams are contracting" and the liberated working mother "depressed at the loss of youth and girlish attraction" and "no longer invested in her husbands ego". Enter the niece or daughter or young girl next door, drawn to play with the man as a cat is instinctively drawn to play with a mouse. She is "learning to transmit the magical vibrations our society requires of the emergent woman", a mixture in transition of the "innocence of the child and the allure of the temptress". The wife is "remarkably oblivious" to these goings on, perhaps not wanting to know who is taking her place as she finds meaning in career or the sedative her physician prescribes. And so the man succumbs in a plot which one wonders Summit might not have conjured had Nabokov not first published "Lolita" in 1955 and Kubrick not adapted to film in 1962. The parallels are striking.

Summits other claim to fame is his own diagnostic construct, "Childhood Sexual Abuse Accommodation Syndrome", published in 1983 yet formulated in his 1970's work, the features of which include; secrecy, helplessness, adaptation and entrapment, delayed conflicted and unconvincing disclosure, and finally retraction after the first brave disclosure.

That is to say, the perpetrator will threaten, seduce, exploit compassion and do whatever is necessary to maintain secrecy. The child will be helpless and aware of the enormous power differential between themselves and the adult perpetrator of sexual abuse. They naturally fall into a state of obedience. To his credit, though inconsistent to the family romance, Summit states that no adolescent is mature enough to consent, however mature they appear. Consequently, adolescents too need be thought of as helpless. Both the perpetrator and the child adapt to the abuse. Given the child is trapped in the situation, they learn to do the necessaries to survive rather than escape. They want to retain power within powerlessness. And yet the drive to disclose and escape is never entirely extinguished. Disclose might be delayed, veiled or cryptic. If and when disclosure is made, this is often recanted out of fear or misplaced compassion for the perpetrator.

Summit would also play into a validation of multiplicity, in describing the possible psychological sequelae from living day after day with sexual abuse and conflict. "This is a mind splitting and mind fragmenting operation" with "inevitable splitting" the child "may develop multiple personalities...."

Channelling the naïve spirit of Despine, the other critical feature of Summits ideology is the premium placed on the testimony of the accuser, most especially children. He has stated "children never fabricate" and "It has become the maxim among child sexual abuse intervention counsellors and investigators that children never fabricate the kinds of sexual manipulations they divulge in complaints and interrogations". Summits worldview was frightening in its confidence, and equally disturbing in the inclusion of the word "interrogation" as something one could do to a child in order to arrive at what might be said, which having been said, is truth. He was essentially proposing that if a child makes an accusation against you, even after hours of interrogation, then you the accused are necessarily guilty. What would you not do to secure a successful prosecution of a child molester if you were certain he (or she) was guilty?

Other psychiatrists such as Judith Herman developed different formulations of incest founded in by her own particularly strong feminist biases. She proposed that it is man's patriarchal rule over the traditional family, this "unbalanced sexuality" that creates within the man the idea that his children are his property. Herman is oft quoted to say "As long as fathers rule but do not nurture, as long as mothers nurture but do not rule, the conditions favouring the development of father-daughter incest will prevail." Which is to say that a man who works and a woman who is homemaker is necessarily an at risk state for incest, remedied only by a reversal of roles and a psychological castration for the father. Only in castration can we assure he is harmless.

The next in the cast are non psychiatric physicians, whose assumptions also played into the panic and whose erroneous teachings sent many people to jail for many years. Bruce Woodling was the family physician who moonlighted as the Los Angeles district sexual trauma investigator. It was the caring Dr Woodling who would attend the emergency department in the middle of the night to see to the examination of women who were allegedly sexually assaulted and compile the photographic and other evidence that would be used by the prosecution. Of acute adult sexual trauma he was an expert. But diagnosing vaginal, anal and other traumata minutes or hours after an alleged violent rape in a rather easy matter to the initiated. What of children making claims of something having happened days, weeks or even month ago? Woodling drew upon assumption to write the 1985 Training Syllabus "Medical Examination of the Sexually Abused Child" and collaborated what he thought he knew about the manifestations of childhood sexual abuse with pediatrician (later University of Southern California Professor of Pediatrics) Astrid Heger. Together they essentially promoted, inter alia, the idea that any anatomical irregularity or blemish to the anus or hymen was indicative of childhood sexual abuse, and that an anus which dilated when stroked was indicative of its adaptation to penetrative sexual trauma. The assumption seems to be something of a romantic projection of the purity and innocence of youth onto the anatomical substance of the youth's body. This idea had not been substantiated in case control studies.

The "science" was accepted uncritically by those prosecutors who would use it as evidence and taken as evidence within the context of the accusation whose veracity was assumed. Even the lack of evidence could be interpreted as evidence, it being all a matter of the play of words. If by chance no anatomical abnormality is found months after an alleged molestation, the fact of the bodies healing can make for the conclusion in the committed witch hunter "the examination is consistent with the child having been molested". Astrid Heger would be one of the key examiners of the children of McMartin, just as Woodling contributed also to many false convictions in the Kern County area in the same period.

Only in the mid to late 1980's did San Francisco professor of Pediatrics Dr John McCann bother to ask the question that ought to have been asked at the outset, i.e. using careful methodology to exclude possibly abused children from study and large sample sizes, what is the normal ano-genital anatomy of the non abused child? To which his answer re the hymen was "We were struck with the fact that we couldn't find a normal (hymen). It took us three years before we found a normal of what we had in our minds as a preconceived normal"

The same he discovered was the case with the anus, which dilated or "winked" in the majority of cases and was very commonly found to be irregular or mildly erythematous (i.e. reddened). Despite this McCann skirts close to coming under the spell of the panic himself when he states. "While medical examiners must maintain a high index of suspicion in this era of unremitting sexual abuse, caution must be exercised during the search for the cause of soft tissue changes discovered in the ano-genital region of a child. If a reasonable explanation is not forthcoming, a more thorough investigation must be instigated if children are to be protected from further exploitation." But how can a reasonable explanation be forthcoming in the face of an accusation, if this not be the faith that what is found is an anatomical variant? What is his basis for the claim of an "era of unremitting sexual abuse"?

Though these and many more seeds of the crisis were sown before in the assumptions physicians and others brought to the table, the McMartin case proper began in May 1983 in the actions of a disturbed woman by the name of Judy Johnson. Judy was a struggling single mother of a 2 ½ year old Billy, her only other child a 13 year old son dying of a brain tumor. She had no other immediate family in the vicinity as her husband had recently walked out on her. Judy was far from the American dream. She was desperate and did not take no for an answer when informed that McMartin enrolments were full. Instead she simply left Billy there one morning with a note of identification and a promise she would return. Her bold move was rewarded with the school not reporting her to children's services. Instead they allowed him to stay that day and return again and again, approx. 10 times in total. Such compassion would be their undoing, as in the days or weeks leading up to August Judy Johnson became increasingly obsessed with her sons anus, which was itchy and red and came to be spotting blood, perhaps from scratching a worm infection (my own guess playing the odds, but we will never know). The blood was too much for Judy, who jumped to the conclusion that he must have been sexually abused. Ray Buckey was the number one suspect, for despite the second wave feminism it was weird that a young man would want to work with very young children. But he was a laid back Californian who wished to live and work close to family in the family business.

And so why not? No one knows how many hours Judy Johnson interrogated her own child to give her the answer her paranoia wanted. In any case, by August 12th she called the police to report her son's revelations, less than a week later she was received for interview by detectives. Ray was arrested September 7th under suspicion of child molestation and released the same day. This is not to imply Ray was off the hook, the following day the chief of police issues an extraordinary letter to approx. 200 parents of current and previous McMartin pupils. It read, in its entirety

"September 8, 1983

Dear Parent:

This Department is conducting a criminal investigation involving child molestation (288 P.C.) Ray Buckey, an employee of Virginia McMartin's Pre-School, was arrested September 7, 1983 by this Department.

The following procedure is obviously an unpleasant one, but to protect the rights of your children as well as the rights of the accused, this inquiry is necessary for a complete investigation.

Records indicate that your child has been or is currently a student at the pre-school. We are asking your assistance in this continuing investigation. Please question your child to see if he or she has been a witness to any crime or if he or she has been a victim. Our investigation indicates that possible criminal acts include: oral sex, fondling of genitals, buttock or chest area, and sodomy, possibly committed under the pretense of "taking the child's temperature." Also photos may have been taken of children without their clothing. Any information from your child regarding having ever observed Ray Buckey to leave a classroom alone with a child during any nap period, or if they have ever observed Ray Buckey tie up a child, is important.

Please complete the enclosed information form and return it to this Department in the enclosed stamped return envelope as soon as possible. We will contact you if circumstances dictate same.

We ask you to please keep this investigation strictly confidential because of the nature of the charges and the highly emotional effect it could have on our community. Please do not discuss this investigation with anyone outside your immediate family. Do not contact or discuss the investigation with Raymond Buckey, any member of the accused defendant's family, or employees connected with the McMartin Pre-School.

THERE IS NO EVIDENCE TO INDICATED THAT THE MANAGEMENT OF VIRGINIA MCMARTIN'S PRE-SCHOOL HAD ANY KNOWLEDGE OF

THIS SITUATION AND NO DETRIMENTAL INFORMATION CONCERNING THE OPERATION OF THE SCHOOL HAS BEEN DISCOVERED DURING THIS INVESTIGATION. ALSO, NO OTHER EMPLOYEE IN THE SCHOOL IS UNDER INVESTIGATION FOR ANY CRIMINAL ACT.

Your prompt attention to this matter and reply no late than Septemeber 16, 1983 will be appreciated.

HARRY L. KUHLMEYER, JR.

Chief of Police

JOHN WEHNER, Captain"

Naturally there is no greater invitation to gossip than requesting people keep a secret. From 8th September onwards in every church house, family house, outhouse, hen house, house of ill repute, street corner and corner store there was one story on everyone's lips, and that story was Ray Buckey and the McMartin School. Parents were understandably immediately placed in a positon of high suspicion of Ray. And like Judy Johnson, some were not secure with their children denying Ray interfered with them. Consequently the interrogated their children again, and again, and again, and informal parents groups formed to discuss the case. Stories were cross pollinated and the natural agitators formed citizens groups with a battle plan for justice against the man they were certain must be guilty.

Judy Johnsons own input continued, became regular and became increasingly strange. Her accusations now inculpated other members of the staff. Despite Billy reporting (via his mother) that Ray et al took him and other children to a Church in which an unholy satanic mass was conducted, a baby was killed in a ritual sacrifice, Ray threatened Billy with a Lion (that is to say a real live Panthera leo) and Ray flew him in a plane, along with Ray levitating himself, the police did not pull back on pursuing the investigation. The Lion was out of its cage in more ways than one.

The police partially outsourced the investigation to L.A. based Children's Institute International (CII), whose funding hunter and front person was social worker Kathleen "Kee" MacFarlane. Macfarlane was a fine arts graduate, who being as employable as her fine arts peers, had to find work in another area. And that she did, in her case a children's home which prompted an interest in children's welfare and master's studies in social work. There she honed her skills as a funding applicant and developed connections in government. Her research took her to the top with a bullet. She had barely graduated in Maryland 1974 before finding herself in an expert role in 1976-1982 for the federally funded National Center on Child Abuse and Neglect (NCCAN) under the title of "Child Sexual Abuse Specialist." These were the early days in child abuse "research" which, like Heger and Woodling, the "expert" was the one working in the role with the (fallacy of) authority invested in them by the state. They were learning and making things up as they went along. And so for Macfarlane the career was from Ohio and Maryland to Washington DC and across the coast to California and CII. Macfarlane and her team, Heger included, seem to have learned their interview techniques in watching American police interrogations on TV, or soaking up what advice she might (I speculate) have been told to her by Department of Justice and District Attorney friends. In the months that followed Macfarlane interviewed at least 360 children, Heger examining at least half that number. Rates of (concluded) molestation were at least 80% (Heger) and closer to universal for Macfarlanes interviewees and those conducted by staff under her watch. The latter achieved this by subjecting the children to gruelling hours of leading questions and puppet play until the child gave the desired answers by appeal to the childrens desire to help, reward and praise or simply to get out of CII and back to where the child wished to be, that is playing at home.

Excerpt from transcript with an 8yr old boy

MacFarlane:

Here's a hard question I don't know if you know the answer to. We'll see how smart you are, Pac-man. Did you ever see anything come out of Mr. Ray's wiener? Do you remember that?

Child:

(no response)

MacFarlane:

Can you remember back that far? We'll see how ... how good your brain is working today, Pac-man.

(Child moves puppet around.)

MacFarlane:

Is that a yes?

(Child nods puppet yes.)

MacFarlane:

Well, you're smart. Now, let's see if we can figure out what it was. I wonder if you can point to something of what color it was.

(Child tries to pick up the pointer with the Pac-man's mouth.)

MacFarlane:

Let me get your pen here (puts a pointer in child's Pac-man puppet mouth).

Child:

It was ...

MacFarlane:

Let's see what color is that.

(Child uses the Pac-man's hand to point to the Pac-man puppet.)

MacFarlane:

Oh, you're pointing to yourself. That must be yellow.

(Child nods puppet yes.)

MacFarlane:

You're smart to point to yourself. What did it feel like? Was it like water? Or some-thing else?

Child:

Um, what?

MacFarlane:

The stuff that came out. Let me try. I'll try a different question on you. We'll try to figure out what that stuff tastes like. We're going to try and figure out if it tastes good.

Child:

He never did that to [me], I don't think.

MacFarlane:

Oh, well, Pac-man, would you know what it tastes like? Would you think it tastes like candy, sort of trying ...

Child:

I think it would taste like yucky ants.

MacFarlane:

Yucky ants. Whoa. That would be kind of yucky. I don't think it would taste like ... you don't think it would taste like strawberries or anything good?

Child:

No.

MacFarlane:

Oh. Think it would so ... do you think that would be sticky, like sticky, yucky ants?

Child:

A little.

Excerpt of an Interview with an 8 yr old Boy

Kathleen MacFarlane: Mr. Monkey is a little bit chicken, and he can't remember any of the naked games, but we think that you can, 'cause we know a naked games that you were around for, 'cause the other kids told us, and it's called Naked Movie Star. Do you remember that game, Mr. Alligator, or is your memory too bad?

Boy: Um, I don't remember that game.

MacFarlane: Oh, Mr. Alligator.

Boy: Umm, well, it's umm, a little song that me and [a friend] heard of.

MacFarlane: Oh.

Boy: Well, I heard out loud someone singing, "Naked Movie Star, Naked Movie Star."

MacFarlane: You know that, Mr. Alligator? That means you're smart, 'cause that's the same song the other kids knew and that's how we really know you're smarter than you look. So you better not play dumb, Mr. Alligator.

Boy: Well, I didn't really hear a whole lot. I just heard someone yell it from out in the _ Someone yelled it.

MacFarlane: Maybe. Mr. Alligator, you peeked in the window one day and saw them playing it, and maybe you could remember and help us.

Boy: Well, no, I haven't seen anyone playing Naked Movie Star. I've only heard the song.

MacFarlane: What good are you? You must be dumb.

Boy: Well I don't know really, umm, remember seeing anyone play that, 'cause I wasn't there, when - I -when people are playing it.

MacFarlane: You weren't? You weren't? That's why we're hoping maybe you saw, see, a lot of these puppets weren't there, but they got to see what happened.

Boy: Well, I saw a lot of fighting.

MacFarlane: I bet you can help us a lot, though, 'cause, like, Naked Movie Star is a simple game, because we know about that game, 'cause we just have had twenty kids told us about that game. Just this morning, a little girl came in and played it for us and sang it just like that. Do you think if I asked you a question, you could put your thinking cap on and you might remember, Mr. Alligator?

Boy: Maybe.

MacFarlane: You could nod your head yes or no. Can you remember who took the pictures for the naked-movie-star game? That would be a great thing to feed into the secret machine [the video camera], and then it would be all gone, just like all the other kids did. You can just nod whether you remember or not, see how good your memory is.

Boy: [Nod's puppet's head.]

MacFarlane: You do? Well, that's remarkable. I wonder if you could hold a pointer in your mouth, and then you wouldn't have to say a word and [boy] wouldn't have to say a word. And you could just point.

Boy: [Places pretend camera on adult male nude doll using alligator puppet] Sometimes he did.

MacFarlane: Can I pat you on the head for that? Look what a big help you can be. You're going to help all these little children, because you're so smart…OK, did they ever pose in funny poses for the pictures?

Boy: Well, it wasn't a real camera. We just played…

MacFarlane: Mr. Alligator, I'm going to…going to ask you something here. Now, we already found out from the other kids that it was a real camera, so you don't have to pretend, OK? Is that a deal?

Boy: Yes, it was a play camera that we played with.

MacFarlane: Oh, and it went flash?

Boy: Well, it didn't exactly go flash.

MacFarlane: It didn't exactly go flash. Went click? Did little pictures go zip, come out of it?

Boy: I don't remember that.

MacFarlane: Oh, you don't remember that. Well, you're doing pretty good, Mr. Alligator. I got to shake your hand.

Excerpt on interview with a 6-year-old girl

Dr. Astrid Heger: Maybe you could show me with this, with this doll [puts hand on two dolls, one naked, one dressed] how the kids danced for the Naked Movie Star.

Girl: They didn't really dance. It was just, like, a song.

Heger: Well, what did they do when they sang the song?

Girl: [Nods her head]

Heger: I heard that, I heard from several different kids that they took their clothes off. I think that [first classmate] told me that, I know that [second classmate] told me that, I know that [third classmate] told me. [Fourth classmate] and [fifth classmate] all told me that. That's kind of a hard secret, it's kind of a yucky secret to talk of-but, maybe, we could see if we could find--/

Girl: Not that I remember.

Heger: This is my favorite puppet right here. [Picks up a bird puppet] You wanna be this puppet? Ok? Then I get to be the Detective Dog…We're gonna just figure it all out. Ok, when that tricky part about touching the kids was going on, could you take a pointer in our mouth and point on the , on the doll over here, on either one of these dolls, where, where the kids were touched? Could you do that?

Girl: I don't know.

Heger: I know that the kids were touched. Let's see if we can figure that out.

Girl: I don't' know.

Heger: You don't' know where they were touched?

Girl: Uh-uh. [Shakes her head]

Heger: Well, some of the kids told me that they were touched sometimes. They said that it was, it kinda, sometimes it kinda hurt. And some the times, it felt pretty good. Do you remember that touching game that went on?

Girl: No.

Heger: Ok. Let me see if we can try something else and -

Girl: Wheeee! [Spins the puppet above her head.]

Heger: Come on, bird, get down here and help us out here.

Girl: No.

Heger: Bird is having a hard time talking. I don't wanna hear any more no's. No no, Detective dog we're gonna figure this out.

By Autumn the interview content was becoming more strange and not unlike that reported by Judy Johnson regarding her own son Billy. Children would speak of trap doors and a network of underground tunnels and rooms under McMartin. They disclosed being placed in shipping boxes and taken on planes and hot air balloons to castles and forests, of also being threatened by staff who sacrificed babies, animals and used wild beasts as tools of fear. They alleged to have been photographed naked and sexually abused in unspeakable ways, of shadowy figures in robes and staff flying like witches (which begs the question why the need for a hot air balloon). The hysterical citizen groups, headed by a McMartin parent Bob Currie, arranged for an excavation of the neighbouring lot to discover "the tunnels". This was an effort soon replicated under the public purse by an engineering firm hired by the district attorney. Police investigated airports, purchased tens of thousands of dollars of pornography in the hopes of finding evidence and staked out dozens of properties and businesses. Enough man power was invested in the case to police a small city.

At the hazard of stating the obvious, by early 1984 Virginia McMartin closed forever a business that went from highly successful for three decades of continuous service to being unable retain enough students to stay afloat. Other day care centres also began dropping like flies over the Los Angeles area, some from being implicated in the alleged satanic network and some merely from the fear of parents at what might happen to their child. By March 1984 the MacMartin seven (i.e. every employee including Ray and an almost Octogenarian Virginia) were arrested and indicted by a grand jury. Preliminary hearings began and both Ray and his mother Peggy remained in jail. Every member of staff was forced to hire their own legal counsel and go up against the might of a state and its district attorney Robert Philobosian, who wished to use McMartin as a spring board to greater political heights. Meanwhile Macfarlane was busy writing funding applications and dating ABC affiliate journalist Wayne Satz, who always seemed to be one step ahead of fellow journalists to the latest scoop. Both the media and the expert industry was having a field day. Pazder had entered the fray, as had Summit. By early 1986 the preliminary trial was over. The new district attorney Ira Reiner concluded there was insufficient evidence to continue a prosecution against all but Ray and his mother Peggy, this despite the fact that the methods used by, and strength of evidence against, these two were identical to the methods and evidence against the seven as a whole. Peggy was bailed after spending close to 2 years in prison. But Ray would stay there. The trial proper (though the preliminary was itself a protracted two years) began July 1987. Not until early 1989 would Rays application for bail be accepted. And yet the trial marched on. By early 1990 the judge was faced with a hung jury, this coinciding with the first signs that the satanic panic might be cracking. Peggy was acquitted, though the state would not yet release its grip on Ray who was held for a second and final trial, this one ending July the same year, again from a hung jury. Thankfully the district attorney did not pursue a third trial.

Only in the aftermath did the staggering costs of the McMartin affair come to light. It remains the most expensive criminal trial in United States history at something in excess of 15 million dollars, inclusive of investigation costs, with tax payer funding of CII during the 1980's adding an extra 15 million. Parenthetically, Mcmartin surpassed the previous expenditure record, that being the case of the Hillside stranglers Kenneth Bianchi and Angelo Buono Junior. Bianchi managed to convince a few expert witness psychiatrists that he suffered from MPD and it was not he who did the killing. Returning tor McMartin, it was also the longest trial, with proceedings in total lasting the better part of 6 years. It chewed through 6 judges, 17 attorneys, 12 primary jurors and several alternates, some jurors spending as much as 560 days in total in the dock, essentially making of their juror role a de facto career. Ray would spend 5 of these years in prison, his mother 2. But none were spared. Babette Spitler lost access to her infant child in the early phase of the trial, and he lost access to her. The matriarch Virginia went from the recipient of many community awards to a pariah, embittered by the community who suddenly turned against her. She died from one too many strokes in 1995. Betty died five years later. Every one of the defendants were frightened, jaded and bankrupt, their homes and every penny of their savings exhausted on legal fees. The day care centre, on a blue chip central corner block, had long been the subject of salivation by property developers, some of which were at the front of the lynch mob. They got the property in the end. And Ray disappeared somewhere to attempt salvage a normal life under a different name. None of the aforementioned professionals faced any loss of liberty or capital.

A Brief Eulogy for Judy Johnson (contra psychiatry)

Judy Johnson was never afforded the opportunity to take the stand and confront Ray and his coven of Luciferian levitators, and not for reason of the prosecution wishing to protect their case from the damage of her testimony. No she died December 1986 from the complications of alcohol dependence. This being no mean feat and not something achieved over night, Johnson dying at the tender age of 42 years must have been drinking for some years. When the panic was breaking she was taken to be what was convenient for those who wished to profit from the destruction of the McMartin seven, that is a brave and caring mother whose story was assumed to be true unless and until proven otherwise. Summit would defend her to the last as someone later made schizophrenic by the stress, and further suggest she had that necessary mix of character and eccentricity to effect such a paradigm shift in public consciousness necessary to reveal new knowledge. But now the panic is over one does not have to go far to see it written that Johnson was an unrecognized schizophrenic. Or so they say, this being the overwhelmingly most common formulation at the turn of the millennium by any who knew anything about the case.

Once again even when psychiatry loses (in the sense that Summit, Pazder and others derive their authority from their credentials) the outcome is psychiatry winning, both in the explaining away of something more complex than a label, and in the use of the label to scapegoat an individual and it being held up as something that exists as a meaningful descriptor. And yet where and what is this thing called schizophrenia as any more existent than the tunnels under McMartin? Johnson was an immensely strained solo mother of two, one of which (her first) was had a brain tumor. And Judy Johnson herself was killing off both brain and liver with alcohol, the realities of these pathologies being something much more real than "schizophrenia". And as she went deeper and deeper into her excursions into her interrogation of Billy her efforts were reflected in the beliefs and behaviors of the greater Los Angeles area, and much of the United States as a whole. Was it her leading questions that make of Johnson a schizophrenic? Was it her belief in the infallibility of child testimony? Was it the belief that a child who shows no evidence of having been abused has a physical examination consistent with having been abused sometime in the past, i.e. a belief in a thing not seen? (at least her child had an erythematous anus). Was it her belief that Ray and the McMartin seven were pedophilic necrophilic zoophilic (and zookeeping) homicidal Satanists with supernatural powers, merely the tip of the ice berg to a vast international ring of the same? But this was a belief ardently shared by hundreds if not tens of thousands of parents, police, countless psychiatrists and psychologists, the judicial machine and the fourth estate at the height of the panic. Are not all these many hundreds if not tens of thousands of persons also schizophrenic? Circa the time of the trial Duke University completed a survey of Los Angeles residents, the finding being a staggering 98% thought the McMartin Seven were guilty, rendering it nigh on impossible to find an unbiased juror. The initial pool required to front court from which the 12 were chosen was approx. 500 persons.

The irony is that a psychiatric witness for the prosecution is an expert in virtue of being a psychiatrist, same is the case for the defense. And the psychiatrist can be viewed through the lens of one who, in virtue of their expertise qua psychiatric credential, can determine if your child has been sexually abused, and you too perhaps though neither you or your child may remember it. Should you or your child come to later believe false memories were "implanted" or you were in any way mentally injured by your interaction with psychiatry, many a member of the public of Manhattan beach took the choice to pursue therapy with, you guessed it, the very species of experts who first bruised them. That is to say that many an American bruised by the panic and its psychiatrists decided get therapy, a conscious leap from the frying pan into the fire, an addiction to therapy. Madness!

But McMartin was a one off?

Whilst it is true the Mcmartin saga was the most high profile and memorable day care case of the Satanic panic, it was far from being the only one. As stated, dozens of day cares centres fell in the Los Angeles area, some from accusation and some by association, for many a parent thought it just too risky to place their child in day care. One wonders if McMartin et al did not contribute in its own small way to the helicopter parenting we observe today. Yet there were many more besides. In California, Kern County was scorched by multiple panicked investigations. Across the fly over states to the Atlantic, in New York at least a dozen preschools were investigated. In North Carolina the Little Rascal case broke state legal records of expenses just as McMartin took the nation. All up across the country the estimate is conservatively in excess of 100 preschools implicated in Satanism. Probably over 10,000 persons had their reputation ruined or brought into danger as a result of the panic and many dozens were imprisoned, some even to this day. No one has really counted their number, and some false convictions may have resulted from false confessions and the faults of coercion within the practice of plea bargaining.

MPD/DID and the Satanic Panic

Heretofore we have been looking at multiple personality disorder in cinema and psychiatry on one hand, and on the other Satanism in film and its panicked interface with psychiatry. Given that both played upon the motif of childhood trauma, the innocence of the child accuser, and repressed memory with dissociation in the victim, it was only inevitable that these two plot lines were to converge on the same stage of what is taken for reality. And converge they did in the psychiatrists and psychologists rooms of thousands of patients across in the US at the height of the panic. Here we will consider a select few.

The Strange Case of Patricia Burgus

Patricia Burgus was an ordinary American mother of a son (John Paul), that was until she had an extremely complicated birth of her second child (Michael), this leaving her emotionally as well as physically bruised, and fearful of her newborns recovery from a delivery that threatened the life of mother and child. He was to have an Erb's palsy for his first 4 years. Additionally, it placed Patricia and her husband, both devout Roman Catholics, in a state of conflict. They both wanted a large family, or such at least was what their public selves desired. But once bitten twice shy after a traumatic delivery, and so she developed what other psychiatrists might jump to call "postnatal depression". By all accounts Pat had some measure of resilience, having recovered from the post traumatic stress of having been previously a hostage in a grocery store armed robbery more or less a decade earlier. Despite this, she was happy before the day of delivery.

Following the birth of Michael, on/off between 1982 to 1984 she sought help from social worker and psychotherapist Ann-Marie Baughman, who it is said, encouraged her to give her various emotional states names, to personify them, this apparently leading to a fracture in the unity of Patricia's psyche and the first emergence of multiple personality, this being Baughmans diagnosis (it being my contention that Baughman could not have made the diagnosis were it not for Sybil and DSM III). Patricia might well have encouraged this in referring to herself in the third person or the collective "we", and we must not judge Baughmans technique so strange, for it was common then and extremely common now in the care of anorexic girls who are encouraged to speak of "Anna" as some alien force in their psyche whom they best challenge and disavow. I have personally seen a couple anorexic patients develop a multiple personality like hysteria as a result of Annasaurus Rex being split off from their own sovereign mind. Anna did this. Anna is telling them that. And yet who is Anna but for a part of them, but an iatrogenic subclinical MPD? Returning to Patricia Burgus, she was motivated to obtain a disability pension, for which psychiatrist opinion was sought. She saw six whom apparently could not agree on the diagnosis. Such is the lot of psychiatry, a broad church only appearing united on the surface. Perhaps revealing something of Pats suggestibility and personality matrix, her 1985 stay at the Menninger Clinic was short, this after they denied her wish to stay with the teddy bears she kept for her child personalities to play with. Rather than choose the Menninger, she remained loyal to her bears. And so Pat found herself at a loss, that was until she called the National Institute of Mental Health (the peak national psychiatric research body), who referred her to Chicago's Rush Hospital, a Dissociation unit headed by psychiatrist Bennett Braun and psychologist Roberta Sachs, both who were also two of the American Psychiatric Associations leading lights and part of the DSM working group on dissociative disorders. By 1986 Pat was an inpatient at Chicago Rush, and the therapy had begun. She was told in no uncertain terms that she must have been abused as a child, and her protests were denied on the assumption she must be repressing the memory. Brauns logic was circular and typical of psychiatry. Childhood trauma leads to repressed memory and dissociation. To be traumatized implies the outcome, the outcome implies the alleged cause. Once you have the diagnosis, the witch hunt begins.

On Satanic cults Braun said "international organization that's got a structure somewhat similar to communist cells". And using language perfectly suitable for demon possession Braun describes MPD thus; "you would never know it existed. Patients develop so many personalities to hide behind …unless they can be coaxed out of the dark shade of the mind you'd never know they were there"

And so at Chicago Rush it was not long before under hypnosis and with what would become countless hours of psychotherapy, Pat was to remember being abused by both parents, in ways unimaginable. And from this she would be estranged from the parents who brought her into the world for the next 6 years. Yet in the Pat Burgus case, she and various of her 300 troupe of personalities were not merely to recall childhood sexual abuse. They, like the other multiples on the ward (hundreds of personalities more than available hospital beds), also began to recall ritual satanic abuse. She would recall being the high priestess of a cult taking in not just her parents yet beyond, a royal bloodline before the founding of the America's. And she would come to believe that her personalities were programming to effect the cult objectives whilst remaining hidden from the world at large, Pat's conscious mind being part of those duped. (The reader might see in this programming the similarity here to another creation of Hollywood, "The Manchurian Candidate"). There would be talk of rituals, sexual, zoophilic and paedophilic, and of sacrifice and cannibalism. both the sacrifice and cannibalism involving babies of course, and I'll leave it to the psychoanalyst readers would to make of this in light of the basic plot of Pats neurosis. Pats husband, who was allowed visitation, at Brauns request even brought in meat from an extended family BBQ to be assayed if it contained human protein. Pats and other patient's dolls and stuffed toys, rather than being seen for what they were, (i.e. objects of hysterical regressions to childhood) were interpreted differently. Instead they were interpreted as replacement objects for the animals and children sacrificed, these stand ins in turn standing in for a recognition of the murders they were responsible for and the children who could never return from the portable incinerators that left the forest without trace of the moonlit witchcraft. The staff, true to the biopsychosocial model, were soon to draw Pats two young boys into the net. MPD was said to be hereditary (bio), Pat was programmed to train her children in the dark arts as she had been (psycho) and she lived within the milieu of witches who also had their designs to protect their own, or trigger a pre-programmed suicide program or assassination rather than risk exposure (social). Pat herself was by now perhaps acting in diminished capacity as she was largely cut off from the rationality of the world outside, in addition to being administered large doses of psychoactive medication (1200mg and 100mg per day respectively of propranolol and fluoxetine, as well as many milligrams of alprazolam and sodium amytal). Consequently, for the alleged protection of the children, both were admitted. First was John Paul followed by Michael. The children were under the care of child psychiatrist Elva Poznanski, who had a knowing yet permissive role in the works of Braun upon the children also, and so the therapeutic team expanded to include Poznanski, Sachs, Braun and a junior doctor, with the hospital executive aware of the general formulation of the cases and what was being treated (satanic ritual abuse). The children were themselves exposed to hours of interrogation and "remembering" their own roles in the cult, of having shot and stabbed people, and Braun would later provide testimony that the children had knowledge of what disembowelment looks and smells like, knowledge that only a surgeon or serial killer could know (though as Pat later thought, such knowledge could have been acquired from a certain scene in any VHS copy of the blockbuster "The Empire Strike Back"). The boys were even provided an unloaded handgun as an aide de memoire, and their revelations rewarded with stickers just as happens when a child does well on a task. Halloween was an incredibly trying time for Rush hospital. What would the children do, or might the Satanists be circling the building? Would there be murder, escape, suicide or perhaps all three?

By 1988 the hospital was approaching the point of scraping the bottom of the families 3 million dollar health insurance barrel, this coinciding with the time Pat Burgus's level of care was reduced from full time inpatient to discharge and to return to day programs. She ceased her medication cold turkey, endured the discontinuation side effects and embarked on a trip back to Iowa. Gradually an idea began to dawn on Pat, that is "where was the evidence?". Not a single satanic artefact hidden anywhere in the home. No talk of missing persons about the town. No bodies in the basement. Pat was in the grip of the paranoids dilemma. The absence of proof may indicate just how wily the conspirators are. But it might also mean that the story wasn't true. She wasn't a high priestess. She was just plain boring Patricia Burgus. It was then that Pat decided lawyer up.

The Strange Case of Mary Shanley

Mary Shanley was, like Patricia Burgus, exposed to her own traumas of the past. In Burgus' case it was a grocery store holdup and difficult birth. In Shanleys case it was alcoholic parents, a rape in the late teens and placing the resultant child up for adoption. Not surprisingly she was and has what we might call vulnerabilities of personality, and her admission to Rush Hospital was not her first. True to Freudian form, Mary married alcoholic Joe and together they had a son Ryan in 1981 before Joe cleaned up his act in 1984. 1987 was a tough year for Mary. Joe wanted more children and Mary had, for some reason, occasion to have a hysterectomy. She was attacked at her son's school and became depressed with panic attacks. Her first therapist, like Burgus, was to suggest MPD and ritual abuse of childhood. And so, via a short stint in another hospital she found herself in 1990 the old Orchard wing of Rush. Much of Shanleys case mirrors that of Burgus. An extremely prolonged expensive admission, hypnosis. a potpourri of ultra-high dose psycho-pharmaceuticals, the diagnosis of MPD and the multiplication of her multiples, the exploration into her involvement in occult Satanism with all the macabre bloody appurtenances of its praxis, the iatrogenic estrangement from accused family and so on. The case is made more bizarre by the one off review by Utah professor of psychology Corydon Hammond, who warned that Shanley was an occultly programmed killer, and the activation of her program was imminent. The move was prompted by Hammond asking her about the Greek alphabet. Shanley could only think of gamma, which Hammond "decoded" as being proof of her unconscious containing a killer program. Anything seemingly innocuous might activate it, a bunch of flowers with a colour trigger, a magazine article with encoded words etcetera. In 1991 Shanley and her then 9 year old son Ryan were spirited off in secret from Chicago to Spring Shadows Glen Hospital under the temporary care and inquisition of Psychologist Dr Judith Peterson, psychiatrists Dr's Gloria Keraga and Richard Seward and psychotherapist Sylvia Davis, all of whom practiced with the same diagnostic formulation to that of Braun et al in Chicago. Peterson, in particular, was said to be an expert in "deprogramming", though not so expert to shorten Shanleys hospital stay, which continued until 1993 (the child Ryan was returned to Chicago Rush after a few weeks). Shanley was held against her will, and was often ambivalent about her beliefs re her role in satanic ritual abuse. She too was discharged circa the time insurance monies were depleted. Upon her release she too lawyered up. An excerpt of her discharge summary reads

"Patient is a victim of satanic ritualistic abuse. Diagnosis of MPD. Apparently someone outside the family is activating her or an alter personality to attempt suicide

... One of the inside parts states that the body will be in danger from March 22nd to April 13th. The right side remembers cult activities such as the rites of spring occurring on March 21st. This is apparently a time for initiation into one of three levels and also a time for blood sacrifice...One of the goals [of therapy] was to teach Mary some self-hypnosis techniques in order to help the alters communicate more appropriately between [sic] each other...by the end of March,

Mary was working quite hard, but some internal parts were sabotaging her progress in therapy...She was struggling with the acceptance of the diagnosis of MPD and dissociation, having a high level of denial, frequently refusing her Inderal, not participating in group activities, maintaining an isolative [sic] and withdrawn demeanor...At this point, Mary was able to identify five generations of cult involvement, going back to Ireland, and an alter named Nura came out..."

Burgus and Shanley; The Aftermath

Having acquired legal counsel and successfully filing suit, the aftermath of the Burgus and Shanley cases had their brief and long forgotten moment on the national news. Burgus settled out of court for 10.6 million dollars (ironically on Halloween). Eventually she reconciled with her parents, who forgave her for the grievous accusations she raised against them, though in their dotage could never reclaim the 6-8 years they lost with their daughter and two grandsons, and only then at the expense of seeing their daughter as a victim without agency in their own demonization of psychiatry (that is to say they could only forgive their daughter by convincing themselves of the lie that she was brainwashed and no part of her chose what the therapists offered). Instead the Burgus family externalized responsibility to the treatment providers. Part of Burgus claim for compensation was, inter alia, the need for finance further psychiatric therapy for the children to treat the trauma brought upon them by the psychiatric therapy they received at Rush. It just goes to show in this subtle Stockholm syndrome, one can escape fantasy Satanism without escaping the more pernicious fantasy that psychiatry somehow somewhere simply must have something meaningful to offer. One just needs more therapy to cure one of the wrongs that therapy has wrought. Madness!

The dissociative unit of Rush was closed in 1998 and Bennet Braun was to lose licence to practice in Illinois for two years, moving his career in private practice in rural Montana and barred for 5 years from working with MPD patients. The self-styled "counterphobic" Braun later sued his own insurance company for allegedly settling the case without his consent, and he remained unrepentant. An unrepentant Sachs also moved into another state and continued to practice. Poznanski's career was also never the same, though she was aging and testified against Braun, essentially plea bargaining her way to walk off stage with dignity. It is to be noted that the children were last to be released from hospital, and Poznanski fought to keep them under state sanctioned (i.e. tax payer funded) stay after the insurance money expired, under the dogged belief that it was not safe to return the children to their mother. Corydon Hammond continued to teach and practice, and no gamma programmed assassin has ever targeted him, or these other arch foils of Satanism either for that matter.

Spring Shadows Glen Hospital Dissociative unit was itself to close in 1994, the hospital renamed and all the aforementioned staff facing charges of insurance fraud, in addition to certain staff on hospital administration. Mary Shanley herself enjoyed an undisclosed though undoubtedly multimillion dollar settlement. Sadly, her outcome was only to be fiscally happy ending. Shanley was never able return to her profession (teaching) as she remained on a national list of suspected child sex offenders. She and her husband divorced, perhaps on account of the drama of the satanic panic though one speculate upon the role of marital problems that predated the Rush admission. Less disputable is the situation with her son, who could never accept she was not as he had been indoctrinated to believe she was. Judith Peterson and her psychiatrist colleagues were unrepentant, and all continued to practice and lead workshops after the end of the panic. Peterson was to give a reply in an interview with Mark Pendergrast that became typical of many practitioners when confronted with the need to control the damage to their reputation, and that is the fall back on extreme philosophical pragmatism.

"It doesn't particularly matter if it's true or not. I wasn't there. The dilemma of true or not true is up to them."

As was the case with day care centres and the satanic panic, Patricia Burgus, Mary Shanley and their respective families were to be just two of hundreds of casualties of the panic, with countless others across the country in the hands of other less illustrious therapists and in other hospitals. In total, other cases from Rush alone were settled to what has been estimated a total of at least triple to five fold the 10.6 million that Patricia Burgus herself received, and one can only speculate on how the insurance companies might have displaced the resultant liability onto patients and practitioners alike. And these were not the only strange cases either. At Rush, there was Elizabeth Gale, who spent near 2000 days in hospital, agreeing to a tubal ligation as she did not wish to be a "breeder" for satanic abuses. Gale was later awarded over 7 million dollars. From Colorado came Kathryn Schwiderski and daughter Kelly Schwiderski known as the "Colorado fetus factory", another family destroyed. The list goes on and on.

Only in America?

There is no denying that the dynamism of the new world was for the Satanic Panic, like many a fad, something that could not be repeated elsewhere on the same scale. And yet in the case of Michelle Remembers we must remember that Canada came before the United States, and the panic found itself also being exported to other Anglo countries, just as MPD was exported from France. The panic reflected back into Canada at a greater intensity before it was finally to end. In the UK circa the same years there were mirror cases of families separated and lives destroyed under the weight of satanic ritual abuse allegations, including Cleveland (i.e. the Cleveland of Englands north) in 1987, Nottingham in 1989, Rochdale in 1990, Orkney in 1991 and approx. 80 cases in total across the UK petering out by the mid-nineties with a post millennial outlier in Lewis (Scotland) in 2003. In Australia, the nation that first not so coincidentally published their own first case of MPD the year The Three Faces of Eve was released and whose psychiatric guild in the early 1980's embraced a Melbourne conference of the International Society for the Study of MPD and Dissociation in the lead up towards the panic, in Sydneys upmarket North Shore certain kindergartens were also implicated in the panic. The local fourth estate wrote of 200 women claiming to be ritual satanic abuse survivors in that city alone. Cases of ritual satanic abuse were also investigated in the smaller cities Perth and Adelaide, the former supposedly having 13 witches covens involved in ritual abuse and the latter provoking such lurid headlines such as "human sacrifice at Adelaide University". In Melbourne the conspiracy included allegations of the Roman Catholic Church being on the villainous side. Insomuch as the international crisis in the reputation of the Latin church was yet to break, one can retrospectively ask how much truth was present in the general notion of institutionalized child abuse, whilst we remain sceptical to the extent to which an undisguised Satan was at the scene of the crime. We must not mock the United States though, for the rest of the Anglo speaking world was saved the extent of the panic only by the unintended benefits of being slow behind its leader. Sometimes the last to catch an idea are the first to be cured of it.

And what of the Psychiatric Guilds?

Todays younger psychiatrists and those trained outside the Anglo speaking world know nothing of the Satanic Panic or the degree to which their psychiatric elders had buy in (at worst), or turned a blind eye (at best). Psychiatric residents are assiduously trained to see the particularly egregious mistakes of the past as having been made at least two generations prior, so as to establish a greater temporal disconnect between themselves and their own professional vulnerabilities. And so we are always living in the age when depravities such as prefrontal lobotomy and many more besides were done by those primitives before our truly scientific, truly evidence based and truly ethically well founded practice came to life in us. The truth is of course that a proper study in the history of psychiatry must pull our pessimistic verisimilitude right up to the moment in which we live, the day in which we work and the patient now right in front of us. Yet this insight, though something which is the spirit and goal of good psychotherapy, is too painful and destabilizing an experience for the profession of psychiatry to bear. And so in the defence of its own ego it fails to confront itself, instead erecting its own fantasy. And we see in the case of Bennett Braun, arguably a scapegoat if ever there was one, that even his penalty was terribly light and was not to become precedent to bring his specialist colleagues into a place of danger, either professionally or financially. Yet where was the vocal public condemnation of psychiatry as vulnerable to its own form of madness, and vulnerable to the present day? Perhaps there was critique from the psychiatrists George Ganaway and Paul McHugh (the latter of whom was to become persona non grata for later opposing the ideology of transgenderism). And there was anthropologist Sherrill Mulhern and psychologist Richard Noll. Ganaway once wrote of those who recovered repressed memories and alternate personalities

"I've Personally encountered "demons, angels, sages, lobsters, chickens, tigers, a gorilla, a unicorn, and 'God'," to name only a few. ". McHugh described it beautifully "MPD is an iatrogenic behavioral syndrome, promoted by suggestion and maintained by clinical attention, social consequences, and group loyalties."

But amongst the profession as a whole, which must have included many sceptics, there was nothing but utter silence. The method is simple and not to be unexpected for a profession thoroughly infused with philosophical pragmatism. Do as much as is possible to maximize the freedom and status of the profession. Do not do anything that might bring the profession into disrepute. Only if absolutely necessary throw a colleague under the bus and only to the extent necessary to satiate the herds thirst for justice. And if possible deflect from, or reframe the interpretation of, the problem or externalize responsibility. And so we have practitioners who behave as if satanic ritual abuse is as real as the nose on their face coming to say afterwards that they were working with the patients truth without commitment into their own. Or we have psychiatry blaming psychology or "untrained" social workers.

And then there is the technique of rebranding and simply forgetting. Formed in 1983, the International Society for the Study of MPD and Dissociation at its height had over 2000 professional members, who were also part of the working groups towards the DSM section on dissociative disorders and many of whom were the colourful figures who rode the panic and many more conspiracy theories besides. By 1994 when the Satanic Panic, false memories and iatrogenic MPD were being exposed, the organization rebranded as "International Society for the Study of Dissociation". And then when childhood sexual abuse was fashionably accepted as real yet detached from its satanic implications, in 2006 the organization rebrands again as the "International Society for the Study of Trauma and Dissociation". To this day it hands out the Cornelia Wilbur award and its guidelines assert that 1-3% of the adult population has MPD/DID.

In the American Psychiatric Association and its diagnostic bible the DSM, the advisory committee for the DSM III (1980) ANXIETY AND DISSOCIATIVE DISORDERS section included the following names; Jean Endicott, Ph.D. George Saslow, M.D., Ph.D. Michael Gelder, M.D. Michael Sheehy, M.D.

Donald F. Klein, M.D. Robert L. Spitzer, M.D. Isaac Marks, M.D. That said, Dissociative disorders were given their own chapter, with multiple personality disorder appearing mid chapter, with a prevalence described thus "The disorder is apparently extremely rare". Like any major publication there was significant work done in lead up to the release of DSM III, the release date being a mere 3 years after the screening of Sybil. On the differential diagnosis, last is listed malingering (i.e. lying) with the comment "Malingering can present a difficult diagnostic dilemma. The presence of secondary gain suggests Malingering. Hypnosis or amytal interview may be of help in resolving especially difficult cases."

That is to say that as recent as 1980 psychiatry thought that hypnosis and the erroneously called "truth serum" of sodium amytal can be a guide to discerning one who lies to the psychiatrist from one who lies to themselves. The premise behind the use of sodium amytal was the lie psychiatry told itself. Ergo the battle was over before it had begun.

By 1987, both the post Sybil effect and the Satanic Panic with MPD as a psychological defence against, or programming by, satanic ritual abuse was at its peak and not yet robustly challenged. The revised third volume of the manual, the DSM III R 1987 included working group members as follows; Bennet G. Braun, M.D., Philip M. Coons, M.D., Richard P. Kluft, M.D., Frank W. Putnam,

M.D., Robert L. Spitzer, M.D., Marlene Steinberg, M.D., and Janet B.W. Williams, D.S.W.

Spitzer was the editor and his involvement in the proliferation of psychiatric diagnoses has been heavily criticised elsewhere (see for example James Davies book "Cracked"). We have encountered the name Bennett Braun above. Richard Kluft, the then Professor of Psychiatry at Pennsylvania's Temple University School of Medicine, Editor-in-Chief of now out of print journal Dissociation (circulation ran between 1988-1997) and Past president of the dissociation society was quoted in 1989 as describing ritual satanic abuse as a "hidden holocaust" and "the average MPD patient is misused twice a week, perhaps 50 weeks of the year for an average of 10 years". Kluft is famous for marathon psychotherapy sessions of many hours. Riding the wave, MPD was placed first in the chapter, the rationale being "increased awareness that Multiple Personality Disorder is in many ways both the paradigm and the most pervasive expression of the spectrum of dissociative phenomenology"

Regarding the explosion in cases, the DSM III-R describe MPD thus

"Within a few years a disorder thought to be rare, apocryphal, or even extinct emerged as a long neglected, underdiagnosed, and frequently misdiagnosed condition, highly associated with significant childhood traumatization, and rather responsive to intensive (and often long-term) psychotherapy. Many patients long thought to have other disorders and relatively unresponsive to the therapies appropriate for those disorders have proven to have this condition"

And

"Recent reports suggest that this disorder is not nearly so rare as it has commonly been thought to be."

Regarding the idea that personalities can be opposites, so limiting the potential of multiplication of the personalities within the given patient to two or three, the DSM IIIR writes

" this reflects an outdated and over-simplistic view of the disorder"

By 1994 the American Psychiatric Association, savy politicians that they are, could see the writing was on the wall for the diagnosis of MPD becoming bad public relations, and many of their intelligentsia becoming liabilities. And so there was a massive sea change in the branding of MPD, all deflecting from what we might speculate to be the real reasons. Not a single one of the original working group were retained, and dissociation buried within a more eclectic working group termed "Psychiatric Systems Interface Disorders (Adjustment, Dissociative, Factitious, Impulse-Control, and Somatoform Disorders and

Psychological Factors Affecting Medical Conditions) Work Group" Names included Robert E. Hales, M.D., Chairperson Ronald L. Martin, M.D. C. Robert Cloninger, M.D., Katharine Anne Phillips, M.D. Vice-Chairperson David A. Spiegel, M.D. Jonathan F. Borus, M.D. Alan Stoudemire, M.D. Jack Denning Burke, Jr., M.D., M.P.H. James J. Strain, M.D.

Joe P. Pagan, M.D. Michael G. Wise, M.D. Steven A. King, M.D.

MPD itself was no more. Instead in its place was the newly constructed "Dissociative Identity Disorder", this returning to being wedged inconspicuously in the centre of the chapter. DSM IV hedges the bet both ways and refuses to state anything as a matter of principle, though do caution thus

"Prevalence; The sharp rise in reported cases of Dissociative Identity Disorder in the United States in recent years has been subject to very different interpretations. Some believe that the greater awareness of the diagnosis among mental health professionals has resulted in the identification of cases that were previously undiagnosed. In contrast, others believe that the syndrome has been over-diagnosed in individuals who are highly suggestible."

In the same year that DSM IV was released, a survey of some over 1,100 psychiatrists and psychologists suggested that almost 100% believed in the reality and commonality of dissociative disorders in general. 80% still took MPD seriously.

It should be noted that the vice chairperson was David A Spiegel, the psychiatrist himself son of psychiatrist Herbert Spiegel, the silent sceptic who described Shirley Mason of Sybil fame as a "brilliant hysteric"

The rebranding and forgetting strategy was to continue into the DSM IV TR (text revision) of 2000. Today, in the DSM 5 (the roman numerals being cast aside) Dissociative Identity Disorder is back to first place in its chapter, and said to have a prevalence in the community of about 1.5%. Can we seriously believe that in a small city of 1 million adults there are 15,000 Sybils, enough for every citizen to know one personally? Does psychiatry even consider the absurdity of such statistics before they toss them around? Perhaps soon with the forgetting of the panic DID will once again become the new black, and everything old becomes new again.

But Why the Panic?

In the current chapter I've put forward the hypothesis that the rise and fall of MPD/DID and ritual satanic abuse was heavily influenced by psychiatry losing the objectivity it never possessed in riding and being ridden by a wave of popular culture, a professional reflection of an inability to distinguish reality from fantasy. This is not to imply that the psychiatrist is the only professional species to which the finger may be pointed when blame is due. As we have seen there were psychologists, social workers, paediatricians and family physicians along with certain members of the police and judiciary all who were involved. And yet it is taken as a given that the world need's its police and its paediatricians, this despite the need from time to time for this or that reform in their practice. But can we take as a given the same putative indispensable need for psychiatry, the same positive value against which we might measure the harms done by psychiatrists in the satanic panic? We have already made clear the sins of omission and pragmatism in the guilds and profession as a whole, and can hardly scapegoat the individuals such as Bennett Braun, in so doing missing the forest for the trees. The current chapter is just one of a dozen blows from which to fell the assumption that psychiatry is necessary. Moreover we must place the tentacles of psychiatry in perspective, not as one amongst equals in the league of the helping professions, and not even an isolated one. When fault is at question in the world of mental health, the profession is minimally if at all influenced by the world of social work, psychology and occupational therapy. On the other hand, psychiatry provides thought leaders and influencers that dominate and contaminate many other helping professions. Boards and clinical teams have a multidisciplinary staff, almost overwhelmingly chaired by a member of the psychiatrist class as the keeper of authority. A professor of psychology may trump a common or garden variety psychiatrist in stature in a court of law, though the same common psychiatrist will carry more weight for the attorney than a common psychologist, social worker or any other allied health worker. And we have seen that Kee Mcfarlane's and others ideology were influenced by the likes of Roland Summit, and a whole cottage industry in MPD was enlivened by psychiatry and underwritten by its guild and publication (what is in the DSM can be billed to the taxpayer or insurance company, along with granting a certain immunity against prosecution to the diagnostician. What is in the book is kosher because it is in the book). Let us not therefore allow psychiatry to diffuse outwards responsibility. Counterfactuals are hazardous to be sure. Yet it is entirely possible the panic would not have occurred if psychiatry were not to have existed. The most charitable conclusion is that the profession of psychiatry did nothing to bring it to its close, and everything to make it worse.

Psychiatry bashing aside, no doubt there are many more contributions to the panic, perhaps something even so vague and stochastic as the publics need for melodrama from time to time, and any old drama will do. There was also not so subtle foundational work done on the political level and the therapeutic state. In the 1970's and 1980's, members of both sides of American politics sought to make their mark and capitalize on the plight of children, concern for children being a perennial tactic of the politician. As Richard Beck writes in his excellent book "We Believe the Children", Walter Mondale was one such politician in seeking to pass his Child Abuse and Protection Treatment Act. Two principal "experts" informing the debate were Professor David Gil, whose research published as "Violence Against Children - Physical Child Abuse in the United States" supported the politically incorrect conclusion that child abuse in toto (i.e. neglect, sexual, and physical violence) is a large scale problem present in those from every walks of life to be sure, yet very much disproportionately more common amongst the poor. Ergo its best indirect remedy was to be in the expensive large scale projects to lift the poor into the more affluent and educated middle class. In the other corner sat Jolly K, founder of parents anonymous, who argued that child abuse was an individual and not a class issue, even a matter akin to an addiction. Jolly K arrived at this belief as her own psychotherapy had stagnated. She could not help beating her children she believed, and so her therapist threw up his hands and suggested she form her own group (hence the modified model of alcoholics anonymous, in drawing upon a higher power). Mondale, arguably not wishing to alienate whole electorates and demonize the democrat voting urban poor, sided against Gil when he stated "this is not a poverty problem. It's a national problem", by which he meant individuals across the nation from all walks of life, a target that was everywhere and nowhere. The resultant was to push child protection further towards the model suggested by Jolly K, medicalization of child abuse and abuser and the growth of the child abuse therapy industry.

The vast majority of MPD patients are single white females who may or may not have been abused as children (for the accuser is always holy and MPD and its assumed traumatic event and the diagnosis dance together in circular reasoning), and over 15% of MPD patients work in the helping professions. Insomuch as the diagnosis is female dominated, in some feminist circles MPD was to be formulated as both the outcome of patriarchal oppression on one hand, and on the other also a proclivity indicative of the special nature of womankind. Of Truddi Chase and her alleged 92 multiple alters in the 1987 book "When Rabbit Howls", celebrated feminist Gloria Steinem speaks of MPD as being a "gift", a proof of women's connectedness with untapped potential of personal expression and creativity. Steinem called for a future when women would be able to live MPD without the antecedent trauma. This was to be a theme played out again thirty years later in the attitude of Dr Fletcher. the treating therapist of the (admittedly male) character in Shayamalan's 2016 fictional film "Split" as she plead for her colleagues to embrace an interest in MPD/DID "and perhaps now they are capable of something we are not. We have brain scans now. DID patients have changed their body chemistry with their thoughts." This is the sentiment reminiscent of Jekyll and Hyde. What a monster Jekyll was to be sure. But what strength and power!

Of McMartin Preschool, the progressive left would see the panic as falling into the hands of those critical of what day care centres might do to the traditional conservative Christian family and traditional women's roles. This speculation can only go so far and cuts both ways. As cases such as Burgus and Shanley and others illustrates, Satanism was considered home grown and intergenerational also. We might just have easily have conceived of the secular state and its separation of powers, secular day care included, as a saviour from Satan at home. And Roman Catholic Pazder aside, many if not most of the mental health community who bought into the panic were supposedly enlightened non believer's, their folly was in believing people were plagued by a religion of a different, Luciferian, kind. Many sceptics were also believers who did not think Satan actually worked that way, and was playing a longer game. As the character Roger Kint said in the film "The Usual Suspects", "The greatest trick the devil ever pulled was convincing the world he didn't exist."

When searching for reasons, we additionally cannot discount the symbolic power of numbers. The panic was coming at a time not merely the end of the century, yet also the end of the millennium, this being remarkable as, well, it only happens once every thousand years. No one will know we ever existed by the time the next one rolls around. One need not be in any away attuned to astrology to attach significance written into the changing of the times. From the second coming to the panic around the millennium bug, protean formulations of both religious and secular eschatology were also there ripe for the picking as the year 2000 drew closer. Occasionally the secular and religious worlds would become blurred, in many Americans seeing communism not as atheistic but Satanic. This was, after all, the rhetoric of Regan. And so Satan was here, there and everywhere. But Satan can also exist in post Soviet void. The height of the satanic panic also came at a time of perestroika, and there were signs aplenty that either the cold war may end in a hot ball of thermonuclear explosion, or the dying out altogether of the USSR as actually came to pass. As there were signs in the late 1980's of the USSR unravelling and Sept 11th 2001 was not yet dreamed of, the United States and her allies were at imminent peril of losing something that defined them for almost half a century. As Georgi Arbatov would presciently say when describing the greatest blow that a dying USSR was to inflect upon the United States, "we have deprived you of an enemy". What better enemy to serve as a replacement object than the perennial eternal Satan himself? He would never let them down.

MORALITY. THE PSYCHOTHERAPY OF DORIAN GRAY

".....because as we know, there are known knowns; there are things we know we know. We also know there are known unknowns; that is to say we know there are some things we do not know. But there are also unknown unknowns—the ones we don't know we don't know....."

Donald Rumsfeld

Aided and abetted by corrupt analysts, patients who have nothing better to do with their lives often use the psychoanalytic situation to transform insignificant childhood hurts into private shrines at which they worship unceasingly the enormity of offences committed against them. The solution is immensely flattering to the patients, as are all forms of unmerited self-aggrandizement; it is immensely profitable for the analysts, as are all forms pandering to peoples vanity; and it is often immensely unpleasant for nearly everyone else in the patient's life

Thomas Szasz

"You will always be fond of me. I represent to you all the sins you never had the courage to commit."

Dorian Gray (Oscar Wilde)

Though both can be, so to speak, a gazing up and into our rear ends, psychotherapy, unlike colonoscopy, is a word without a sense, without a denotation. It may once have had a chance of indicating an asymmetrical relationship between two persons where one takes the role of navigator or tourist into the inner world and life of another, to arrive at a place of understanding of who the latter is and how they arrived at the current state of being. Such is an already impossible task. Just as mental health is subsumed within a model of the mind in its abstractions which is lacking an answer (see chapter 3), the explanation of who I am and the journey I have taken through life must necessarily be subsumed within an ever expanding realm of social, political, metaphysical and a/theological life. The larger picture really does matter towards the goal of the well examined life, and we are stumbling and tumbling over vistas of what we do not know and can only speculate upon as articles of faith so as to arrive at our understanding. Needless to say though say it I shall, any thoughtful person must surely acknowledge that the subjectivity of the therapist is an insoluble obstacle to the confrontation of the patient with their objective selves, to say nothing of the patient. If such a thing as the objective self actually exists, surely the only psychotherapist worth their salt is the divine if they exist and if not, then we always have the solace of despair. And so either in our ignorance or to defend against despair we return to a faith less troubling than it deserves to be by the collapse of the will to truth into the contentment of embracing idols of our own making. That is psychotherapy in a nutshell.

Unfortunately, those deep torturing doubts that are my constant companion never seem to trouble the mind of the proverbial ninety nine point nine recurring percent of psychotherapists, and scarcely ever does it pass through their minds if they really can know anything about the person so as to give licence to having discovered what they have claim to have found in the depths of their psyche.

These sandy headed ostriches can be sympathized with, though not forgiven for therefore inventing fantastic models of the psyche and schools of psychotherapy to treat the one who would be patient. The behaviourist school, in its more radical excursions, was taken to deny if not the value of exploring the mental (a reasonable, though cowardly defence), to denying the existence of the mental altogether (an absurdity). This absurdity is approached in the third chapter. And contra the behaviourist school may be various readings of the analyst Freud who proposed that mind and behaviour, though ultimately materialistic, is operationally governed by the cognitive and emotional features of mind, albeit not the surface mind as opposed to that construct known as the "unconscious". Thus analysis too was a retreat of a kind from mind as we experientially know it. And whereas the behaviourists denied what cannot be denied (i.e. mind), the analysts and their heirs invented what cannot be falsified. Both in their way became cults.

And between the two there are innumerable schools, each to varying degrees kissing cousins or the chalk to the others cheese. Each may be said to lay claim to the model of the psyche, and thus the model of psychological suffering, and thus the model of recovery. Ironically the closer they are the fiercer may be the battles between them to claim the knowledge of the person, knowledge I have concluded is a priori impossible. There are the pure Lacanian Freudians, object relationist Kleinians, so called middle school, Jungians (pre and post having been influenced by his narcissistic pseudo-psychotic occult phase), humanists and so called existential psychotherapists, family systems and cyberneticists, cognitive behaviourists, gurus of many mindfulness approaches, fusion and eclectic psychotherapists, attachment theory universalists and so on and so forth. The numbers of the various psychotherapeutic schools can be as great or as few as one wishes. Insomuch as they are, after all, nominally different schools, they number at least a hundred. Insomuch as divisions may be (mis)placed, some may schematically number them in as few as four main groups (e.g. cognitive behavioural, humanistic, mindfulness and analytical). This too is problematic. For example, the cognitive behavioural school, narcissistically considered the "scientist practitioner model" and erroneously linked to Socrates and the stoics, is fundamentally deeply analytical in it being predicated on discovering the gnostic "core belief". Pray tell how deep does the core go? What is its origin? What is its architecture or topography? Is not the discovery of the core belief a telling to the therapist what they wanted to hear, and what the therapist hinted at finding all along? And from what source come the drives towards these contrivances? Aaron Beck himself arrived at his CBT through an analytical approach and a reasoning necessarily contaminated by the same, and he left his creation to a daughter heir, just as Freud did with his. Insomuch as we might be inclined to heap negative criticism on psychoanalysis, if the trunk is rotten, is not the branch also? And let it not be lost on us that all the mindfulness schools are, to be frank, dissimulations, plagiarisms and permutations of various of the more contemplative schools of religion, leaving behind what those religions would say is the most important thing to grasp and practice.

Some would say of all of this that none of it matters. They would say that the key feature of any good psychotherapy is the so called "common factors". That is to say, whether the patient sits across from a Freudian exploring their Oedipus complex or the existentialist exploring their anxiety as borne from fear of personal meaninglessness and mortality, each will languish or triumph on the basis of variables such as regularity of appointments, mutual commitment, mutual trust, unconditional acceptance and the therapists caring intentionality directed towards the patient.

And that dear reader, leads us to the greatest rot up from the roots of the tree of the psychotherapies. All of the above fluffy caring common factors sounds like delectable fruit for sure. Yet this is a distraction from the corrosive implications. For starters, a therapy that can be anything (providing it contains the common factors), is indeed a therapy of nothing at all. Certainly all therapists in one fell swoop lose the status as authority figures, that is unless they cunningly attempt to reify the common factors as a special technique of an expert intelligentsia. Indeed, some do just this, kicking up a fuss about the therapeutic frame of regularity of time, place, even location of the chairs in the therapist's rooms. But this political power play won't fly. One can just as well achieve the common factors in a caring conversation with a friend over coffee, or with ones caring grandmother or pastor or spouse. Even a stranger at a bus stop may do as one off therapy, providing love pierce through alienation. And therein also lay a sinister implication of the role of therapists as proxies for what ought to be already in place in the community. Each therapist ought to feel a sense of dread that they are a living and sad indictment on the state of the world, which out sources what ought to be insourced. Why are they even needed? They are the pathos of the world as much as the patient, a sign that the community either does not care or has divested itself of common or good sense. Moreover, in virtue of being there to be used, they are an impediment to the community being forced to confront its deficiencies and find the remedy within itself. To wit, perhaps the best psychotherapy is the one that simply ceases to meet with patients and allows itself to die into the pages of history. For only in that death can a community confront what requires confrontation, complete its own psychotherapy, and finally grow up.

Secondly, if it is true that the common factors are the operational force towards recovery and not the specific theoretical schemata of mind and its maladies that each of the therapies clings to, ought we not consider an active destruction of those therapies themselves as an affront to truth, or at least for reason that we have not appropriately acknowledged their (highly) possible falsity? But what would a therapist say, if to tell a patient that the therapy is just a play with metaphor? Could they say that their interpretation of the patient is a convenient story towards an end? Would it not lose its power, the mystery lost like a shaman who reveals that the dance is just a dance, the talisman is just wood or stone? The commitment to therapy itself would then be a suspension of the will to truth, a commitment to pragmatism. And this, as I argued in a previous chapter is morally fraught.

And finally for now, discussion of the relative truth value of the therapies versus one another and versus the notion of the common factors, all this serves as a diabolical red herring. Which therapy is more effective than the other is the distracting question? We can pursue such a debate throughout this century as we did in the last, I would predict with surety against any prospect of resolution. Yet the question is not which therapy works. The question is what it is for therapy to work, what "recovery" is and ought to be. Where are the boundaries between symptom alleviation as morally neutral and morally charged? Surely these are the questions that ought to be resolved in the mind of every budding therapist before sitting across from a patient. These concerns are borne out in a thought experiment. Let us imagine the patient is a serial rapist. And let us imagine that he has convinced us as to the error of his former ways, and that he is a changed man. So changed in fact that he is plagued by the pain of conscience. This is not pain of unwanted temptation of his previous drives as he is cured of temptation. The pain has no utility and he shall rape no more. No the pain is instead a painful manifestation of memory pure and simple, and needless to say a challenge to ego strengths and that greater evil known as "self esteem". Now our ex rapist wishes to forget, and let us imagine you are the therapist, a hypnotherapist of renown. You have the power to make him forget. You have the power to relieve him of his symptoms and effect what could be considered a recovery. So what do you do and why? Your answer to this question, and indeed every psychotherapeutic encounter at least to some degree, is a necessary encounter with morality. What is the value of memory? What is the value of anxiety? What is the good life, the well examined life, and how are those with whom I have lived to be remembered? What part did I play in where I am? What is it best to be and become? To such a hypothetical patient as our rapist you may refuse to offer your services and have your own moral reasons. Or you may accept, again with moral justification. Or you may accept simply on the basis of being a mercenary, alleviating symptoms and going where the money takes you, where the patients values are your values. To wit you are in the land of a morality whether you like it or not, and in any direction you turn questions may be rightly raised against you, perhaps more than your "client". Are you comfortable being a mercenary? You see pragmatism is a many headed Hydra. And it rears its ugly heads again and again and again in every school of psychotherapy. But arguably no head is more grotesque and mystifying than that otherwise known as Intensive Short Term Dynamic Psychotherapy, or ISTDP. It is the worst symptom of the disease that is psychotherapy.

What is ISTDP about?

For this chapter I draw primarily upon two introductory articles in the American Journal of Psychotherapy, Vol. 69, No. 4, 2015 by Catherine Hickey,

M.D, along with another by the same author in Psychodynamic Psychiatry, 43(4) 601–622, 2015, and finally the published journal articles by Allan Abbass and texts of ISTDP circa the same years and before. All are faithful to the metapsychology and practice of ISTDP at the time of my own writings. Know this dear reader, lest in time they are bruised by my critique and attempt rewrite history.

ISTDP's unstated predicates are simple enough, and shared with many other schools of psychotherapeutic thought and practice. Just three of these will be mentioned for the benefit of the lay reader. Imagine all the machinations of your conscious mind. What this mind might be was discussed in chapter 3, yet includes all the interior world your awareness, i.e. the stream of conscious thoughts infused with emotions as the collective modus operandi behind your deliberate behaviours as observed by others. Or all this would be the modus operandi were there not the alleged unconscious, the real master of who you think you are. The content is different "down there" in unconsciousland, often symbolic in its representation and the conflict often more dramatic. Yet its conceptual geometry is thought to be much the same form. Your surface mind has interior mental action. It thinks about things. It feels about things. Sometimes it thinks and feels too much or in unhealthy ways. It plans and deliberates. And so does your unconscious. The only difference is that one is largely contingent and you are aware of (conscious) and the other is largely determinant and something about which you are unaware (unconscious). The machinations of the latter are purported to reveal itself only in tantalizing lifts of the veil such as in dreams or slips of the tongue (Freud) or in something as benign and indirect as a sigh or becoming distracted when certain themes are being discussed (ISTDP).

And so Freud may say that your surface fears of failure and anxiety, your frustrations and poor assertiveness stems from, in the cliché oedipal example, the unconsciously held desire for sexual union with your mother and the fear of being castrated, if not killed, by your fathers unconscious were it to become ascendant. This is a conflict hidden from the conscious mind since childhood when it first became manifest to the unconscious, hidden on account of it being too threatening. (Melanie Klein of the so called object relations school was even more radical in believing unconscious dramas to begin in utero, where every foetus is a proto Shakespeare floating in its own stage of collective unconscious, the collective unconscious in turn partly a pagan occultist construct and partly informed by the proto fascist formulations attempting to account for degeneration of the inferiors of society). It is this fear within powerlessness that may explain why you are not all that you could be, and your trepidation to take the leap to make it so. Or it is perhaps this fear why you were anxious to follow in the footsteps of your father, for to become the father can sometimes be the closest thing to victory over the same (if you can't beat them, join them, if you can't join them, become them). Whether you are especially anxious to become your father or especially anxious to run in the opposite direction, both can be interpreted to mean the same thing, a convenient plasticity of interpretation which ought to raise suspicions in any critical thinker. Where Freud might have made libido (contra popular interpretation not entirely synonymous with lust) the primary driving force of the unconscious, other psychodynamic theorists are more brazen dissimulators of Nietzsche and the Teutonic soul than Freud was, in seeing power and domination the primary drive. Others, more from softer sentiment and equally borrowing on wishful thinking than any evidence, conceive of love to be what makes the unconscious go round. But not ISTDP. As we shall see later, love is not what they are about.

The second predicate, as exampled above, is that the unconscious conflict creates conscious (i.e. surface) neurosis, neurosis being an eloquent and now outdated term of art for a mixed bag of painful thoughts and feelings, potentially leading to maladaptive behaviour and general misery. To the extent none of us may lay claim to be Christ or a Bodhisattva, all of us to a greater or lesser extent are touched by unconscious conflict. The proportion naturally approaches one hundred percent of those seeking help by the psychiatrist. After all, why else are they there?

The third predicate is a practical one, that being that the way to rectify the conscious neurosis is via a raising the unconscious to the surface. Freuds authority afforded him a more or less genteel approach. He essentially informed the patient of her unconscious machinations. Like Moses come down from the mountain, the information alone was proffered as sufficient to convey truth and effect recovery. For some reason it was lost on Freud and his heirs that when Sophocles tragic hero Oedipus acquired his own insight, that this was just the beginning, not the end, of his woe.

Intensive short term dynamic psychotherapy is further predicated on the following

Firstly, ISTDP supposes that surface neurosis is caused by, and holding back from, the release of powerful emotions. Overwhelmingly in ISTDP literature the emotion in question is rage, pure primitive murderous rage directed at significant others from the past or present. Often the rage is sexualized, and by extension therefore often necessarily incestuous in that the significant figures of childhood is the family. It is murderous rage that makes the unconscious world go round.

Secondly, ISTDP relies upon an assumption that may be considered an unstated metaphor from either physical chemistry (almost an unstated application and perversion of Boyles law), or on the other hand a metaphor from economics. The idea is that the patient's unconscious will be resistant to releasing the painful shameful murderous rage. And so if the therapist applies extra "pressure", the number of required sessions can be made fewer. They don't quite quantify how the proportionality is scaled, yet it would not be a mischaracterization to say that if the therapist doubles the pressure the sessions ought to be (at least) halved to maximize therapeutic efficiency and bring the patient sooner to a point of recovery (whatever recovery is). The logic seems sound enough. Yet does this guarantee automatic translation to the world of human relationships? Can we get to marriage with half the dinner dates, providing a languid course gives way to forced torrents of passion?

A glimpse into an ISTDP session or two

ISTDP is structured similar to other talk therapies. The patient sits in one comfortable chair and the therapist in the other, each chair facing or oblique to one another, each close enough, yet not too close. The ISTDP session will be videorecorded, for this is exceedingly important (more on this anon). The therapist will ask questions about symptoms, about relationships past and present, the basic pedestrian stuff of any explorative psychotherapy. When supposedly painful and important material begins to emerge the patient will "resist", where resistance might be a sigh, a drifting off or distractibility as an unconscious tool of avoidance. Never mind the reader's intuition that sometimes, as in the leitmotif to Casablanca, "…a kiss is just a kiss, a sigh is just a sigh….". No, a sigh is always more than a sigh. And never mind that not all distractibility is dissociative, and how the therapist, that great gnostic exploring the inner world might possibly objectively discern the difference. Another psychiatrist might say the patient has ADHD. I might say the patient is just distracted per se, bored (perhaps with me) or has smoked too much cannabis today. In any case, our ISTDP therapist knows better. Resistance can also be manifest in muscle tensions, fist clenching, a tight throat and the like. At the right time the therapist will probe deeper as to the themes arising during these bodily revelations, eventually bravely meeting resistance head on, exploring feelings without retreat. ISTDP even has a technical term of art for this dramatic moment, the "head on collision". Hickey also writes as to the attitude the therapist must take towards the enemy resistance

"the therapist must also convey a considerable amount of disrespect for the patient's resistance"

The challenge to the resistance must not be prematurely applied however, as this will result in a failure to "unlock" the unconscious. I'll refrain from what the Freudian what make from such a description of technique. Suffice to say a therapist wishing to satisfy their patient ought not to suffer from premature investigation.

The whole dance of the therapist asking questions, encountering resistance, pulling back and sometimes increasing pressure is known as the "central dynamic sequence" or CDS and has the following stages; inquiry, pressure, challenge, transference resistance, direct access to the unconscious, systematic analysis of the transference, and dynamic exploration into the unconscious.

Sounds like sophisticated stuff indeed, for what is essentially an exercise in psychological "button pushing".

The buttons being pushed are naturally seen as there within the patient from the beginning, though ISTDP has a remarkable talent for publishing cases in which the transcript clearly described what we in the trade call "leading questions", that is to say a case of the therapist stating "these are the facts of the ugly truth, don't you think?" The outcome of the button pushing is what is also known in psychotherapeutic circles as an abreaction leading to catharsis, and what the undisciplined laity might describe as losing one's temper, having a cry and feeling much better afterwards, though hopefully a little guilty. The ISTDP community does not use the archaic terminology of abreaction and catharsis themselves. Such I assume would be to diminish their claim to novelty and discovery.

What is distinctive about ISTDP, and I'll grant it to be internally coherent to its theory, is that it's abreaction of primitive murderous rage is itself full of murderous rage. This is manifest in what I can only describe as a therapist guided patient generated pseudo-dissociative role play of fantasy ultra-violence. That's a mouthful and I shan't dignify it with an acronym. Essentially what I am saying is that the patient is responsible for being coached to whip themselves into a frenzy to imagine themselves as brutally killing another human being who is to blame for their neurosis, and even coached in how to kill them. Below is an excerpt from the transcript of a therapy session in Hickey's first paper between a patient "PT" (of whom it is implied is actually a medical doctor in ISTDP training herself,

as she is a professional therapist with a knowledge of surgical terminology) and
"HD", the discoverer and doyen of ISTDP himself, Habib Davanloo.

"HD: How do you experience this rage?

PT: I have a knife—I start attacking.

HD: But that doesn't show how the rage goes.

(At this point, the patient has the full activation and experience of the
neurobiological pathway of murderous rage: She physically gestures as
though she has a knife in her hand and is slashing the therapist.)

HD: Don't close your eyes. Don't move too much. That's not how you
hold a knife.

PT: Down and down (repeatedly).

HD: Go on. Go on. Let's see how systematically you go. Go on. Go on.
Go on. (Here the patient has a massive passage of guilt. She is extremely
tearful.)

HD: Look to my eyes.

PT: I see my grandmother and mother together.

HD: Could you describe my eyes?

PT: They are green/blue. Why did I do this to her? Why? How could
I do this?

HD: Look to my murdered body. You said my eyes were
green . . . face with the feeling. Face with your feeling.

PT: I love you. I love you so much.

HD: You are talking to whom?

PT: My grandmother

HD: How does she look at you?

PT: She loves me too. I love you.

HD: How badly the body is damaged?

PT: There's blood. I have carved. There is a big incision down her
head and down her neck and her abdomen is filled with blood. I'm so
sorry. I'm so sorry. I love you.

HD: Obviously you are loaded with the primitive murderous rage.
Look, you have to face the truth of your unconscious. You say you love
her but at the same time you have murderous feelings. You see the two
sides? A part of you wants to destroy her but another part of you loves
her. But you have to face the two sides of the ugly truth of your
unconscious. You have to face it.

PT: I have to face it.

HD: One part of you wants to torture her even worse than this.

Another part wants to love her. This is the ugly truth of your unconscious.

If you want to examine it we can examine it.

PT: I want to.

HD: There is a massive primitiveness, and it is extremely important

you examine . . . this.

PT: Yes, there is.

HD: You carefully want to examine it? If you want to put an end to it,

and I put emphasis on if, if you want to put an end to the suffering . . . ."

In a subsequent session the abreaction is even more graphic in its violence

"HD: How do you feel that anger towards me?

PT: I would punch you in the face with a knife—go right in to your

eyeball, slash down your eye, down your face, and down your chest

and abdomen. I would take a knife and put it up your rectum until it

comes out of your abdomen—it is a curved knife. I slice down and

mutilate you. I tear open with massive claws your abdomen—down to

your backbone, and there is a river of blood coming out.

HD: And then what is my situation? If you look at me I am disastrously

mutilated.

PT: (Appears to have massive waves of guilt-laden feeling). I'm sorry."

ISTDP; How did it evolve?

ISTDP literature waxes lyrically and sycophantically about its founder and pioneer into the unconscious Habib Davanloo. The story goes that Davanloo started out in the 1960's as a Boston psychoanalytic trainee of Elizabeth Zetzel, Eric Lindemann and Helen Deutsch. Davanloo was driven to discover why some patients recovered and some did not. Fortunately, over time and with advances in technology he was able to amass a huge library of filmed therapy sessions. Having settled into Montreal, Davanloo poured himself over the video footage to observe what occurred during those sessions that were allegedly successful, what was said and not said so as to "unlock the unconscious". From this came hypothesis testing based on what was observed, resulting in new video-recordings of new patients, new viewings of video-recordings and ever greater refinements of technique with ever greater elaborations of the "discoveries" made as the fruits of "research". Davanloo was said to accomplish what Freud never could, that being reliable recovery in a timely manner and with avoidance of the dreaded "analysis interminable", i.e. psychoanalysis that goes on forever without any satisfactory therapeutic end point. The apogee of his "discoveries" was a metapsychology bloated with terminology and many an acronym (e.g. MUSC or multidimensional unconscious structural changes and the aforementioned central dynamic sequence or CDS), spiralling into elaborations only surpassed by other masters of fictional omphaloskepsis such as Ken Wilber and Carl Jung. The distillation of Davanloo's metapsychology was not so great a departure to Freud in the inner conflict being partially guilt ridden masochism (what Freud would call superego) fused with primitive murderous rage (what Freud would see is clearly a variant on his id construct). That's where the similarity ends.

The video-recording persisted and transitioned to become a necessary motif for ISTDP to this day, and held up as a necessary presence in every therapy session. Nowadays pilgrims flock to Montreal and other training Mecca's to be trained in the art of ISTDP and unlocking the unconscious to fantasy murder and mayhem in intensive immersive and expensive workshops. And as Hickey notes, trainee therapists are very often participants in recorded sessions themselves, both as fledgling therapists and patients.

ISTDP; A critique.

Does the unconscious exist, and how is it structured?

When I was a junior doctor in psychiatric training, we were at one point asked about our opinions on psychodynamic psychotherapy in general, and Freud's psychoanalysis in particular. As it turns out I did take issue with the lot of it, and said so. "Well you wouldn't deny the existence of the unconscious would you?" came the reply from our instructor, as if to imply that from a belief in the Mediterranean Sea must follow a belief in Atlantis and her treasures submerged beneath it. What followed after some debate was some concession to the science as having moved on since Freud, though how such a "science" might have advanced when the unconscious in all its alleged forms is non falsifiable is beyond me, and only "science" in the most expansive and classical use of the term. Psychodynamic psychotherapy is a science in the sense that almost anything can be argued to be a science. In what way does the use of a word (i.e. science) entail legitimacy?

Now much older, I'm neither about to deny the existence of the Mediterranean or the complexity of the person from which we might grope for metaphor of what lay beneath the metaphorical surface. Now that is hardly a salve for my own ignorance, or an invitation to fill a vacuum with a lie.

Dreams, qua an alleged window into the unconscious, can mean anything and nothing and only have value as tools to explore what might be consciously held opinions and conflict. Some esoteric practitioners use tarot cards to accomplish the same, not as divinations to the future yet as themes to be explored. Disclosures during hypnosis are as good as worthless. Now I'm not about to commit the sin of the radical behaviourist or radical materialist. Just as some may deny the conscious, I'm not about to deny the existence of something deeper in the mind when the epistemological going gets tough. Yet I am neither about to convert it into some great gnostic puzzle, develop a mendacious metapsychology of the unconscious and in so doing raise myself to the station of the great seer into souls. People are complex and very often more than meet the eye. People have faith in their faithlessness and faithlessness in their faith. They both want and don't want. Something they often don't want is to know what they don't want to know. We lie to ourselves. We are always and often in some degree of tension between acknowledging our sins and wanting after a place in ourselves where we may be more comfortable, even if that comfort is self-punishment. We might see in others what we deny in ourselves (projection). Others may remind us of those of the past, leaving us behaving in a way "as if" the person from the past were there in front of us (transference). We may like others to feel what we feel and in so doing solve our problems for us (projective identification). We may have our own neuroses and enter into the career of psychology or psychiatry such that our profession may vicariously heal us (also projective identification, just don't tell the patient we are more screwed up in psychological knots than they are). We may have difficulty seeing others as persons also of mixed motives and mixed virtues and sins, tending instead to black/white judgments (splitting). There is nothing revelatory about these and other psychotherapeutic terms of art. Great psychoanalysts have always been with us, and draw their power as analysts from our ability to identify with the lesson they are teaching, for some part of us knew the lesson all along. In Sophocles Oedipus, both the protagonist and Jocasta his mother/wife/queen from early in the plot both know yet do not want to know. Deep into his own "psychotherapy" and in his letter to the Roman Church St Paul writes "For I do not do the good I want to do, but the evil I do not want to do, this I keep on doing". Christ spoke of projection and so did Shakespeare in King Lear, both within the context of puffing up one's moral vanity via punishing a prostitute. The list of great analysts proceeds down history into Dostoevsky, Tolstoy, Nietzsche and Orwell. This is nothing new.

The unconscious itself is a metaphor without location or a clear extension. Is it to be seen as existing within the individual alone? If so where is it, and brain scans are, a priori not going to provide a sufficient phenomenological and philosophical answer. Actually they are entirely unhelpful to the question as mind has never been observed in any brain scan, let alone sub mind. Or is it in the driving force behind collective activities and habits of the group, as was exploited by Freuds nephew Edward Bernays, the propagandist who ought to have joined the pantheon of twentieth century super villains. Is it within or at least connected to some spiritual realm from which comes symbolic representations in the proverbial angel and devil on my shoulder? Can the reader be sure that there is nothing but superstition behind these symbols? Or is the unconscious a post hoc and pragmatic explanation for what we do and feel consciously, without the unconscious "being" anything or anywhere at all? Or is the unconscious a disavowed conscious wish, held once fleetingly at the edge of thought before being ignored, as suggested above. In this sense the unconscious is not necessarily some churning magma pushing up from below as much as possibly something someone does not wish to be responsible for being pushed down from above. And what is "down" and "deep" and "up" and "down" anyway when applied to such a construct, except as geometrical metaphor? I'm herein guilty of such non-sense use of spatial language myself, for lack of a better way to describe it.

So much for the form and location of the unconscious. But what of the content? The list of hypothetical dramas deep in the unconscious is as endless as the dramas of the surface self. Indeed, it's deeper still as we have what the conscious thinks and feels, what the unconscious thinks and feels, and insomuch as each may be symbolic representations of the other there is a third conceptual space wherein lay the interpretation. In what quasi platonic space can the symbol and the therapy be found?

It is to be made clear to the reader, and this being the confession of one who has invested in being a therapist, that I cannot lay claim to stating as a matter of fact that the unconscious exists at all, much less its form and content, its location, extension and dynamics. Yet ISTDP practitioners in their naïve hubris do not know what they do not know. And that is that they also know nothing. Nothing!

Which brings us to the question of how and why traditional psychodynamic psychotherapy and its intensive psychopathic child have acquired the language of the unconscious as being there, psycho-subterranean, to be raised, to be unlocked etcetera etcetera etcetera. Why are they even interested in raising or unlocking anything? Why not just pour tonnes of psychological cement on the nuclear reactor and move on with life? To even countenance such an idea is to be met with accusations of that second greatest of psychiatric sins, i.e. to stigmatize. They will accuse you thus "do you expect them to just move on?". Well yes in fact. Much of the time that is precisely what I suggest. To love, work and to play is both the evidence of recovery and the means by which it is to be achieved, if it ever will.

To answer the question of why this drive to raise the unconscious (and construct it as a thing to be raised) I would of course be speculating and guilty of even more imaginative elaborations than that of ISDTP. But oh well. When in Rome….

Firstly, catharsis and letting it out are natural to every human with powerful emotions. There's nothing sophisticated and scientific in such imminent intuitions. So what? More fool psychiatry to have discovered the obvious.

Then there are doctors as doctors, of which Freud was, so is Davanloo and so am I, at least in the sense of our original academic training before beginning on the journey of forgetting real medicine. Incising abscesses and draining out the pus is incredibly satisfying to both patient and physician, and only in the most recent decades has medicine been about putting stuff into the body as opposed to taking stuff out. Take as a further example the case of George Washington, likely killed by his army of presidential physicians letting out the supposed bad blood and collectively exsanguinating him in the process. I cannot help but to wonder if it is the sirens call of unreleased pus that transforms and bewitches the psychiatrist into wanting to play real doctor and take to the patient with a metaphorical scalpel.

But for the psychiatrist to achieve the zenith of narcissism and identify with the full historical suite of authority figures, they need not simply be doctor, surgeon, magistrate and self-proclaimed philosopher kings. They also need become priests and exorcists. This was outlined in a previous chapter and expanded here.

For the reader unfamiliar with a good exorcism or the film genre, these are the following steps in the drama. Initially the demon possessed host presents either calm or not, yet always with a soul pregnant with the demon within. The priest will begin the ritual (central dynamic sequence of unlocking the unconscious), with a frame or stance towards the spiritual patient and invocations to combat the prince of lies with the king of truth, much as Hickey or Abbass or Davanloo himself makes appeals to "truth". All this is to say that the exorcism will be supposedly a confrontation with the reality of being, all the lights will come on and all that is hidden and unclean is to be brought to the surface and cast away. During the exorcism there are explorations, made through prayers and questionings, the goal being to know the name of the demon, the discovery if you will of the core traumatized little creature that was cast out of heaven and now just sits stewing and plotting in in primitive murderous rage. Does this sound familiar? Naturally such a creature will make moves towards remaining hidden and misidentified. It will conscript the surface consciousness of the host to "resist". Minus Hollywood's dramatic licence of spinning heads and superhuman strength of any exorcism film worth its salt, "resistance" and the "unlocking" is much the same in ISTDP. There will be sighs, great muscle tensions and writhing and churnings of the body and its viscera. This is "somatised resistance" and "striated muscle tension". There may be judgments and projections towards the priest "complex transference feelings". All the while our intrepid priest moves forward applying "pressure" to know the demons name and have it cast out. And out it will come, perhaps through sigh and shortly after a clenched and tight throat (often a behavioural motif in ISTDP) to our demon shrieking itself out into the night and off into the nearest herd of gentile pigs. Or in the case of ISTDP out comes the primitive murderous rage as discharged affect and good ole fantasy ultraviolence. Either way the demon or "demon" manifests.

The Moral Price of ISTDP

When I first heard about ISTDP it was from enthusiastic colleagues who had attended (expensive) workshops from the travelling apostles of Davanloo. In their eyes danced a sparkle of having discovered something new and exciting, not the usual dying embers of one who long entered the space of therapeutic nihilism and attempting preserve their narcissism by convincing themselves their usual therapy "works". The faithlessness in their usual therapies (i.e. standard long term dynamic psychotherapy, CBT and DBT to name but a few) was betrayed by this undeniable sparkle of their new love. Still, when they first spoke about the fantasy killing my first impression was that they were surely joking, if only because they seemed not to be in the slightest bit conflicted by what they had seen and what they intended to do with patients themselves. Or I thought perhaps it was an artefact of the workshop example being a patient with an unusually depraved character. And so I obtained the few review papers of the time, titles as mentioned above and several more besides. Lo and behold each mentioned the rage and each mentioned the killing and mutilation. And then I obtained a couple of the lead ISTDP texts, opening pages at random in disturbed bibliomancy, hoping to see that such cases are an anomaly. Once again in each chosen case transcript was the description of a brutal crime scene, primitive murderous rage. It was as they said.

And so I once again embarked on an informal survey of psychiatric colleague's attitudes to the therapy. The response almost universally took one of two directions. They either slumbered in amoral pragmatic oblivion, simply not caring or thinking about the moral question "as long as the patient gets better" they would say or "I too have fantasized about killing someone" several others would say as if normality is moral normativity. Or they found the idea of such a therapy distasteful, though I hazard to add this was only after I made the error of asking the question with my own judgment written on my face. Probably all but one or two like minded individuals feigned distaste for my benefit. Yet rather than take a stand against it and hold their colleague's feet to the moral fire, save for one single colleague even they instead turned the blind eye. Psychiatrists only attack psychiatrists who attempt to bring the profession into disrepute (hence my nom de plume), and psychiatric training is a process of deeply entering into post pragmatic ethical relativism. Most horrifying of all was the fervour with which the true believers embraced it with each successive workshop, and how they sailed beyond the horizon where I thought I could reach their moral sensibilities. This was something approaching the cult mentality I had not seen in twenty years, proving the obvious that premillennial apocalyptic zealots, age of Aquarian hippies, ideologues of all stripes and supposedly erudite critically thinking "scientific" psychiatrists all share similar DNA, and identical vulnerability to cultism.

I only recall this story to alert the reader who may, like I, reflexively adjudicate that ISTDP is evil, that we are most certainly not necessarily in the majority and have our work cut out for ourselves. Like any moral argument it can only be made quasi-deductively after an invitation to empathy has been accepted, or the argument will be unconvincing. I will try anyway

The informal premises are as follows

Major premise; "providing no one is physically hurt, all is morally neutral or morally good"

Minor premise; "providing recovery is achieved (whatever that is), all is permissible or even the moral good, providing the physical non-aggression premise is not violated"

Let us apply it to a few particular cases. Do these premises hold fast to your moral intuitions?

Case 1; imagine you are the grandmother of the patient in Hickey's published case vignettes, for she is the latest victim of fantasy killing. She is described as being quite feisty, authoritative and stubborn, a "queen bee". She was a widow from an age before its due, and likely as a European lived during a time of war. There is no description of this grandmother being in an any way an abuser of children, the patient included. Now imagine yourself as the grandmother, and somewhere sometime your granddaughter does this to your reputation and your memory. The reader can if they wish obtain the original papers to find the grandmother arraigned in this fantasy court without the basics of jurisprudential decency. Did the events and relations of the past occur as alleged to have occurred? Upon what pivots the scales to weigh the burden of proof? Is there a dialectic whereby the grandmother is offered any robust defence at all, even a defence of mitigating account for who she was and what she did or did not do? Is the punishment consonant to the crime?

Case 2: Imagine you are one half of a married couple and all that this is meant to entail. Like any human you have your personal insecurities and like any couple you have your shared conflict. The ISTDP patient would assent to the belief that at least some of the conflict is informed by transferences from the past, and even unconscious thoughts and feelings about your spouse in the present, and vice versa. And so there you are in the kitchen one night, your other half returns home and you enquire as to how that psychotherapy session went. And what you hear is that they feel much better now, thank you, a bit guilty yet better nonetheless and ready to move forward into the spirit of love that the therapy has opened them up to. And what occurred during this therapy you ask? "Well", they say, "the climax was truly cathartic. I discovered an intensity of emotion heretofore not experienced". Your curiosity is piqued and ask to hear more. They continue; "the climax was a kind of pseudo-dissociation. I was angry, muscles tense and the therapist asked if I wanted to proceed and let it out. I started imagining like it was really happening stabbing someone repeatedly, tearing at the open wounds. I even stabbed at and up their genitalia. At first I thought it was directed at the therapist but the eye colour didn't match". Then who were you killing and mutilating you ask? "it was you dearest" comes their reply, "It was you".

Case 3; case number 3 is identical to the first, except the mutilated, defiled and tossed around object of a self-centred pragmatic catharsis is a child, for as any parent knows children can be the catalyst of much angst, and so they too are liable to some ole fantasy ultraviolence. Remember what the morality of ISTDP demands, or why would the therapist partake in it i.e. what is not done to the flesh is morally neutral. Now do not flinch. Imagine this scenario of fantasizing in a substantial way (with role play) torturing and killing a child. Get out your claws and knives. Do your worst. Release also the sexualized content of the rage. No one is really hurt. Is this a price worth paying to "feel better"?

So I ask the reader what their moral impressions to these cases are, not as a crime of thought the like of which ought to be instantiated into the criminal code by the legislature, for such an inclusion would be another kind of evil, and contra the conditionally libertarian thrust of this book you are kind enough to read. No what I'm asking the reader to be is the judge in their own court of the heart, of the mind and of the family. If you were the physically unscathed spouse or co-parent of the child what would this disclosure do to the relationship. What would it say about it? And what if you did not even ask that evening in the kitchen. What does it mean that it happened? And what does it mean that psychiatry simply does not care about these questions?

But ISTDP works?

Does it? I'm not convinced on its own terms or that of so called evidence based medicine, and my own philosophical commitment is that it is absurd to attempt quantify and measure the human condition and purpose of life. For those persons who attempt to couple the idea of psychodynamic with psychometric I can have only pity, this being the best I can do. In any case the evidence of effect is a distraction and the value free appeal to evidence is itself a sign of utter moral famine. But let us grant it actually worked, in the sense that the patient comes in with anxiety or emotional instability or OCD or somatised pain or whatever and walks out utterly cured of these symptoms, along with all the attendant dysfunction in their social and occupational now restored. Now the question becomes a more nuanced one, one where I cannot avoid returning to the analogy of the priest and the metaphor of exorcism once more. Faithful or faithless the reader may be. It does not matter. The moral sensibilities are the same. Here we approach the question of just what is therapy of the psyche. Should therapy be a confrontation with one's character and cultivation of the better virtues? Or should it be the atomized consumerist want to feel happy and void of unpleasant thoughts and feelings? Are we to take a leaf from the book of Seneca or of Crowley, the latter of whom would say "Do what thou wilt.

That is the whole of the law". Here we approach the question of what would it profit a man (or woman) if s/he inherits the world and loses their own soul. So you feel better. That's nice. You sleep better at night. That's good too. You cross the street without trepidation and jump into the pool of life without casting the toe in first. Bravo. But has the demon been cast out? No, for the demon is you if you are the patient, not now in a herd of pigs heading for the cliff, and not in the fantasized corpse of your parent or grandparent. The demon, if you will continue indulge me the metaphor, is now an alleged unconscious sated of its desire for murderous discharge, that is until another supposed loved one irks it. It remains within you after the initial miracle of ISTDP sessions and those "top up" sessions usually deemed necessary down the track (so much for an advance on analysis interminable). Insomuch as the unconscious is the stuff of speculation and the conscious is the stuff of undeniable interior reality, the question is who consciously chose the therapy? You. And who consciously assented to the pseudo-exorcism as an exploration of the unconscious as being a killer who ought to have his kill? You. That is to say who consciously constructed themselves as a choice to be what ISTDP says you are, without a shred of evidence? You. Who is making a living statement about what other humans are as depraved killers varnished with a thin coat of conscious neurosis? You. Who fantasy killed someone without any access to fantasy due process for the victim? You. And who propagates this ontology of the person. If you are the therapist? This too is you.

You see the religious metaphor rings louder still. I'm reminded of a warning from an exorcist of old. When the demon is cast out we must be cautious it does not roam about and soon return to the newly cleaned house with a legion of friends, all more cunning, covert and evil than the next. ISTDP is both the pseudo-exorcism and this stronger repossession with a damaged character even more deserving of condemnation, all rolled up in one seamless package. The prince of lies indeed.

A Return to Genealogy of ISTDP

What is curiously lacking in all of the gospels of Davanloo, as far as I can tell, is what Davanloo himself was exposed to in the days before video. You see Davanloo was a trainee of Erich Lindemann, who in turn was no ordinary analyst. Erich Lindemann was the attending psychiatrist following the Cocoanut Grove Nightclub fire the evening of November 28th 1942. Cocoanut Grove was the closest mainland United States came to the flames of war that raged across

Europe at the time, a terrible taste of transatlantic daily life, and just about the only thing that knocked the war off the front page of the newspapers. That November evening the club was packed beyond capacity with almost one thousand souls, flammable faux palms and even more flammable drapery from floor to ceiling and across the top, some of this drapery even concealing potential exits. And with hopelessly inadequate observable exits to cater for literally hundreds of terrified patrons clamouring in flames and smoky darkness for a way out, by the end of the night almost five hundred were scorched or dead from carbon monoxide poisoning. Scores of others were horribly burned and scarred for life. This is trauma with an upper case "T" before the construct of PTSD was developed as it is now, and long before Kubler Ross developed her stages of grief. And what did Lindemann discover? Lindemann discovered deformed and injured club patrons and surviving loved ones in extremis of grief and emotional discharge. Often this was delayed some days after the event. Yes, there were clenched muscles and throats held tight against the release of screams that would come in their due time and season. And yes Lindemann encountered much survivor rage also, with the club, with fate, with God, with oneself, with the ignoble irony of being a wartime casualty of peacetime frivolity, and even anger with the loved ones themselves for being there that night of all nights. The similarities between the somatic reactions and abreactions bear almost identical similarity to Davanloos ISTDP as if the latter were a dissimulated trading on the echo of the screams from Cocoanut Grove down to this day. I can't help but wonder if ISTDP is not Davanloos way of saying that if there is no fire to be found, one might as well pretend there was one anyway and light it from the sparks of the patient's imagination. The crucial point for one with moral sensibilities is that anyone of common decency can empathize with the loved one left behind after the Cocoanut Grove, along with their moment or moments of rage after such a tragedy. Were any to leap on the grave with fists thumping who could say this was anyone other than a suffering human. However much the behaviour might be inappropriate it would at least be meaningful and evoke pity. There but by the grace of God or the luck of the void go I, that their grief is not mine. It is this same empathic hook that drives the fans of the vigilante film genre. We can tolerate gratuitous excesses of cinematic violence to be inflicted on a depraved criminal who deserves it from a victim who alone carries the burden of vengeance upon them. But stabbing little old grannies, even little bad grannies, to feel better. This simply won't do.

A Return to Training; An Eye on the Eye Makes the Whole World Blind

Psychotherapy training has long valued the place of role play and observation of therapy sessions. One can hardly fault the reasoning behind this. Seeing and doing are axiomatic to any form of training. Neither can one fault the inclusion of technologies such as videorecording and access of archival material to the same end of teaching the novice. And neither can a critic so quickly draw a negative conclusion from a therapy that would ask the trainee receive therapy themselves, though universalizing this may be a praxis ad absurdum (or medical students would graduate with many surgical scars, no uterus or appendix and having had every orifice explored). Indeed except for Freud himself (who self-analysed), all apostles and disciples of apostles of psychanalysis were expected to take to the couch, this being an anointing into themselves becoming analysts. However, all of these common sense conventions of training serve to provide cover for what may be another sinister side to ISTDP's immorality and to cloud the therapist from insight into their own trespass against decency. As was clearly stated in Hickeys papers, trainee therapists themselves are filmed not simply in role playing patients, but as being bone fide patients. Imagine if you will that the therapist might at some point hear the whisper of that small voice of conscience suggesting the moral arguments as I have in this chapter. You see it is easy for me to heed the moral voice as I have never allowed myself fall sway to the cult of Davanloo. I have not, in the way of Davanloo, found fantasy blood on my hands. But what if I had been in the chair itself, stabbing and slashing away at my own dearly departed grannies while that little light on the videocamera glowed "recording", a nest of voyeur trainees looking on? What if I had facilitated others in committing the same fantasy ultraviolence, again, and again and again? And what if in the camera I had the symbolic presence of the all seeing eye of Davanloo in each of my sessions as therapist, no matter where I roam around the world? Would I not then be disinclined to wish to see my own moral crimes? This reminds me of that grainy online video of the Ba'ath Party conference when Saddam Hussein gave one half of his ministers pistols and instructed them to coldly shoot the other half of their comrades. Just how can you extricate yourself from a monster after such an immoral buy in, when you have become the monster yourself? The execution initiation into a group is as old as man.

What's the alternative?

Once at a presentation I was asked what the alternative to psychodynamic psychiatry in general and ISTDP in particular might be, as if to imply there must be something and I ought to have it ready on a plate. That's also a question asked when I might be on the verge of convincing another that SSRI's should all be thrown into the trash. But why do they ask this? Who after having squashed a cockroach feels compelled to go grab some less offensive bug to occupy the home? The ready and welcome answer against psychotherapy for many a biologically minded psychiatrist is to recourse to medication. But in the proverbial nine times out of ten, psychotropic medication has non-specific salutatory effects, adverse effects that the psychiatrist assiduously downplays the significance of, and medication fails utterly to engage with the patient's personality and challenges within their life. It is, to borrow that overused metaphor, a "bandaid solution". Regarding psychotropic medication, these are heavy statements made without evidence, yet others have argued the same more comprehensively than I and the reader can explore elsewhere if they wish not to take my word for it. Moreover, as any reader of Huxleys Brave New World is aware, psychotropic medication can dull the mind against the pains which might be the drivers towards necessary change in the patient's own life, in addition to that of the world around them.

And so we cycle back to the question of psychotherapy. Even here the question is not one in which psychiatry ought to assume it's need to live on in some form, for Freud himself paved the way to analysts without medical degrees (arguably so as to give his daughter and heir a royal road to his throne). In answering the question asked of me "what do we do without traditional psychotherapy" I'm impressed with the subtext. The want is not, I suspect, for the patients good, as opposed to a replacement for the viability of the profession as being masters of the mind. And so it will only let go of one rung of the ladder if it has another to grasp hold of. Here we approach what psychiatry as a profession has in common with ISTDP patients, i.e. the willingness to kill off the other providing it (psychiatry) walks away unscathed. But why is the blade never turned towards the self? The dearth of fantasy self-killing in ISTDP is extremely telling. That and the whole superstructure of psychiatric guild and practice speaks of a covert (and often overt) narcissism held even when some less than convincing humility and guilt is placed on display. In the final chapter I'll propose what such an alternative psychotherapy might be, though I warn that you will find it all too laconic. Suffice to say for now that whether we be patient or psychotherapist we ought not to be architects of our own Dorian Grays, where the superficial psyche is restored to the appearances of beauty at the expense of corrupting our true selves. At least Gray had his portrait as a yardstick to his own need for redemption. This chapter is the portrait of psychotherapy.

BIO-ALCHEMY. TABULA RUINA.

'When I use a word,' Humpty Dumpty said in rather a scornful tone, 'it means just what I choose it to mean–neither more nor less.'

'The question is,' said Alice, 'whether you can make words mean different things–that's all.'

'The question is,' said Humpty Dumpty, 'which is to be master–that's all'

(Alice and Humpty) Lewis Carroll

Choosing Sides

It is said by some that the road to hell is paved by good intentions, whilst others (myself included) when receiving an inappropriate gift will sincerely respond "it's the thought that counts". Being strongly disposed to the view good intentions are a good in themselves, this is not to imply that the outcome of an intended good is a good in fact. Perhaps it is better said that the river to heaven can be flowing with the blood of the victims of good intentions. To all people of conscience whose intentions fall short of the goal, it would be a personal hell to have that much blood on one's hands. To wit like a scarred and singed Icarus we fall headlong from heaven to hell, the latter especially inescapable if the outcome is both foreseeable and poor. It is at escaping this fall and certain vicious moral spirals that the current chapter is addressed.

And so the question is this; a child or adolescent presents claiming to be a boy trapped in a girl's body. In one corner there are those psychiatrists and psychologists (and other species of the "helping" professions") who would say that child is, in any essentially meaningful sense it is to be, a boy. And vice versa, a child claiming to be a girl trapped inside a boy's body will be declared to be a girl. What follows are further acts and rituals of (trans)gender affirmation. These include, yet not limited to the following if the child desires it;

a name in keeping with its "realized" gender,

clothing congruent to the gender the child identifies with,

an assertive call to others to relate to the child as being the gender he/she/it/they/ze identify with (bathrooms, personal pronouns, identity documents etcetera). This also includes a prohibition against "conversion therapy", i.e. therapy that in any conceivable way is aimed at challenging the child against it the gender it claims to be.

and at the appropriate times pharmacology to prevent or arrest puberty will begin followed by....

Even more powerful pharmacology to begin to steer the bodies secondary sex characteristics towards the gender the youth identifies with.

The final steps are surgical procedures including replacing as best as the surgeon can a penis with a vagina or vagina with a penis, and mastectomy if the identity trapped inside the female body identifies as being male.

Every single one of these steps is shepherded by adults following an ideology informed and endorsed by the guilds of psychiatry +/- guilds of paediatrics and family medical practitioners.

In the other corner are those who would say such a practice is a kind of mad perversion. We are the sex we are, this being the sex which we were discovered (not assigned) to be the day we were born, or the days to follow in extremely rare ambiguous cases. And if someone's psyche, a child especially, does not align with the biological facts of the world then whatever this psychological state is, it is not insight into an inner gnostic truth of their personhood. This corner would say that the adults a priori ought to know better. This corner would say it is the (trans)gender affirmatives who are practicing the real conversion therapy.

Now psychiatry cannot weasel its way into talk of diagnosis as a construct and its application to the person as evolving and revealing itself over time, forever dissolving the sins of the present as they can be argued never to have been fully formed. This is a most slippery strategy. Real life isn't a romantic journey towards verisimilitude without ever reaching a destination. The destination is the "now" within which each person lives, a case in point being that in lobotomized patients the damage is done. They cannot be cured by looking back through the retrospectoscope and saying we now know better now. Nor can psychiatry say there are various even mutually exclusive ways of formulating a case, all of which are acceptable and true in themselves in some queer truth-fluid pragmatic way. No, the matter must be put more bluntly. The stakes are very high here. In this debate (and I wish a debate was not stifled from the more powerful pro-trans side), one side are protecting the interests of the child and the other are not. One will be the villain of denying the child the ability to be who they truly are inside. This side will simply prolong, if not create, the suffering and stigmatization of being trapped in the wrong body, perhaps inciting the person even onto suicide.

That would be the villainous camp into which I would belong if I am wrong. On the other hand, us trans critics will claim that our opponents are frankly psychological, chemical and physical mutilators of children, placing their politics and deranged ideology before young lives, a Munchausen by proxy on a grand scale. I can only hope posterity looks back upon us through the eye of truth. Whomever the villain is proven to be, whether you or me, he or she, they or zee should be given no quarter. Which side will you be on and what will you have done about it when the dust settles and the lawyers begin soliciting for clients?

A Note on Assigned Gender

All guilds, professional bodies and governments the anglo world over have radically changed the definitions with which to construct our a priori's at a truly revolutionary pace. Once it was a given that the midwife, obstetrician, paediatrician and all the village would look to the genitalia of the baby and discover as a datum of nature, a fact in the world, what the babies sex is. In cases of ambiguous genitalia this knowledge would come soon after with genetic or other testing, at least in the contemporary setting where such investigations are available. Now the language has changed seemingly overnight. Everywhere one reads they will hear the call of the state censor towards the use of the term assigned gender, if not refraining from mention of gender at all until the child is old enough to tell us who they are. That is to say, biological sex is no longer determinative of whether the baby is and will be girl or boy, a woman or man. Instead in the use of the word "assigned", the gender is given as a provisional diagnosis in an otherwise epistemologically ambiguous state. We cannot know if this newborn with a penis and testicles is a boy until it grows old enough to tell us what "it" is when we encourage it to "explore gender identities" or be "creative" with gender. It is to say if it walks like a duck and quacks like a duck we pencil it in as being a duck until later when it can tell us it is a chicken, a chicken duck or not a bird at all, perhaps a fish or a tree.

Amidst the assigning a supposedly uncertain gender, we also have the appropriation of terms heretofore the province of the hard science of organic chemistry. The initiated will know that certain compounds may have certain arrangements of molecular groups attached on the same side (cis) or opposite side (trans) the main chain of carbon, this arrangement to significantly affect certain properties of the molecule as a whole. And so from this we have the inspiration for the terms cis gender (what I will usually refer to as the anatomical male/female) and trans gender (whose gender identification is misaligned with initially assigned biological sex). By use of such a psycho-linguistic tactic the person is rendered thus a conglomeration of functional and structural subunits, the metaphorical equivalent of the contents of a test tube.

"Assigned gender", cis/trans gender, gender queer, gender fluid, pan gender and on it goes. All these neologisms, like Bonnevilles revolutionary la langue universelle de la Republique, a necessary violence against all the old language to usher in the new utopia. In the process of the birth of the new republic of sexuality both women and men, girls and boys, and certainly ladies and gentlemen all face the linguistic guillotine. And the vast majority of conservatives in their cowardice of self censorship march their own language to its death. For shame.

On the Genealogy of Genderosis

So how did this all begin. Our genealogy can begin with Magnus Hirschfeld, the German Jewish (and consequently exiled) gay activist living in the dying days of a libertine Weimar Germany. Hirschfeld mostly fought for gay rights, and is said to have coined the term transvestite as equivalent to cross dressing. It is also said that he was supportive of transgenderism qua living as another gender, though in believing there were essentially an infinite range of sexualities he effectively sought to dissolve all boundaries. Anything goes was essentially his motto and he was more romantic and political than analytical in his approach.

Next there is David Cauldwell, the surgeon with a lifelong interest in sexual anatomy who coined the term transsexual. His autobiography strangely points out that from a young age ""I all but made a fetish of my study of the genital and related organs". This is a strange use of the word "fetish" by one who would presumably know the technical application of it, as a split object that is not in itself the person with whom one has sexual congress, yet necessary for arousal and orgasm nonetheless. Caudwell fell out of favour with his American professors (plural) and was to finally graduate from a medical school in Mexico, before going onto a career in surgery and a self-styled career as a psychiatrist and sexologist. He wrote his essay Psychopathia Transexualis soon after the second world war, and was one of the first to promote the idea that psychological sex can differ from biological sex as a valid alternate state of identity. Because he figured that changing the biological sex to align with the mind was not possible given technology of the day, along with his belief that psychological sex was plastic, his entirely pragmatic conclusion was to pathologise the mental aspect of the disharmony.

Harry Benjamin was one of the first to take up Cauldwells idea of transsexualism and promote it, though also claimed to be the first to coin the term. In truth both were wrong, as a better translation of Hirschfelds work reveals it was he to first use it, or a close equivalent in the concept of 'seelischer Transsexualismus' or "transsexualism of the psyche". Benjamin, a family physician, was born in Berlin and knew Hirschfeld who introduced him, it seems as only an observer, to Berlins homosexual bars and drag shows which were flourishing at the turn of the Twentieth century. It was not until after the second world war that Benjamin collaborated with Kinsey in what both saw was a very rare thing, a young man in his early twenties who wanted to fully and completely transition to become a girl, indeed to be the girl he was inside. Let it not be lost on the trans critic that the young man's mother desperately wanted the same. The fact these two sexologists both saw such an occurrence as exceedingly rare underscores the fact that the current spate of transgenderism in childhood and adolescence is socially constructed and socially amplified. The young man, who was named Barry, was discouraged from transitioning by psychiatrists yet affirmed as female at an early age by his mother, who was as equally obsessed as Barry that he be transitioned. Despite the Barry case being oft written as unique and formative, some sources state that Benjamin had encountered other adult transgender like individuals before and after the extreme case of Barry, amounting to many hundreds over the course of a long career. Yet given Benjamins career was as long as any could be, and given he was a veritable magnet for alternative sexualities, the reader ought not think his many hundreds of cases amount to anything but the tiniest dot on the population landscape. All of Benjamins cases are worth a careful closer look by those who would wish to ignore the question of psychopathology in trans childhood, and think that all trans children are an uncomplicated case of being "x" trapped in the body of a "y", with any psychological problems entirely after the fact as a result of persecution by a transphobic oppressor. His first patient Otto, as an unselected example, was an anxious boy of a widowed mother. Grist for the mill of both the Freudian and Fliessian (for those familiar with Wilhelm Fliess), he slept with his mother until age 14, was used as a dress model from early childhood, and fantasized that his nosebleeds were menstrual bleeds. Otto dressed as, and identified with, being more female than male. Otto, like many others, would also begin a life of closet autogynephilia, which is to say he was sexually aroused by the image and kinaesthetic feel of himself dressing as a female and would masturbate with himself qua female Otto as the object of sexual desire. Needless to say, autogynephilia is not a normal part of the life of the anatomical girl who is to grow and identify with being a woman, even a lesbian woman. Nor is it normal for the anatomical boy who lusts for the female that is not himself to use himself as the object of desire. Others such as the Canadian contemporary psychologist Ray Blanchard have to this day attempted to make clear this potential psycho-developmental road towards transgenderism to be at play in at least a sizable fraction of cases, with the predictable resistance by the trans-activists to silence his voice.

Benjamin was funded in part by the exceedingly wealthy transgender female to male philanthropist Reed Erickson, as was Johns Hopkins University, where John Money worked. (A similar ideological contamination into academia is now being injected by the male to female transgender billionaire Jennifer Pritzker). One may speculate the eccentricities and agenda of Erickson might have been in lockstep with that of Benjamin, or influential and biased in any case. Erickson was also heavily involved in the new age movement. Despite his wealth and his transition which was said to be successful, Erickson died an unhappy woman become man from the consequences of drug addiction in Mexico whilst a fugitive from narcotics police.

Harry Benjamin was to live long and die at the age of 101 years. He is remembered by all as being an unusually caring and empathic physician, though one that any critic of the transgender movement would say was nonetheless horribly misguided in the scope of his care and as a foundation stone to the new trans hysteria. In his twilight years an association carrying his name was founded, later to be rebranded WPATH, the World Professional Association for Transgender Health.

Next we have John Money, the New Zealand born Harvard educated psychologist who became famous (and later infamous) for the idea that from the perspective of sexual identity children are born tabula rasa. That is to say the hypothesis of which he was convinced was that a child could become either woman or man as a result of rearing and regardless of the biological starting point. Of Moneys many contributions there are two which bear mention here. The first was that it was Money who first entangled the word gender into human sexuality. Before Money there was simply sex, and sex was binary in the human world and divided on male and female lines into girls and boys, women and men, ladies and gentlemen. Gender, on the other hand, was something used in the world of language and linguistics and alien to human life. For example, in Spain and Italy one lives in a "casa" (female) and in Germany "Haus" (neutral).

In France "la maison" is female. In Russian the "dom" (transliterated from the Cyrillic) is male. It appears the further into the east one travels the greater the degree to which the place in which one resides transitions gender. In English of course an inanimate object such as a house is almost always gender neutral, though it is common to think of particular objects or classes of animal in terms of gender. One may hear for example of a ship as "setting sail on her maiden voyage". In Spanish a bridge "Puente" is male whilst a German bridge "brucke" is female. Though I heard once that German literature tends to quasi anthropomorphize and describe a bridge in female terms (e.g. as gracefully extended) and Spanish literature often describes a bridge in terms of masculine strength to carry, no one seriously considers either a bridge or a house as a sexual or asexual being. The beauty of a language used over centuries is that it is what it is without category errors or people taking leave of reality. Nonetheless John Money succeeded in changing the psycholinguistic landscape by taking gender out of the languages and driving it into human psychology (and ontology) as a complicating variable, such that conceptually someone could be the female gender despite by all other accounts being a genetic and anatomically sexual male. Moneys victory was literally an enormous re-engineering of language over reality, this adjusting on a grand scale what people believe is the concrete nature of the world. Now decades after Money, to those readers who might reflexively take for granted that gender "is a thing" and is separate to biological sex, we ought to take a pause that previous centuries would have been thought you insane. And with future adventures in engineering language to the end of inverting reality, future generations might see a human in other radically alien ways, alien even to what a human ipso facto is. The whole affair is akin to a magic where incantations (mere words) can invoke a perceived something out of nothing, with tangible effects in the world.

Moneys other infamous place in history was the testing out of his tabula rasa hypothesis on vulnerable children. All babies were fair game, including those babies who were clearly male and suffering only from a delay of the testicles descending from the abdomen into the scrotal sack. The case that drove Money into posthumous notoriety was that of David Reimer, though not nearly as much into the infamy Money deserved. For an experimental psychologist such as Money, David was the perfect subject. He was an identical twin with a brother raised in the same home. And David (born under another name), required a non-elective circumcision as a baby, presumably for phimosis. Tragically there were complications from the surgeon using a cautery device that was too powerful in a hand that went too far, and during the procedure David's penis was burned into a state of complete ablation. What followed was David being socially and surgically (later hormonally) transitioned from infancy to become a girl, and he would be none the wiser until his adolescence. But try as he might, and despite the herculean efforts of the adults around him, he never thought himself to be a girl. Eventually he was told he had in fact been born male, whereupon he immediately sought to transition back to his natal sex. It was then he adopted the name David, an allusion to seeing his persona as battling the Goliath forces of John Money and the cruel fate of the world. David's surgeons and endocrinologists tried their best to realign David's body back to his natal sex and he attempted live a normal life as a normal man in the years to pass. Unfortunately, too much damage had already been done, much yet admittedly not all of this damage can be attributed to his role in Moneys experiment. He was always troubled by his sexual inadequacy and had irreparable psychological scars from being forced into the role of a girl for his formative years. His brother Brian had later suicided age 37 years. With trust in the world seriously eroded, he had a troubled relationship with his birth family and also with the woman he had married, and he had been conned out of a substantial amount of savings, this to be another blow by another Goliath which whilst not being Money, was an object to which he was sensitized after having been a victim of an experiment. Someone with more favourable formative experiences might have weathered the financial storm better, the death of the brother and challenges of adulthood. David himself chose suicide two years after his twin. From the part of Reimer's childhood when the tide turned against Moneys hypothesis, Money assiduously and deliberately ignored the follow up and reporting the failure of his experiment of the boy who was turned a girl, resulting in at least two generations of psychologists and psychiatrists educated to believe Moneys tabula rasa hypothesis had been proven. In reality the exact opposite was the case.

It is arguably from Money and his ilk that we have inspired the gender bread person (now obsolete as a genderbread "person" was considered to appear too masculine and was historically linked to the gingerbread man story) and now the gender unicorn (which a trans critic would reasonably see as a path towards transhumanism). In their gender creativity and exploration, the child is now asked to look at the gender unicorn and other pictographs, and further expected to believe that a) biological sex re anatomical sex, b) perceived gender, c) gender expression (style of dress and toy preference) and d) sexual appetite (who you are attracted to) are each and all completely independent mix and match variables.

This is not and has never been true. That "Cis hetero" is the overwhelming norm is a biological fact.

Next we have Alfred Kinsey, the PhD entomologist and expert on wasps, who as a university academic was asked to teach a course on human sexuality, this being a formative step in a career making him a household name as the world's most famous sexologist of his day, and ours also. Kinsey's interest in human sexuality was as broad as his own personal sexual paraphilic proclivities and the huge variance of sexual escapades in the animal kingdom with which he was acquainted. The belief and promotion of the idea a boy/girl could be trapped in a girl's/boy's body was a minor part of his career and trivial compared to a knowledge that some animals could be different sexes at different stages of the life cycle or different sexes at the same time. This is to say nothing of the fact that animals are not fettered by incest and other taboos. To the libertine Darwinist all that is not red and tooth and claw is to be permitted and man can be whatever the animal is, for man is an animal like any other. Kinsey is only of oblique interest to us here in the question of trans children, in the sense that he was a leading light in an anti-conservative tide in middle twentieth century America and symbiotically connected to the above mentioned early transactivists in breaking any and all taboos. Kinseys name is steeped in controversy. There is, for example the infamous tables 30-34 of his text the "Sexual Behaviour in The Human Male". In table 34 for example, the timing from manual and oral arousal to orgasm (or rather what was taken to be orgasm though it might have been tortured affect) of samples of males of various ages down to infancy are precisely quantified. Were these results concocted? After all, Kinsey was a methodologists nightmare, passing off data on the sexual behaviour of prisoners, perverts and prostitutes as if they were representative of the population norm. Was Kinsey merely the recipient of data about which he did not check the veracity? Or was Kinsey himself a participant in the paedophilia, even just as an observer? Were the paedophile "researchers" who provided the data one or many? And in the sense in which the soliciting for, and reporting of, this "data" was at least partially prospective, did Kinsey protect the anonymity of monsters before and after the fact of the paedophilic crimes? Any one of the possibilities leads to a damning indictment. In any case, one thing is clear. Kinsey endorsed paedophilia both in the tabulated substance of the text and other direct quotes he had made. To quote one example, this from the companion volume "Sexual Behaviour in the Human Female", he states

"The adult contacts are a source of pleasure to some children and sometimes may arouse the child erotically and bring it to orgasm. It is difficult to understand why a child – except for its cultural conditioning should be disturbed at having its genitalia touched."

There are many Kinsey fanatics out there who simply cannot bring themselves to see that there was more to the man than being a methodologist of the poorest scientific quality.

The subject of paedophilia is neither a digression nor to be seen as a censorious accusation against the morality of the trans movement. Rather the question is more analytical than that. To my knowledge Kinsey did not ask himself or us an horrific question (I could not stomach reading the whole corpus of his work, bad data being a waste of time). Yet I smell in Kinsey and the trans children movement of today the formation of a question that to be fair almost all have not asked except in subtext, with implications that will surely emerge at some point. The trans movement so far as children are concerned would have us believe that a child can know that it is a boy/girl trapped in a girl's/boy's body. Fair enough we might say. After all, non-trans children do come to acquire a stable sense of what it is to be a boy or girl at a fairly young age, though we must be cautious not to over-interpret a concrete statement by a young child without further exploration and elaboration. A four year old natal boy might say he is a boy yesterday, today and tomorrow. Yet that same four year old boy might believe that placing him in a dress makes him a girl. It might not be until age 7 or 8 that the child might really understand what they are as biological boys or girls, though certainly not to the degree of sophistication as that of seen through adult eyes. In any case, we might ask what it is for the anatomical boy to say he is really a girl, or vice versa. Putting aside for the moment accepting the notion of radical gender fluidity, let us imagine each human being can be only one sex/gender, and this be binary, even if it is different to that "assigned" at birth. An anatomical boy is seen to have meaning qua boy as there is an implied continuance between what he is now and what he will be an adult man. This is an anatomical (and scientific) given and ought not be considered a controversial statement. We would see that recognizing (not assigning) the child's sexual identity at or soon after birth implicitly contains within it the telos of the boy as a man to be. And insomuch as 99.9 recurring percent of the time this is borne out to be true, under a classical or Bayesian probability calculus we trans critics have the numbers well and truly on our side. We do not need to ask a child its concept of adult man/woman and need not factor this into any decision making process. Trans critical people such as myself would simply let the girl become the woman, the boy become the man.

Yet the promotor of trans children needs ask themselves this question. In order for a seed to know it is a tree of a different kind, the seed needs see further than the beingness of the seed that it is. It needs to know what it is to be a tree of both the kind it thinks it is not, and more importantly it would need to know the beingness of the mature tree it thinks it is.

Yet can the child see into themselves what adulthood is so as to make the informed choice to be the opposite sex? Even if we are to accept, as I don't, that the anatomical boy can know that "he" really is a girl inside, that "he" really is a "she", this is necessarily attached to what the telos of the girl, i.e. what the girl will be in becoming a woman. The boy cannot give informed consent to transition to be the girl the child claims to be unless this same child knows what womanhood is and what it is to be a woman qua an adult. This is in turn complicated as a woman qua adult is in all likelihood a sexual being. What I am saying is that in order for the boy to know he is a girl he needs to know he will be a woman, and this surely is to know what woman is in her variables, including looking at sexual behaviour through adult female eyes. I cannot see how it is possible for the trans movement to grant children the sophisticated knowledge of selfhood of sexual identity and the selfhood of the adult, without dragging into childhood also the implication that sexual behaviour can similarly be consented between child and child and between child and adult. And so just as I predicted the move to legalize gay marriage (rightly or wrongly) would rapidly be followed by an explosion of the adult trans movement, I predicted also the adult trans movement would be rapidly followed by an explosion of the childrens trans movement. The final step, more difficult though inch wise to progress nonetheless, will be the trans movement in children as a bridge towards the greater sexualisation of children, without anyone really knowing why. This is already happening with so called mainstream media completely oblivious to the obvious when clearly sexualized drag or trans children are paraded on streets with giant phalluses, or dancing in strip bars with the adults cheering on their celebration of diversity.

WPATH
WPATH (World Professional Association for Transgender Health)
(See also the section to follow on guild and other professional body guidelines.)

WPATH was previously named after Harry Benjamin and borne from a transactivist movement, this being the primary criteria for membership, with academia and appeal to science attached and detached where this might be suasive, and members coming to occupy the hierarchy of a cause already decided. It is fair to say that almost all the above mentioned US based luminaries of the twentieth century have been heavily influential in WPATHS thought and practice. In fact, many current members are no more than three degrees of separation from having been academic apprentices of these founding fathers of transgenderism, and so the mission and ordination of the fathers could be said to live on in WPATH, if not become more extreme. And we can see in the biographies and published work of WPATH chairs, that this ostensive health organization sees political activism as part of its heavy artillery towards social change. On the website circa late 2019 (this may later be edited) we have for example the child and adolescent committee being headed by one who WPATH introduces as "Laura Edwards-Leeper, MD", though Leeper is actually a PhD psychologist and not a physician (not that this matters except as a digression to trivia and perhaps a clue that WPATH do not care about the details, as letters at the end of one's name are just something to market the argument from authority). Dr Edwards Leeper is convinced of the view that watchful waiting to see what the child will think is its gender when it grows to maturity is not neutral and indeed harmful, contributing to suicide. Ergo the gender affirming approach as young as possible is the way to go. And we have WPATH's Sam Winter, PhD; an academic psychologist at Western Australia's Curtin University. His bio on the Curtin university website makes clear the activist element of the trans question in his own area of interest, and the degree to which this has become a metric of virtue for a university to be aligned with the trans cause

"We are looking forward to building up research student numbers in sexology, and I am especially looking forward to supervising research students in gender diversity, transgender and transsexual health and rights, as well as in other areas of sexual and gender development, diversity, education, health and rights. In 2015 Curtin was ranked the top university in Australia for LGBTI equality in the annual national 'Pride in Diversity' awards. This was the third consecutive year! And it was judged third best employer nationally. So if you want to research sexual and gender diversity this is a great place to do it."

Third and last from this unselected sample of the first three names, we have Dianne Berg, PhD, a University of Minnesota psychologist, also a strong advocate of the gender affirmative approach, having authored the apt named "Gender

Affirmative Lifespan Approach", a trademarked education program which in the fact of it being trademarked is also a commercial product. Her interests cut across transgenderism in all ages, including those described as "gender creative children". Is sexual identity a play thing with no more gravitas than finger painting and Lego?

Guild Current Guidelines

World Professional Association for Transgender Health (WPATH) Guidelines.

Much can be achieved by use of, and implied authority in, an acronym. This along with strategic positioning have resulted in WPATH cited the world over as the experts. In many ways, the anglo speaking guidelines in the guilds of paediatrics and psychiatry are rebranded endorsements of WPATH, though we should not allow this be an excuse for these guilds to disavow in future what seismic shifts in the social fabric that they have wrought and to which they were fully complicate. WPATH's official guidelines might appear to represent the organization as prima facie guarded about affirming transgenderism in children and adolescents. The guidelines for example acknowledge the transition rates are low (i.e. trans children tend not to become trans adults if gently managed without affirmation), and in the section on early childhood WPATH does acknowledge this area is fraught with uncertainty. Nonetheless they invite parents thus

"parents may want to present this role change as an exploration of living in another gender role rather than an irreversible situation" and also state that practitioners should be supportive in "exploring gender identity" and prior to puberty refer the adolescent "for additional physical interventions (such as puberty-suppressing hormones)".

The call is also to advocate and educate family, schools etcetera in transgender affirmation. In the section "Psychological and Social Interventions for Children and Adolescents" it is stated "Psychotherapy should focus on reducing a child's or adolescent's distress related to the gender dysphoria and on ameliorating any other psychosocial difficulties". That is to say the psychotherapeutic approach should not be affirming the natal sex. The guidelines continue (I've included their references within the quote)

"Treatment aimed at trying to change a person's gender identity and expression to become more congruent with sex assigned at birth has been attempted in the past without success (Gelder & Marks, 1969; Greenson, 1964), particularly in the long term (Cohen-Kettenis & Kuiper, 1984; Pauly, 1965). Such treatment is no longer considered ethical." and

"Mental health professionals should not impose a binary view of gender. They should give ample room for clients to explore different options for gender expression. Hormonal or surgical interventions are appropriate for some adolescents, but not for others." There is the call to support social transition "For example, a client might attend school while undergoing social transition only partly (e.g., by wearing clothing and having a hairstyle that reflects gender identity) or completely (e.g., by also using a name and pronouns congruent with gender identity)."

To the extent that the guidelines make mention of low transition rates (i.e. trans children tending to not to become trans adults), this contribution can be credited to Dr Kenneth Zucker (see Zuckergate, vide infra). The reader will note that the current WPATH guidelines were issued 2012 and long overdue a revision. In this rapidly evolving unveiling of ideology, 2012 is ancient history. The practice and ideology of the WPATH has now become even more extreme and any tiny sliver of conservatism or caution that might be found in the WPATH of old is long gone. Truth be known it was never there to begin with. Kenneth Zucker is now anathema and the train is going all the way affirmation and transition at increasingly younger ages.

As an example of change, more recently in November 15, 2017 WPATH issues the blanket statement, further breaking the binary into a multiplicity of genders held by otherwise undifferentiated individuals, and age to no longer matter.

"WPATH advocates that appropriate gender recognition should be available to transgender youth, including those who are under the age of majority, as well as to individuals who are incarcerated or institutionalized. WPATH recognizes that there is a spectrum of gender identities, and that choices of identity limited to Male or Female may be inadequate to reflect all gender identities. An option of X, NB (non-binary), or Other (as examples) should be available for individuals who so choose."Note the word "choose".

And with the proliferation of the lucrative trans industry and gender clinics (from 1 to several dozen in this century alone in the United States), WPATH refers to other influencers such as genderspectrum.org which assert

"the concept of insistence, consistence and persistence to help determine if a child is truly gender-expansive or transgender." and

"If your child has identified as the opposite gender since early childhood, it is unlikely they will change their mind. Most people have some sense of their Gender identity between the ages of two and four years old. For most, this awareness remains stable over time. For example, a 12 year old child who was assigned a male gender at birth, but has consistently asserted "I am a girl" since the age of three, will most likely remain transgender throughout life."

A similar philosophy is to be found at genderdiversity.org and imatyfa.org (i.e. trans youth family allies), the latter of which promotes

"Anyone who will enthusiastically nurture, support, respect and validate a trans, gender variant or gender questioning youth's inherent right to self-identify and self-express, regardless of their age or where on the gender continuum that expression may fall, or more importantly, may lead."

It ought not be lost on the reader that all these organizations, like the guilds are 501(c)(3) non-profit organization, and as such are exempt from tax, an industry in collusion with the state.

The American Psychiatric Association or APA (USA)

The American Psychiatric Association is the professional guild of psychiatrists in the United States. In a beautifully pragmatic move of plausible deniability, the APA publish material they officially deny is official APA policy, yet nonetheless use the APA platform to vigorously promote transgender affirmation by WPATH as the body that they endorse to be the experts. To this end they even sell a trans affirmative online course. The APA additionally cites their own publication, the DSM 5, and the inclusion of gender dysphoria of childhood as a valid diagnosis in itself and a path in childhood towards transgender affirmation and transition. If the APA acknowledges any controversy, it is that inclusion of transgender persons in DSM 5, albeit only if dysphoric (i.e. emotionally distraught), increases the probability that transgenderism per se will be stigmatized by the trans-critics whom they demonize.

"The Gender Dysphoria diagnosis functions as a double-edged sword. It provides an avenue for treatment, making medical and surgical options available to TGNC (trans gender non conforming) people. However, it also has the potential to stigmatize TGNC people by categorizing them as mentally ill."

This is a strange statement, as dysphoria is by their own conceptual schemata a mental state which is not one of wellness (i.e. it is illness), and so the term is not a stigma but a statement of an unpleasant fact. To reify the diagnostic construct is, one could argue, the makings of a stigma. Yet even this does not make sense as it is seen as secondary to the persecution from others, even if indirectly. It is no more stigmatizing than the diagnosis of "adjustment disorder" which might apply to anyone having difficulty coping with very hard times that are not of their making. In any case, this is simply an analogue of whatever echoes of concern are leftover from the time pre DSM III (i.e. pre 1980) when homosexuality was officially removed as a mental illness, and before the time when psychiatry in its pragmatism decided take it off the table (and rightly take it off the table they did). Now the pendulum has swung in the opposite direction. The inclusion of gender dysphoria in the DSM is a mixture of reluctance, ambivalence, opportunism and power politics. Transgender dysphoria in the DSM is a means to retain political power and codify the issue in a way that validates insurance claims and intellectual authority over the subject where psychiatry still has a seat at the table. They want to say that trans is normal and they have the authority in declaring it so, and assist the patient realize its normality in the face of a hostile surround, i.e. the cure of the dysphoria. But of transgenderism itself being a sane and valid state of being, the APA are fully sold on the notion that a woman can be trapped inside the body of a man, and a man can be trapped inside the body of a woman. They will say that the psychological malady is only in those who do not accept this as fact. Note that the DSM 5 was released in 2013, and like the current WPATH guidelines is also ancient history in the evolution of the rhetoric.

A 2017 special issue in the journal Psychiatric Clinics of North America is an example of how quickly a revolution can move, the editorial being an explicitly political call to activism. The editorial calls for

"a trans-affirmative treatment paradigm that celebrates the broad spectrum of gender identities and the range of treatment options and outcomes. The editors talk of being "cis gender" and having "gender privilege and unearned advantages", and later state they "recognize that we have gendered identities implicated in and affected by gender-based oppression"

Such declarations of oppression are pregnant in implication with a call to force the non-believer to heel.

The UK. (Royal College of Psychiatrists)

The psychiatric guild of the UK issued a position statement March 2018. This also affirms the concept of assigned gender, and invoke the only other alternative diagnostic nosology to that of the DSM 5, i.e. at the time the World Health Organizations International Classification of Diseases version 10 or ICD 10 (though the reader will note both DSM and ICD are likely become integrated into a globalist nosology in the coming years, the now updated 2019 ICD 11 being a bridge towards this). The RCPsych goes on to say

'Gender identity disorder' is the umbrella term used in the 10th edition of the International Classification of Diseases (ICD; WHO, 1992) although it is expected that the 11th edition will adopt the new term "gender incongruence". The term 'conversion therapy' has also been used to describe treatments for transgender people that aim to suppress or divert their gender identity – i.e. to make them cisgender – that is exclusively identified with the sex assigned to them at birth. Conversion therapies may draw from treatment principles established for other purposes, for example psychoanalytic or behaviour therapy. They may include barriers to gender-affirming medical and psychological treatments. There is no scientific support for use of treatments in such a way and such applications are widely regarded as unacceptable."

In other words, there is to be no attempt whatsoever to challenge the adult transgender person that they may not be as they claim they are. Of the trans child or adolescent RCPsych begins by being notionally more reserved and cautious in stating

"Long-term follow-up studies of young transgender people are needed." And

"....the College believes that a watch and wait policy, which does not place any pressure on children to live or behave in accordance with their sex assigned at birth or to move rapidly to gender transition, may be an appropriate course of action when young people first present."

Yet read again that amidst the watchful waiting any attempt for parents to be, well, paternalistic and align the trans affirming child with their natal (i.e. biological sex) is professionally discouraged and indeed watchful waiting is redefined as anything but watchful waiting. Rather it is an affirmation to social transitioning. Professionals are encouraged to advocate thus

"These include tackling bullying, effective safeguarding, parental concerns, and practical considerations (such as appropriate language, use of toilets and changing rooms, and uniforms)."

And the RCPsych cites WPATH and US guilds for legitimacy with the comment

"World Professional Association for Transgender Health (WPATH), the American Academy of Child & Adolescent Psychiatry, and the American Psychological Association, that psychological treatments to suppress or 'revert' gender-diverse behaviours are unscientific and unethical."

Along with all this is use of UK legislation in a rather sinister threat against those who would oppose trans affirmation in adults and children.

"…use of conversion therapy with transgender and gender diverse (or lesbian, gay or bisexual) people may be an act of discrimination under the Equality Act (2010)."

Australia, New Zealand and Oceania (including the Royal Australian and New Zealand Collage of Psychiatrists)

In 2018, The Medical Journal of Australia published the position statement "Australian standards of care and treatment guidelines for transgender and gender diverse children and adolescents" in which it is claimed that 1.2% of Australian children are transgender, citing a New Zealand paper in which a further 2.5% of children are said to be unsure of their gender (the implication being that even they might not be their natal sex). Given that these 2.5% of children will be invited to explore their gender ambivalence, this essentially creates a picture unprecedented in history, and surely raising red flags to any who might suspect transgenderism is the result of social contagion and suggestion as opposed to the discovery of a real state of nature heretofore underdiagnosed. It essentially creates a prevalence of 1.2-3.7% where every classroom has a gender insecure or incongruent child, thus establishing a beachhead from which can be launched further erosions into the other children's perception of sexual identity as binary and in accord with biology, and undermine all parental attempts to insulate themselves from exposure to the ideology. Just as it only takes one peanut allergic child to alter the menu of all (and fair enough), only one supposedly trans-child forces an ideology upon each and every child, including yours!

In the MJA position statement, it is further implied that the distress experienced by these children can only be due to persecution by others, not some underlying psychoneurosis driving both the gender dysphoria and general distress as an alternative explanation.

This statement is endorsed by the Australian and New Zealand Professional Association for Transgender Health, the Oceanic branch of, you guessed it,… WPATH. Essentially the approach is child driven. If the child says they are a different gender to their biological/natal sex, this is not up for debate by the adults in the room. This is to be affirmed and the child is to be placed on the path to transition as the child sees fit. There is not the slightest suggestion that the pro trans beliefs of the adults around the child might influence what the child will desire as the driver of their own transition, be it slow or fast, partial or complete. Those family members and professionals who do not support affirmation and transition are seen as requiring education, the implication being that failure to support affirmation reflects professional incapacity or personal bigotry. The positon statement also perpetuates the myth that pubertal suppression is completely reversible and harmless.

The Royal Australian and New Zealand College of Psychiatrists issued a positon statement in March 2019 in which the difference between homosexuality and trans-sexuality is acknowledged through a prohibition of efforts to change sexual orientation (qua homosexuality). And fair enough for history is littered with failed, immoral and sometimes painful attempts to attempt to convert gay to straight. However, the final opaque paragraphs seem to conflate the two into "alternative sexualities" and recommend acceptance, support, and identity exploration of all alternative sexualities and a prohibition against "sexual orientation change efforts of any kind". Elsewhere in position statement 83 issued Sept 2019 the RANZCP uncritically cites the NZ study mentioned above, and conflates alternative sexualities (i.e. LGBTQ+) into one group, the grouping having no sense except in political terms as a coalition in opposition to so called cis gender heterosexuality. What is the evidence for equivalence between a unfounded suspicion of the validity of adult homosexuality and incursions against the liberty of the same, and reasoned horror against the child who doubts its own natal sex? Absolutely none. This position statement is explicitly trans-affirmative for children.

A Critique on The Transitioning Process

Social transitioning

The trans activists would have us transition a child from as young as the child can communicate gender incongruence, though most will add the qualification that the claim to be a different gender to the natal sex must be "persistent, consistent and insistent". These three catch phrase criteria are seen as evidence in favour of the capacity of the child to know who they really are, and a signal to the activist masquerading as health practitioner to begin the transition process. As noted at the opening to the chapter, transition is often elaborated to be whatever the child wishes itself to be, with themselves and their own satisfaction to be the driver to change. This change might include a change in name to that which is traditionally associated with the opposite assigned sex, a change in the type or style of dress and all the ingredients of which the reader would imagine the appearance of things to be when he becomes she, and she becomes he. The critical observation to make clear here is that social transitioning is just that, social. As such it depends upon the surrounding social actors to either agree with being part of the transaction of transition, or to be forced and coerced to play their part. This is both deeply illiberal and deeply anticonservative. Should the trans advocate face opposition they will tell those that oppose, be it family, teacher or whomever, that opposing the child will lead to greater degrees of gender dysphoria and probably death given the high rate of attempted suicide. Ideally the opposing actor might, in their want to be compassionate and avoid being a harm to the child or adolescent (or adult), consider themselves re-educated and liberated from their previously held bigotry. They will then change their tune and join with the party in the march towards the trans-inclusive utopia. But what if the opposing actor continues on the wayward path, either in the life of the child or that of the adult, either in the life of the individual at hand or on the political stage? It usually does not come to that. Usually fear of group exclusion and self-censorship is sufficient to effect the social change in the cowardly many by the strident cries of the few who have the political power. Social ostracism until the transphobe corrects themselves is a minimum criterion, such that the child is shielded from perceived bigotry. Yet if opposition persists, the transactivists will then bare their teeth with threats of loss of employment and the like if there be any hint to fail to comply with the trans-affirmative approach. Any effort to cultivate within the mind of the child an acceptance of their biological/natal/anatomical sex will be considered "transphobia", to be an example of "conversion therapy" and as such unprofessional, unethical and immoral. It cannot be overstated that in small ways or large, directly or in our political assent, all of us are being compelled to partake in social transitioning of the trans child (and adult). Only certain privileged individuals have the luxury to oppose it if they dare, in virtue of being successfully and independently funded and employed, or protected by a herd immunity such as the Muslim faithful enjoy. But what of the trans-critical teacher, the doctor or nurse, the psychologist or psychiatrist? If one of these is confronted with, for example, the natal boy who insists he is a girl what are they to do? If they discover, once again as one example of many, that this boy has been bullied by his father and other boys and found solace in the company of girls, or if he likes what natal girls usually likes, the conservative practitioner might conclude that he is the boy that he is, with his "gender dysphoria" informed by adverse events in the world in over-identifying with being female. They might then like to steer him towards his natal gender by affirming him to be a boy, by encouraging him to join a less bullish boy peer group. They will likely then in their gentle insistence that his identity conform with the biological reality of the world and the traditional convention of the village be consequently labelled a transphobe and accused of practicing conversion therapy. In the eyes of the transactivist this approach is bundled into the same nefarious basket and seen as no different to those of the mid twentieth century who would imprison the adult male homosexual, chemically castrate him and deliver painful electric shocks to the genitals were he to be aroused by a male image. For the transactivist, any manoeuvre no matter how meek and mild to steer the child towards the natal gender is forbidden upon pain of career death. And the reader ought to make no mistake. Many a career has died and will die by their hand.

Puberty blockade

Puberty can be a psycho-developmentally challenging affair at the best of times, though seen to be a psychological trauma of the highest order in the trans preadolescent. And so it must be stopped at all costs. Another more positive way to frame puberty is as being formative to character, and the transactivists projecting outwards a terror of a confrontation with the rites of passage into maturity, similar to that of some anorexic girls who wish to terminally forestall womanhood by starving themselves into preadolescence. More on puberty as character development anon. To begin, let us look medically at the treatment itself, and its risks. Puberty suppression usually relies upon use of a medication that actually stimulates the release of the pituitary hormones that in turn drive sex hormone production and puberty, though in the consistency of the stimulation the medication quickly exhausts the physiology into a state of inaction and puberty comes to a grinding halt before it begins, that is if it were allowed to occur. Some trans gender clinics have been known to commence puberty blockage in natal girls as young as 8 years old, for well-nourished western world children tend to begin puberty relatively earlier, this being out of pace with their psychological maturation. On suppressing the production and release of what the laity might ironically call male and female hormones, the role of these medications has traditionally been either to starve cancers that normally feed on these sex steroids, or they are used in the case of the girl (or sometimes boy) with precocious puberty, i.e. pathologically early puberty. The goal is to simply slow down the course of nature and actually facilitate a normal puberty, with the drugs removed within the range of age at which puberty normally begins. Treating precocious puberty by temporarily suspending puberty actually improves upon the final height of the child, whose growth would be stunted without puberty suppression. The rate of complications is consequently low and harmonious with the developmental trajectory of the cohort of the patient's peers, and is an attempt to align with what community has made a community standard, and more importantly the standard of nature also. Yet even here there are some girls whose menarche (first period) is delayed up to a couple years after drug removal and the endeavour of suppression of a precocious puberty is only to be supervised by those who are specialist paediatric endocrinologists. These are not benign drugs.

Slowing puberty in the precocious female is not at all equivalent to that of arresting it in the normal natal female, and one cannot extrapolate the results in the former to that of the latter, though trans activists often do. Neither is it true to say that developmental windows can be suspended indefinitely. Needless to say there is no long term data on the effects of puberty suppression in the trans child, and any differences found would be decades down the track and conveniently confounded by any other endocrine and surgical excursions made thereafter. And it is simply not possible to conduct the crossover experiment where the same child can be compared as having had puberty suppression that is subsequently released, versus never having had puberty supressed at all. The simple fact is that if a child has a few years of puberty suppression and then the child changes their mind, neither they nor their parents can ever know if they come to attain to height, shape and bone mass they might have otherwise achieved. Have they merely suspended the future or altered it?

Two arguments are employed in favour of puberty suppression, and neither are coherent with each other on closer inspection. The first argument is that the preadolescent needs time to "explore" and mature so as to make the decision if to continue transitioning, and that puberty suppression is a harmless and reversible intermission between the first act of life, and what to do next. As we have seen above, the claim that it is a harmless interruption is factually wrong and medically minded transactivists know it is, yet nothing further will be stated here save to call them out on their myopia at best, or mendacity at worst. The second pro transition argument is that secondary sex characteristics are deleterious to the final outcome the transactivist seeks, both aesthetically and psychologically. For the boy to become a woman he ought not pass through a nasty stage of looking like a man, as Adams apples and male chins, wide shoulders and narrow hips are phenotypes difficult or impossible to surgically correct for.

The matter is this; what is the value of more time to explore and decide? And from this, what is the truth that the transactivists believe in their own argument? We are expected to believe, as they allegedly do, that the prepubescent child who is consistent, insistent and persistent already knows who they are. Granted a child may change its mind and children often do. This expanded duration of self reflection would render the transactivist vulnerable to the claim that most transchildren are passing through a phase.

And so the second argument need be ready at hand, i.e. the avoidance of developing incongruent secondary sex characteristics. And yet we cannot escape the first argument. Granted it is not difficult to find sympathy with the individual who finds themselves looking well and truly like the sex with which they do not identify. And sure enough no one would advocate we be exposed to everything in life before we adjudicate that it is not for us (such as leaping off tall buildings). Yet we must ask ourselves if watching for the terrifying first signs of puberty in order to suppress it is at least partially an iatrogenic cultivated fear of something that ought not be feared. We must also ask ourselves how the child can explore its natal sex so as to reject it if not exposed to the very experience which largely defines the target of exploration and the beingness of its natal sex, and this exploration necessarily requires going deep into the territory of puberty. What if the bullied little boy who thinks he is a girl finds himself in a few years growing taller and more powerful, and likes the feel of himself in his own male body. And he might then like those sideways glances and little flirtations he receives from those who are of the opposite, or the same, natal sex who like the look of his body. Despite the oft present trepidations and clumsiness of youth and whether he be chaste or not, he might like the idea of the what this body can do and be in doing and being with theirs. And the same would apply to the natal female. Like many a girl she might hate the growth of breasts and the onset of monthly cycles. Yet she too might come to feel puberty is worth it when the world starts seeing her as a young woman and she feels this is something that is perfectly fine to be. No one can know themselves without a certain quanta of confrontation with themselves and with life. Puberty suppression is not an exploration of sexual identity. It is an insulation against it.

Puberty suppression is not simply the suppression of outward sexual characteristics and with it the dialogue between mind, body and world. There is evidence to suggest that gender identity development, far from being a one step process complete in utero (from a neuroscientific point of view), has the potential for a second minor phase in adolescence. In example of such evidence lay in the outcomes for XY boys with a deficiency in the enzyme responsible for producing testosterone in utero, along with other hormones down the biochemical chain. These babies are born with ambiguous or female like external genitalia and brains that might similarly be under virilised (under masculinized). Yet regardless what gender they are reared, they tend to become adults identifying as being male. One hypothesis to account for this is that the brain in utero is exquisitely sensitive to what androgens are present and only a little will do. Another, and perhaps the most parsimonious, hypothesis for such an outcome is that they are additionally virilised by testosterone in adolescence that can be synthesized by other pathways. Once again, depriving a child of puberty deprives them of the neurodevelopmental experience that could be considered natures "exploration of gender".

The trans lobby appear to miss the other point that suppression of puberty for purpose of exploration puts a pause on the other non-sexual aspects of development keeping trajectories with age matched peers. Imagine yourself remaining outwardly a child for an extra few years as your friends leap forward in the beginnings of their man/womanhood. The trans-activist only appears to miss these and other crucial points as they have decided from the outset that transition will and ought to happen.

It is these and other dirty little facts (see Zuckergate below) that make for a trans-ideology that is desperate to halt puberty as soon as possible. The strategy is to make the child blind before they might see.

Cross sex hormones

If puberty suppression persists without exposing the body to sex hormones, growth suppression will sooner or later certainly occur. Additionally, if the child is not released from puberty suppression back to the hormonal milieu of the natal sex, and this be followed in lock step instead by cross sex hormones, the patient rapidly passes from a zone where permanent infertility is increasingly possible to a place where irreversible infertility is guaranteed. Only those adults who passed through puberty before changing genders and who retained their ovaries or testes or who had gametes frozen have any hope of fertility should they change their mind. The reader will see the thread of my argument that the harms of any given stage of transition under the current guidelines are thus defined by the harms of the plan as a whole. Ergo this is an ensemble plan that aims to sterilize the child whilst they are a young child themselves, the process in a sense beginning at the social transition phase. Each step simply makes it harder to go back and perverts from natures plan. And needless to say the exposure to cross sex hormones irreversibly alters the appearance of the body and face. The use of hormones incongruent with that of the natal sex (i.e. cross sex hormones) is not to be considered equivalent to the natural release of sex hormones congruent with the natal sex, if for no other reason than that the physician of the hospital who prescribes specific doses at specific times is a much poorer conductor of the orchestra than the physiology of nature. Thus there is the potential for long term adverse outcomes, these being realized over time and which would obviously be higher if the (cross) hormone replacement therapy is begun at a young age. Nonetheless it remains to be seen if female to male trans children treated with testosterone will reach middle or later ages with an unacceptably higher risk of deep venous clots, stroke or various cardiac problems. It remains to be seen if the male to female trans treated with oestrogen will have unacceptably higher rates of the same cardiac and vascular events, to name but a few.

Surgery

Constructing a vagina in a patient with a penis, or vice versa, is needless to say a very complicated affair fraught with risk of complication. Transition requires more than one surgery and surgical transition cannot be considered reversible. Usually a vagina can be constructed by slicing the penis and turning it inwards, often with additional flaps of tissue taken from the scrotum or elsewhere. Yet often the new vagina need by lined with a short segment of bowel, this either in the first or subsequent surgeries. Complications are legion and include damage to the bladder and fistula (channels) forming between the bowel and the new vagina where faecal material can flow from the former to the latter. No neo vagina can be considered equivalent to the indigenous anatomical form, and the construction of the new vagina needs be supported by the insertion of material such that the structure does not scar down and close. Similarly, the new vagina need be anchored internally like a tent that needs be held up from above, or it risks falling and protrusion. That is prolapse can also be a complication, these complications collectively being but a tiny sample of problems that can arise. Needless to say, normal sexual function is far from a forgone conclusion and far less likely than what would occur had the anatomical boy been allowed grow into a man.

What of making a male external genitalia? The labia majora can be stretched outward, and in it placed prosthetic non functional testes. Half of these patients suffer complications, chiefly the prosthesis wandering about like a walnut in a cushion and failing to stay in the right place. The patient may opt not so much for a penis to be constructed, as for a clitoris to be surgically more exposed and brought out further. If they opt for a penis, the vagina cannot simply be grabbed and pulled outside like turning a bag inside out. The skin must come from somewhere and generally comes from the abdomen. The substance of the neo penis itself historically has come from bone (some animals achieve erection by way of a bone that descends into the penis, though in humans who have evolved a different erectile mechanism and bone implant often resulted in death to the surrounding tissue), cartilage, and other material including most recently non biological prosthetics with or without urinary outflow. Making a penis that can urinate is an option that requires a catheter that places the patient at interminable risk of urinary infection, and so the new penis may not be an organ of urination at all if complications are to be minimized. Forearm muscle may also be used for penis construction. Surgically crafted penises are difficult to attach to the pelvic wall, and great post-surgical care must be had so that they do not lose position, twist or point off in the wrong direction. Needless to say neo penises are not spontaneously able to become erect and non -biological erectile structures implanted within the penile shaft have a lifecycle poorer than some organ transplants. No more than approx. 60% achieve organism, which would likely be less than that that could have been achieved had the genital mutilation not begun in the first instance and the girl allowed grow up as an anatomical female.

Mastectomies need be seen as the first phase of a surgical approach including breast augmentation with implants, with its own long list of risks. Placing children on the affirmative path can be said to compel them to risk all these complications.

More On the Metaphysics of Identity in Trans Children and Adolescents

A lot of what passes for argument in the trans camp can be formulated as "I am a woman because I feel like a woman", this said by an individual with a penis, testicles and an XY chromosome compliment. (Or conversely "I feel like a man", in the case of female to male or "F2M" trans). This is a statement groping for a sense of itself and a ground to stand the claim upon. What is it for the anatomical man to feel like a woman? How does he, an anatomical man, know he is feeling like a woman? Has he been an anatomical woman in some previous incarnation and come to access the consciousness of a past life, holding both present and past consciousness's before himself, the adjudicator some third entity that is also himself (or herself or themselves as the case may be)? And if so, is he simply reliving similarities in personality between he and the woman he was in a past life, a kind of transcendental nostalgia? Or does our man who feels like a woman possess some peculiar telepathic power to fuse consciousness with an anatomical woman and verify within this fusion state the validity of his claim? Now I am no Susan Blackmore, though I've also become jaded with any claims to the existence of psychic phenomena the likes of which this anatomical man would need to support his claim. And putting all this aside, what is the essential feeling state of womanhood that he identifies with? Might he just be identifying with this woman or that woman as opposed to womanhood as such? And what is womanhood as such, some Platonic ideal form perhaps? And the reader will bear this in mind on talk about X "identifies with being a woman". Identity in a philosophical sense most often relates to the individual and a strong argument for sameness. When does X become Y, when in any meaningful way Y is defined as X, and X is defined as non Y?

So how does he know what he feels he knows? And how do we know what he claims to know is true? And if we are to say that by simply asserting that he feels like a woman that "he" becomes or is in a strong sense "she", as asserted by the trans movement, then this is an exercise in begging the question, a circular reasoning, a fallacy in petitio principia. If I feel like a woman, what am I? Answer is a woman. And how do I know I am a woman? Because I feel like I am one.

I might say I feel like an astronaut, this without ever having piloted a plane and without ever having received so much as a phone call from NASA, let alone having seen the inside of a rocket ship and seen the Earth from on high. Or I might be an athlete committed to the belief I feel like a gold medalist, visualising myself standing centre of the dais with my anthem playing. Neither aspiration can change the fact that the measure of the astronaut or the gold medalist are external criteria which are either objective or intersubjective across time and place to achieve a level of stability the likes of which can pass for using the term "objective". Were this not the case I could demand a place in history alongside Yuri Gagarin and Carl Lewis. I could even be a God if I feel like one. I need no apologetic to silence the atheist. I just need make the claim as a fait accompli. I feel like God. Ergo I am God.

Might it not be better said that the human with a penis, testes and XY chromosomes feels what it is like for a man to imagine himself feeling like he is a woman, or to put another way he is imagining what a woman experiences and applies it to himself as a category error of identity. This is altogether immaterial to the question of being itself. He is, was and forever will be a man with a fertile imagination. There are tell-tale signs of this, for example in certain celebrity male to female trans self-descriptions of internal mental states as being a little too close to what the stereotype is of what men think a woman's inner worlds to be.

Now you might challenge me thus; "but what if a community of anatomical females quiz the anatomical male and find in this XY being a kindred spirit, a woman trapped in a man's body?" This too is a nonsense, for such an adjudication is not merely in what the male thinks of himself as not "he but "she", nor what a group of females think of him, but would involve an ignoring biological facts and a stretching of a community standard that can then become fluid and entirely arbitrary. These anatomical women may just as well admit into the club and without consent the most effeminate anatomical males and kick out of the girls club most of the tomboys or even an anatomical female who likes action films. There is no logical compulsion to include the subject's self identified gender when making the judgment based on a groups consensus without an objective biological referent, for the group might merely conclude that the individual lacks insight into who they are. (This lack of an objective referent is, parenthetically, the grave problem of almost all psychiatric diagnoses, and this is why transgenderism and psychiatry are guilty of the same epistemological crimes). The whole affair might become a farce where the group of "women" with the power to decide these matters of womanhood all have an XY chromosome complement and a penis, when all women's jails and sorority houses are filled with anatomical men and all women's sports are fought and won by athletes born with testes and penises. And then where will the anatomical woman go to find the purity of her kind, and more importantly where will she locate her true kind in the halls of power?

And what of temporality? Can I not say today I feel like a woman and thus I am a woman, whilst tomorrow reverting to being a man? Where is the ontological premium on consistency to define the now of being? And besides, in this transgender Turing test no anatomical woman can know what is in the inner world of the anatomical man who claims to be a woman, only what he says is there. How did you, a woman, know he is not lying to you, after first of all lying to himself? And so finally such an exercise in feminine empathy might come back to bite the caring feminist hand that feeds it. If a man can decide what it is to feel like a woman, might this not be formulated as the gender construction imposed upon women by men, this being every bit what Simone de Beauvoir and the other radical feminists alluded to when saying gender is oppressed upon them. Of course it cuts both ways you might say. The XX anatomical woman might feel like a man, become a man, and be imposing her feminist vision of man upon the enemy sex. Yet in the process of becoming the man she seeks to become, one woman is no more. In being recognized as a man "she" immediately ceases to be so says the trans ideology. Indeed "she" never was there in the first place. And so one man creates woman from himself, diluting true womanhood with dissimulation. And one woman annihilates herself in becoming a man. This is not a symmetry of destruction, as in the eyes of the feminist the predicate is a history of things as a political power play, with men the architects of the asymmetry from which other asymmetries flow. Ergo the feminist can say with transgenderism we only move from asymmetrical oppression to asymmetrical gendercide, from holding back women to annihilation of women. The trans ideology is a war against both reality and feminism, this being said by a cisgender heterosexual, and a conservative one at that.

We can take things one step further, this being hardly an argumentum ad absurdum. Or if it is, it finds itself in absurd company. As any scholar in the field of differences in the brain between the sexes knows, the data does not point to us having any ability to type the sex of a human from brain substructural differences. But as any anatomist knows, there is that old euphonious dictum of embryology by Ernst Haeckel "ontogeny recapitulates phylogeny". This is to say that during development in utero the human foetus has certain anatomical similarities with those animals from whom we are thought to have evolved. Although many of Haeckel's claims have not stood the test of time, certain example cases remain broadly true. All vertebrates (humans included) pass through a stage where we have structures that resemble gills and tails. We all pass through a stage when our hands are webbed like a tree frog, our heart is not always four chambered and so on. Some people even have third or fourth nipples, or a line of moles along the arc where in other mammalian species multiple breasts grow (imagine a sow and her multiple suckling piglets for example)

So what is it to stop an ostensive human claiming that they are, deep in their gnostic selves, a fish, a frog, a monkey, a pig or for those of feline character a common house cat (though I'll grant humans did not evolve from cats)? Nonetheless here there is at least a biological argument, however tenuous. With it we can add what the organism claims to identify with as a statement of being that other animal. I am a monkey or cat trapped in a humans body, albeit a bipedal intelligent one with a drivers licence. I am cat. Hear me purr.

Or what of age or race? I have often thought I identified with those of the older generation rather than my peers, and often lamented at being born fifty or so years out of place. Take me back to the inception of modern dentistry I say, and damn the internet and the smart phone. And I have known a few Anglo persons who strongly feel to have found their own people in that of the Japanese or Jews for example, and can see the appeal of both. What is to stop some outwardly young white anglo saxon male stating they identify with being a senior and demanding to collect a Japanese or Israeli age pension? Why limit them if they feel like it? And would you entertain the deluded beliefs of an anatomical human who thought they were a Japanese house cat if they threatened suicide on account of your nippono-feline-phobia? Would you be bigoted if you did not assent? Would you be culpable for their suicide?

Obviously the whole issue becomes amplified to the point of terrifying farce in the case of a child or adolescent, where adolescence is in part defined by an identity in statu nascendi, this being an axiom of all schools of developmental psychology who might otherwise compete for explanations of how the child becomes the adult. To restate what has been said before, the trans movement will rest their argument on the notion of insistence, persistence and consistency. Which is to say if the child sticks to their guns and affirms being the opposite sex then they are truly what they claim to be. Have these supposed experts never met a child who sticks to their guns in wanting to grow up to be a policeman or superhero or astronaut? Have they never encountered the adolescent or young adult who dabbles for years in a cult, counterculture or alternate politics they will later abandon or even regret, looking back then and saying how foolish and immature they were? The zealots become the apostates and the sceptics become the zealots. We often have known these ideologically concrete fifteen year olds, lost contact with them only to find them waiting at the bus stop fifteen years later, having happily embraced conformity down to their very marrow. Or we have all known those who madly yearn to be a concert pianist. Later find them at thirty not having touched a key in years, and not the slightest desire to. And has it not occurred to the so called experts that the child is heavily influenced by the social milieu without, including pro-trans ideology. Of course they have and we saw the vulnerability of children in the nonsense they spouted in the satanic moral panic of a previous chapter, just sacrificial pawns in an adult political game.

The child's lack of self-knowledge is why the efforts to transition are so frantic, and the suppression of debate so fierce.

What about Disorders of Sex Development (DSD) or Intersex?

The trans lobby often makes the claim that so called disorders of sexual development make sex (and gender) a spectrum. These are persons whom might formerly have been called the hermaphrodites, later termed intersex conditions, and to whom might also be ascribed the term disorders of sexual differentiation. From the fact of these disorders existing and before the fact of knowing anything about them, the laity will then almost be asked to imagine a vast cohort of people out there with penis, testes, vagina and ovaries all in the same body, with half the brains cells in some sex determining region carrying XY and the other half XX chromosome complements. And so they might be asked to imagine what is so special about the conventional anatomical woman or man save for being a place where some of the balls of nature by chance fell in one place, and where in others no balls fall at all. The balls of nature could, and do, fall pretty well anywhere in this stochastic chaos. Or so they might be expected to believe, and expect you to believe the same.

This claim can only be made in complete ignorance of what a spectrum conceptually is, along with ignorance around the prevalence and nature of disorders of sexual differentiation. Below I will outline some of these extremely rare conditions, making clear that things are not so opaque.

Klinefelters Syndrome; these babies represent about one in six hundred to a thousand live births. They might have a female type couple of X chromosomes (i.e. XX). Indeed, this is typically the case, though they may even have several X chromosomes. Regardless how many X chromosomes they have, they all have a Y also, and some have two. They might have smaller testes and they might have delayed puberty. They might unusually develop female like breasts if left unchecked, as many obese or anabolic steroid abusing men also grow boobs without losing their sexual identity as men. Yet Klinefelters boys are boys. These boys cannot be used in any meaningful way to construct an argument for sex (or gender) being a spectrum. Even the belief that Klinefelters boys were hypermasculine in their behaviour (especially those with two copies of the Y chromosome) have been put to rest.

Turners Syndrome; These babies are effectively born with only one functioning X chromosome, and this might be represented as XO. The condition is also common relative to other so called disorders of sex development, yet only about one in a few thousand female babies have Turners syndrome. This is a disorder of sex development only in the sense the disorder involves sex chromosomes, the puberty is often delayed and they often fail to fully develop female secondary sex characteristics. Turners babies with the additional complication of having degraded fragments of Y chromosome are exceedingly rare. All Turners patients are girls, and these girls cannot be used in any meaningful way to construct an argument for sex (or gender) being spectrum.

Virilisation of genetic females; The majority of these cases might be specified as having congenital adrenal hyperplasia, though there are other causes besides. These are genetic females (XX) who represent approx. one in fifteen to twenty thousand live births. These babies typically have genetic mutations that alters the hormonal milieu towards a male like hormone bias such that they are born with ambiguous genitalia. The clitoris might be enlarged to resemble the head of the penis continuous with the labia minora (the inner folds) which might have partially fused to resemble the root of the penis. Either side of this sits the labia majora, which might be so enlarged and partially fused as to resemble a scrotum within which no testes sit, the absence of testes being a clue as to what might be the underlying condition. These babies are girls and almost always resolved to be the case, with the best outcome being medical and surgical management to this end, and a recognition of who they are as girls. 95% will then grow to identify as women, this majority not being trivial. Many of these women will be lesbian relative to population norms, though this will remain a minority and of only indirect interest to the question of gender identity. Should these genetic females diagnosis be missed in infancy, they may be raised as males. Medical and surgical management to this end will follow. In such cases some continue to identify with being male, though the rates of success on such an occasion are sufficiently poor to encourage correct diagnosis as females as early as possible in infancy. Such lamentable outcomes make it such that raising these girls as boys is not the outcome of an option so much as the outcome of a missed diagnosis, however forgivable it might be. Such a stance is not controversial. This diagnosis cannot be used in any meaningful way to construct an argument for sex (or gender) being spectrum.

Androgen deficiency or insensitivity syndromes; These are under-virilised genetic XY males. The default state of nature is for the embryo to develop into the female (I say embryo as sexual differentiation begins before the foetal stage and often before the mother might even know she is pregnant with her child). The Y chromosome plays a part in a genetic cascade towards being a male through production and action of so called "male" hormones, these being hormones and other factors that are either orders of magnitude higher in levels in the male, or male specific. This cascade is only as good as the biochemical production line. If the various genes on the Y or other chromosomes for the various male sex hormone production and action go awry, this biases development away from virilisation and towards the default female plan. The baby is usually born with testes, though these have not descended. The external genitalia might appear ambiguous or as per that of a normal female baby. These babies are not a homogenous group. Dozens of genetic lesions contribute to androgen deficiency or insensitivity as a class, each of which are individually very rare and variable in their presentation.

The extreme case is complete androgen insensitivity. All male hormones might be normally produced, yet receiving tissues are unable to recognize the lions share of them. These XY babies have normal external female genitalia, whilst lacking internal female anatomy such as the uterus, ovaries etc. This will remain unnoticed until years later when as females they are assessed for infertility and amenorrhea in adolescence or adulthood. Then the undescended testes will also be discovered on imaging and the discussion had if to remove them as they carry an increased risk of cancer. Often these women will likely pass through all the formative years identifying as female and none the wiser of what sex chromosome complement they carry. Does the existence of these women challenge the view that sex is binary? Not at all. This extreme represents no more than about a couple dozen adult females in a city with a population of a million persons. Many a paediatrician, endocrinologist or gynaecologist can go a whole career without encountering such a patient. These are women and for various reasons it is absolutely reasonable to consider them women. For starters it is a hypothesis of considerable strength that the brain was just as under-virilised as was the anlage to the genitalia. This is to be predicted with a very high level of inference based on the knowledge of the cellular biology involved, and does not depend on the identification of a sex determinative multicellular region of the brain. Then there is the fact that in the external female genitalia there is indeed a biological referent to the individual being female, a referent that was present at birth and which the community recognized as an objective marker of being female. This was not something "assigned" so much as simply observed ipso facto to be the case, and all assumptions and practices within the life of the girl resolved around this fact from the day of her birth onwards. Further, there is the fact that when the diagnosis is made in the adult or late adolescent the past cannot be changed, and the past has fully determined the present without human ideological intervention. Both nature and nurture worked as harmoniously as was possible together towards a common end. Now we have an adult identifying as female and who, if challenged, could mount a strong argument as to why this is the case and why the community ought to share in acknowledging her self-identification. And so these exceptionally rare cases do not challenge the binary view of sex.

Neither is this challenged by another extremely rare condition known as Swyer syndrome, where the functional sex determining of the Y chromosome is either mutated or lacking. Indeed, this is more the case as the undescended testes are also underdeveloped, the external genitalia are female, and the internal anatomy female also often present, perhaps even to the point of sustaining an ability to become pregnant by artificial means. These too are girls and women.

Gender identification of other cases with only partial androgen insensitivity or deficiency and partial under-virilisation is less clear, yet not entirely vexed. For example, genetic XY males with 5α-reductase deficiency are lacking the hormone largely responsible for in utero development of male external genitalia (which is separate to the case of additional development of the genitalia in adolescence). Not surprisingly they often have ambiguous genitalia at birth. Yet these genetic males most often grow to see themselves as male, irrespective of whether they were raised as males or females. The same applies even for those genetic males with 17?-hydroxysteroid dehydrogenase-3 deficiency, the enzyme responsible for the production of testosterone itself. They are males who mostly come to identify with being males. Steering these boys to being raised as girls was perhaps historically biased by the fact that surgically it is easier to resolve ambiguous genitalia to something resembling female anatomy than male ("easier to dig a hole than build a pole" some surgeons did say). Nonetheless medicine and science has every reason to pursue a course of action towards assisting nature in its "intentions", diagnosing the correct sex early and rearing accordingly. Once again raising the child as female or male is not an arbitrary option. The sex is not to be assigned so much as discovered as best as one can, and nature supported.

Genetic Chimerism; The usual occurrence is for the fertilized egg to divide into genetic copies of itself with (genetically speaking) each cell in the body genetically the same, the exceptions being the production of sperm or ova and certain cells of the immune system also being genetically dissimilar in specific ways not germane to the current discussion. Extremely rarely things go awry whereby a single individual embryo is actually a fusion of two fertilized eggs that would otherwise have developed into two fraternal twins, a brother and a sister, an XX and an XY. These fusion embryos carry some cells with the XY male and some with the XX female pattern of chromosomes. There are other mechanisms how this outcome can come about, that might through these other means be more properly considered genetic mosaicism. Collectively chimera and mosaics might amount to no more than one in fifty to one hundred thousand persons, though the exact numbers are not known, and so reliable findings about psychosexual development are not clear either. In any case, such a chimera/mosaic can conceivably come to have a mixture of male and female sexual anatomy or genital ambiguity, though this is an uncommon outcome. Although there are some cases termed "true hermaphroditism", nature does not perfectly split the baby down the middle. Nature does not produce a baby with a perfectly formed ovary one side and perfectly formed and descended testicle on the other, a uterus in the centre and both a perfectly formed vagina and penis below both, and a half female half male brain above the lot. And nature has never ever produced a human who is a self contained reproductive unit, able to get themselves pregnant.

Usually the outcome of such genetic admixture is an unambiguous male or female. Of those cases that are ambiguous, once again the question is whether the baby is a diagnostic and management challenge to conquer, or a simple case of normal variation and diversity. Common sense would fall on the side of the former conclusion, though this value judgment is a harder road to take. Yet take it we must. An individual raised male with internal tissue capable of menstruation might have painful bloody urine in adolescence and adulthood. An individual raised as female with internal tissue of a testis might develop a testicular cancer. Both might develop inguinal hernia. These are but a few of many examples of complications of mosaicism that point towards these states being pathologies within a person who has value as a person, not diversities to be celebrated as the source and location of a persons value itself.

XX Ovotesticular Disorder; These are extremely rare genetic females, who might have tacked onto one of the X chromosomes the region that ordinarily sits upon the Y chromosome and which largely activates male development. They might have variant anatomical abnormalities including ovarian and testicular tissue in the one person, similar to the genetic chimeras and mosaics mentioned above, and with similar challenges to diagnosis and management.

Persistent Mullerian Duct Syndrome; these are very rare genetic males with male genitalia. The only thing that they have in common with the woman is the persistence of the embryological structure that gives rise to the fallopian tubes and much of the uterus. They do not actually develop fully formed internal or external female anatomy and are boys in any meaningful sense. They are only of interest to infertility specialists, the surgeons and the paediatricians if the testes remain undescended.

Cloacal exstrophy in the XY male. These can be genetic XY males with testes, though unfortunately lack a penis or the penis is excessively small on account of a congenital defect where a more primitive structure (the cloaca) that ought to have separated into part of the rectum and bladder is instead retained and impacts on the development of the external genitalia. As stated above, it is easier in these cases to surgically construct female genitalia and raise the child as a female. Such an approach was driven not simply by practical ease for the surgeon, as by the tabula rasa philosophy of John Money as outlined earlier in the chapter. Yet such an approach would be a mistake. To quote just one paper of patients with cloacal exstophy in XY males with testes; "14 of 16 subjects were raised as females, Of these 14, 2 were living with "unclear sexual identity" though declared themselves males, and an additional 8 had been living as males. All 16 subjects had moderate to marked interests and attitudes that were considered typical of males". These babies are best seen as males and medical surgical expertize brought to bear on complete harmony of external genitalia with the other sex characteristics. In the XX female, the cloacal exstrophy results usually in either a bifurcated vagina and a clitoris which also appears partially divided. Females with cloacal exstrophy are females. The existence of this genitally challenging condition is in neither case the basis for argument of gender as a spectrum, and is included here only as an additional refutation to the ideas of John Money.

Concluding remarks on Disorders of Sex Differentiation

When we pass light through a prism, we have refraction into the various colours that we also see in the rainbow (red, orange, yellow, green, blue, indigo and violet). Yet even these colours are only rendered discrete by the physiology and perception of our own vision, with clear graduation of change between differently perceived colours. These colours exist within a continuous range with a wavelength approx. 380 to 740 nanometres, the range extending beyond this into the non-visible expanse of electromagnetic radiation. We call this continuous range within which something might be found a spectrum, and electromagnetic radiation is a worthy example. Now when sperm and egg are refracted through the prism of the bedroom and sexual intercourse, there are only two bands of great thickness, with nothing outside of this range. One band is XY with testes and male external genitalia and the other is XX with ovaries and female external genitalia. Between these two bands is a vanishingly thin line, which in our analogy would be too thin to see with the naked eye. And within this vanishingly thin line most of what might be ambiguous can be resolved as an epistemic problem with an ontological solution of boy or girl being the case. Of the remainder even this is not necessarily a third category, as its members are not homogenous save for the quality of having an anatomy and physiology which is disharmonious with the almost universal norm. Only the most procrustean argument can make of these malformations and mutations a celebration of diversity or normal variation as opposed to disease. Now disease is a harsh word I'll grant you. Yet disease is not an open and inevitable door to stigma and persecution. And the want to save someone from stigma is an attitude that cannot extent to a denial of biological fact. And this is the politically incorrect crux of the argument. None of the colours of the visible light spectrum could be considered physical aberrations. With disorders of sex development, the same cannot be said. Whether one invokes the mind of a divine creator as designing an ideal body plan qua female and male or one sees biological sex the outcome of a Darwinian evolution as towards to a harmonious reproductive end, we arrive at the same conclusion. We must similarly face the reality that a couple who visit a fertility clinic, where he cannot produce sperm and/or she cannot be fertilized by non-technological means have a fertility disorder, a disease. These are problems with which to be sympathized much less persecuted, yet are not normal variations or diversities to be celebrated. Similarly, sex determining genes mutated away from purpose are gene lesions, not gene variation. An undescended testis is an embryological process failure, not diversity, any more than endometriosis or a congenital hole in the heart is diversity. A disharmonious combination of brain, sex chromosomes, internal sexual anatomy and external genitalia are similarly all diseases of a kind. And they do not inform the trans argument which as far as the evidence goes, is personally and socially constructed.

In any case and as stated, biological sex is as far as one could imagine a departure from the concept of a spectrum. It is an almost pure binomial (binary) distribution. And conceptually the term intersex implies the categories between which the inter resides. The validity of the suffix "sex" is proved by the prefix "inter".

But wait? Gender as defined by internal psychological identification is different to biological sex you might say. Is not this the gender that exists upon a spectrum? Not so. Much of this chapter is devoted to this idea being nonsense, illogical and a misapplication of a term better left in linguistics. Until the most recent few years of our collective unravelling into madness, biological sex and gender identification has throughout all of human history possessed such a tight correlation as to suggest unity. That is to say the anatomical woman in almost all cases would have identified with being a woman, an anatomical man would identify with being a man. This correlation does not allow for the invocation of the descriptor "spectrum". I am proposing as a matter of simple fact that biological sex is the only place in which any concept of gender has any meaning as a statement of identity. We might speak of the anatomical man as possessing certain features of personality often found in the anatomical woman, and vice versa. Yet tomboys and effeminate men do not amount to a finding of identity rightly defined by other criteria.

Brain Sex

One such criteria by which sexual identity might be defined, and one in which there is immediate implied scientific legitimacy, is brain sex. The trans activist might make move towards the innards of the skull, and simply state that genitalia, chromosomes and the like be damned. They may even strategically ignore the psychological and social world as first causes and legitimate grounding as to the truth of sexual identity, at least for a time to slip and slide to other suasive territory. They would say the mental world is a representation of the biological world of the brain, and posit that in the trans person that the brain has the indelible stamp of the sex opposite to the body in which it resides. Brain is all that matters then, and the brain is the sun around which the world must orbit. Very well then. Let us be brutally scientific and get the modal logic right before we start.

Let us remind ourselves of the gravitas of the proposed intervention. Social transitioning is a major event that necessarily impacts on the lives of all in society, and will be psychologically harmful if not grounded in reality. Similarly, all pharmacology that tinkers with the endocrine system has risks and any medication is a poison if not medically indicated, just as surgery the likes of which occurs in transitioning is mutilation without an extreme argument in favour of it being indicated.

So what evidence might we need before exposing a child's developing body and brain to powerful hormonal modulators and hacking off breasts and balls?

Firstly, we would need have a specific valid and reliable marker of differentiating the sex of the brain as male or female. Now it is obvious that there are on average sexual differences between the brains of the sexes and that these differences have bearings on behaviour. We know this by inference from animal models and the human also (see the section on intersex for example, or read the early work on rodents where exposing newborn female rats to testosterone has them growing up mounting female rats just as a male does). About this fact much has been written. Yet it is not enough to infer that female and male brains have been feminized or virilised in some undefined way with differences between the means. We would need point with a scrupulously straightened finger to something in the brain that validates the claim, this being either a discrete structure, a pattern of organization or whatever. This marker would need be something specific and identified on first principles as being meaningfully related to sexual differentiation and identity, i.e. something that is theoretically meaningful. A large male might have a larger volume of the post central gyrus related to skin sensation than that of the petite female, this obviously in turn related to the differential surface area of skin. And so what? Male brains are often on average larger than female brains and this tells us nothing about intellect any more than we could say the same of a blue whale's brain being larger than a human. Similarly, the area of the brain that is involved with primary somato-sensation of the skin or activation of skeletal muscle has nothing to tell us of the question of brain sex qua gender identity. The brain sex marker would need be determined as further specific to sexual identity itself, and have discriminative validity vs that of identifying sexual appetite for example, as this co-variation of identity and behaviour seriously complicates things. It would not be possible to construct a meaningful argument if it were found, for example, that male to female transgendered persons have a female type insula. Why? Because I can show evidence of the insula being involved in basic proprioception, body perception, depression, disgust and social compliance, sense of self in social acceptance/rejection scenarios, attention and so called ADHD, nurturing behaviour, inhibition of sexual temptation, anorexia nervosa and so on and so forth. Same for the amygdala (anxiety, fear, sexual arousal, exposure to novel non threatening stimuli, happiness etcetera). Such a difference within a brain region would be only the beginning of the debate as to the meaning of the difference.

Having been identified, the marker would need be without significant overlap between the sexes. This is to say that the predictive marker is not meaningfully defined by averages. If behind the screen we are told is an unidentified adult with height 155cm we might have the odds firmly on our side to guess that our unknown person is a woman, though they might also be a short man. Any putative sex identity region (or pattern) in the brain ought not to just be generally different between the sexes if the question is to biologically argue for sex identity and transition. The difference must be of a quantity that is never seen in non trans members of the natal sex of the subject in question. A 155cm adult person can only be necessarily a woman if there are no 155cm adult males in the world. And from this finding of class difference the strength of the marker must be such that the prediction can be made with reference to the marker alone and blinded to the other particulars of the individual. For example we would need see the brain imaging result of this marker alone and be able to say that this region with this measured quantity (volume of area for example) predicts with a very high confidence that the unknown individual is either a natal female/trans minded female in a male body or a natal male/trans minded male in a female body.

Next, the brain marker identified would need be a measure of trans as defined as the sex of the brain that the individual identifies with, and not a third category. This is to say by way of a simple and silly thought experiment that if male brains are blue and female brains are pink, if we were to open the brain of an outwardly anatomical man who says it is a woman inside, we would find a pink brain (or a blue brain to disprove the brain sex hypothesis). We would not find a green or a purple or a rainbow coloured brain. To find a green or purple brain would then define the trans brain as a third category. And it would not be possible to successfully argue that this third category is not pathological. Why? Because the argument was that the trans XY person with penis and testes has a female brain, and their identity argument is bound up in this hypothesis. Further, the finding of a green or purple brain would have thus been proved to be a marker of incongruence itself. And given that the question is attached to the question of what to do about it, surgically and medically correcting the incongruence only remains coherent to the outcome of a pink body to a pink brain. All this is heavily value laden and cannot avoid both ethical and moral debate.

Next there would need be evidence of differences in the sex determining/correlative region of the brain of the trans person that are unequivocally not confounded by environmental influences. That is to ask have we created a brain difference (say with xeno-oestrogens) only to say we have discovered a natural kind. Now no one by sheer force of will and wearing a dress can magically turn their penis into a vagina. The brain on the other hand is quite plastic within the modules and distributed patterns of function. For example, the brain area devoted to the fine muscle activity of the hand is greater than the comparatively clumsy and oafish foot, and will be greater still in its volume and elaboration in the concert pianist than the musical philistine. Yet in the double arm amputee who learns to paint and type with their feet, the area devoted to the hand will regress and atrophy and the area devoted to the feet will become unusually prominent, essentially an inverted hand. Does this argue for a constitutional difference (i.e. primary causative difference) in the brain of the pianist or the double arm amputee? Not at all. It was the behaviour and environment that altered the brain from what would have been the default natural state. In a similar sense, any study related to the brain sex typing of the trans individual must address the question of the effect upon the brain of living trans and countless other environmental inputs. It would need to go beyond that achievable within the boundaries of the brains plasticity to environmental influences both on theoretical grounds and in the life of the patient. Finally, any studies purporting to have identified a difference in the trans brain would need rely on extremely rigorous controls and not patient report of their lifestyle. Most prima facie controlled studies in humans are not as controlled as the investigators would like us to believe, for the simple fact that the investigator is not present in the life of the subject of their investigation. The use, for example, of non-prescription cross sex hormones is as rife and as underreported a problem in the adult trans world as performance enhancing drugs are in the world of the athlete and bodybuilder, and easily obtained by the user who is motivated, connected with the appropriate in group and has a modicum of social skills.

Next, it would need be proven that the marker applies to the age of the individual in question. It would not be enough to find a brain sex difference in adults and then assume that the same difference explains trans in children in general, much less a specific child or adolescent before us who claims to be trapped in the wrong body. There would need be robust prospective evidence that the marker can blindly predict in advance not simply that the child is a trans child, yet have predictive power that they will certainly be a trans adult and not desist (i.e. not decide as a late adolescent or young adult that they are comfortable in their natal/anatomical sex)

Ideally there will also be natural ablation experiments supporting the hypothesis. For example if there is a rare cis gender adult who suffers a rapid onset gender dysphoria, have they been found to have some stoke, tumour or injury to the area of the brain that is thought to determine sex? If not, then we need revise our model of what constitutes the trans brain. The same is the case if approached from the opposite side. If we have a transgender patient with a brain disease the likes of which by chance results a brain made congruent with their natal sex, does this correlate with a rapid reversal of the trans mindset. If not, then once again the model asserting X region of the brain as gender identity determinative would be wrong and require serious revision.

And next and vital to the above, each of these discoveries would need be replicated, i.e. repeated once or twice in separate experiments and the same results found to be the case. This is an extremely difficult challenge in the case of rare "disorders". But science is what it is in the demands it places upon us. Neuroscience and social psychology is rife with studies either which are not replicated or in replication the original findings fail to be repeated the second time round, and social psychology has been plagued in recent years by multiple occurrences of outright fraud. Journals are notoriously averse to publishing replication studies of failed experiments, resulting in an ever present and justified suspicion that the disconfirming evidence is sitting in a drawer somewhere.

This chapter was to contain a paper by paper review of the literature on brain sex re the question of trans in general and children in particular. In the end this ambition was abandoned as there wasn't the evidence to critique. At this juncture the trans lobby would do as well to take a step back from the brain and look to other strategies, as they might not like what they likely will not find. On my survey of the literature I can assure the reader that we are not even remotely close to being within a country mile of fulfilling such criteria of evidence as outlined above to warrant the ideological and chemical poisoning and surgical mutilation of the adult, let alone the child or adolescent. The trans lobby simply do not have the evidence. But let us fantasize and grant the opponent enough rope. If brain sex is ever proven in a way that accords with the trans world view, this would not provide a posteriori vindication for what the ideologues do today. If one executes a free citizen who is then after the fact found guilty of a capital crime, the execution remains a murder in not having first passed through the jurisprudential gates of due process. The same is the case in science. One is not proven to be right all along by being lucky or intuitive. The rightness only has its being in the proof.

It is worth illuminating upon the construct incoherence of psychiatry in this regard, this incoherence kept afloat by psychiatrists being expert pragmatists and sophists. In order for psychiatry qua a self styled neuro-scientific enterprise to endorse trans kids its needs knowledge of the brain it does not have, and in not having this knowledge psychiatry ought to be painfully hoisted on its own petard. Neither can it slither sideways into the world of descriptive criteria as a justification to diagnosis. You see psychiatry has long divided delusions into delusions in general, and various eponymous and descriptive subtypes of specific delusions. One subtype is the so called "bizarre" delusion. Technically speaking, a bizarre delusion is not simply a belief that is false, fixed, not factual etcetera as per the usual definition of the term. A bizarre delusion is one that is not possible given the knowledge of the physical and biological universe as it stands. So someone might be deluded into thinking their partner is unfaithful and this be driven by a psychotic illness. Yet infidelity is possible and so the delusion is not bizarre. But if a patient were to say that their spouse is both sitting aside them in the consulting room whilst being simultaneously at home sleeping with the pool man that would be a bizarre delusion in the physical impossibility to be in two different places at the same time. Now we might ask ourselves how psychiatry ought to formulate an individual who claims to be (to be in a strong sense) female when almost every cell carries an XY chromosome pair, and from whose body hangs a penis and two testicles. Is this not a wonderful example of a bizarre delusion? In endorsing such an idea as true, is not psychiatry obliged to diagnose itself by its own lights as suffering from a bizarre delusion? Or might it just reveal its hand as philosophically pragmatic, where truth is always what it wants it to be as measured by the ends it wishes to achieve.

Zuckergate (with a Brief Historical Digression)

Kenneth Zucker was, and is, one of the worlds most pre-eminent sexologists and arguably the worlds leading expert on what might be described trans in children and adolescents. Based in Toronto, Zucker headed up the Child Youth and Family Gender Identity Clinic and was a thought leader in the formulation of the relevant section of the DSM and also the 2012 WPATH guidelines before being cast out of the trans Eden of the WPATH. His tale of woe has been summarized in numerous articles by the investigative journalist Jesse Singal, whom I might add has himself been thrust into the same controversial orbit as Zucker for the audacity of being sympathetic a trans heretic.

Zuckers work revolved around prospective studies on trans kids, with the incendiary finding that most trans children, if approached with a therapeutic attitude that could be described to "help children feel comfortable in their own bodies," will indeed come to feel comfortable in their own bodies. Zuckers work has been criticized for allegedly being bias by non trans kids who were simply gender atypical. However roughly two thirds at the time did satisfy the diagnosis of gender identity disorder as per DSM IV TR and the remainder with the subthreshold diagnosis would have met criteria under the DSM 5 for gender dysphoria. And all would have been the very kinds of children targeted by the trans movement for affirmation and transition. Other researchers such as Thomas Steensma have found the same results as Zucker, if not more so. A conservative estimate of desistence often quoted is around 80%, i.e. 80% of boys thinking themselves to be girls will have a natural history such that they will reach young adulthood being comfortable with being men. This is a fact that the trans lobby is determined to silence

I have read some of Zuckers work, and also parts of the doctoral dissertation of his protégé Devita Singh which, strangely, is available in the public domain. No work of this kind is completely immune from methodological critique, yet these are works of quality orders of magnitude greater than the trans activists and trans in house journals with ideologically bias peer review. I caution the reader against taking anything to be legitimate simply from invocation of the words "scientific journal" or "peer review" or "evidence based". Five angry drunkards in an ally can also be an occasion of peer review and the term does not guarantee a rigorous dialectic with attorneys for both the defence and prosecution of a hypothesis. Real science and real philosophy are intellectual blood sports where only the ideas that cannot be killed off are permitted to survive. Zuckers findings have also been replicated, replication being something rare in the social psychology, and his work is the best evidence to date. It ought to be the basis for best practice, and an argument that transgender affirmation and transition is the real nefarious practice to which ought to be ascribed "gender conversion therapy".

And what was Zuckers penalty for such heresy? In late 2015 whilst on vacation, the university arranged an external review informed by trans-activists and further arranged the findings to be released in a (more or less) publicly available report. This included patient reports into his conduct, two of which were negative and included the allegation that he told a young trans female (natal male) that she (I would say he) was a "hairy little vermin". This being Canada, Zucker was afforded no due process of the American jurisprudence of his birth, i.e. he was not assumed innocent until proven guilty, and he was not permitted any reasonable defence against a prosecution that was assiduously weaving its web with him unaware and in absentia. He was simply fired from his post 9 days out from Christmas Eve, in the very meeting he was informed of the reports existence and its imminent release. Subsequently both negative allegations were found to be false, with substantial evidence that they were concocted to the goal of removing Zucker. And in his person being removed, removed also would be the last bastion of academia against the trans juggernaut. By the alleged complainants own admission, someone called him "a hairy little vermin", yet it was certainly not Zucker.

Zuckergate is equally illustrative of how savage and rapid ideological shifts and moral panics can erupt upon a society seemingly oblivious of themselves sleepwalking toward a radical future. In 2012 Zucker was part of the intelligentsia informing when you the reader are sane or mad and what we are to intellectually make of your sexuality whatever it is. His was the only spirit of temperance in the 2012 WPATH guidelines, a call to watchful waiting and not automatic trans affirmation. In 2015 he was dismissed from a unit he headed for 34 years with without trial for unfounded professional misconduct. Yet the tide of acceptable thought and opinion had changed even more. As I write this chapter at the close of 2019, Zucker is a pariah with trans zealots systemically freezing him out of the universities, the expert advisory panels and succeeding in de-platforming him from conferences where he was previously welcomed.

Zuckers approach can be formulated as more than simple watchful waiting, which would be equivalent to no intervention at all. He did encourage a thorough evaluative process including an exploration not only into the gender affirmed by the child, yet also into the reasons why the child might affirm the incongruent gender in the first place. Such an approach is now seen to be loaded with implications as to motive, and is all too easily interpreted by the trans lobby as a "conversion therapy" away from the gender the child claims to be, and is assumed to be in this begging of the philosophical question to the natal gender. The trans lobby have proven themselves terrified of what a clinician such as Zucker might find, that is that the gender incongruence might stem from psychologically destabilizing experiences of childhood and that the criterion of "persistence" might not be so persistent after all. As such they have been determined to silence him, and have been most successful in their efforts. Others have been silenced also, and it worth pointing out in this drama what is typical in the trans debate. In the articles I reviewed, the pro trans community were unabashed in being identified so as to be quoted contra Zucker. Yet those who would defend him had to be quoted anonymously, for fear of losing their jobs also. The reader may ask who are the victims here. Those transactivists who claim to be the downtrodden against the conservative Goliath, or those sober minded scientists or conservatives who rightly intuit they must censor themselves.

Another more sinister implication can be made from the systematic silencing of Zucker, this being admittedly speculative on my part. Though the vast majority of anatomical boys who think they are girls trapped in the wrong body grow to become comfortable with being young men (i.e. they desist), a large faction of these anatomical boys grow to become homosexual young men. Lesbianism is also overrepresented in adult females who as children believed they were boys trapped in a female body. This ought to be not entirely unexpected. In 1962 Karl Urlich described his homosexuality thus "anima muliebris virili corpore inclusa" or a female psyche trapped in a males body. This was millennia after homosexuality became known to man, though only a few years before the term homosexual was actually coined by another Karl, that being Karl Maria Kertbeny.

Zuckers work opens a Pandora's box that can be interpreted in more than one way by both sides of the political divide viz a viz homosexuality. On one hand we might imagine it points the way to homosexuality being (at least in some individuals) the outcome of adverse events of childhood that result in some with trans confusion also. The "homophilic" thing to do would not be to affirm trans in childhood at all. Quite the contrary it would be seen as proto homosexual behaviour in a child who does not yet know, nay cannot yet know, what he is as a sexual being. The homophobic formulation of the same approach would be to interpret trans in childhood as one of the many manifestations of adverse events that define the latter emergent homosexuality as psychopathology. On the other hand, the psychoanalyst or amateur political analyst in me can readily formulate the silencing of Zucker and the push to affirm as soon as possible as the trans lobbies attempt to cure the world of homosexuality by converting male children destined to be gay into heterosexual females, whilst also undermining the identity and power of the feminists as women. In one fell swoop the trans lobby thus would take the reins as the supreme sexual minority to be favoured and protected. In a political sense, LGBTQ+ is an informal coalition which must fight two battles. The first is the battle of the group in opposition to cis gender heterosexuals, and the second as factions within the group in opposition with themselves for party power. It is not simply the silencing of Zucker that might be formulated in terms of a, perhaps unconsciously driven, trans vs homosexual politics. Part of the trans argument is that the current explosion in clinics reflects a prevalence in the community that was heretofore until the twenty first century sent underground from extreme persecution and bigotry. What to make then of the fact that there were pockets of time and place when alternative sexualities were able to raise their head and not having their existence challenged. And yet within these times, with the homosexuality as the archetypal alternative sexuality (and cross dressing cis gender persons), fully fledged cross gender identifying persons were still exceedingly rare. Take for example ancient Greece, notorious for homosexuality and pederasty also. Yet where was trans as trans ideologues currently define the person as being, as X trapped in a Y body? Or what of turn of the century England. We know of Oscar Wilde and Wilde was persecuted for his homosexuality. But where was trans? And what of the sexually liberated quarter of a Berlin in a pre Weimer and Weimer Germany and the equivalent even more libertine Paris of the fin de siecle. From years before Bismarck decriminalized homosexuality in 1922, the cosmopolitan elite was homo-tolerant, this being much more the case in the land of the heirs to the Jacobins. Trans was there in Western Europe for sure, yet so exceedingly rare as to make homosexuality look pedestrian. Equally this was the case in Moscow and Leningrad where the social experiment was even more violent in its liberation from church and tradition. From the first years of the twentieth century when revolution was fomenting to just prior to Stalins triumph over Trotskyism, the avant-garde was hell bent on destroying all conservative sexual identities, consigning the traditional family to history and undoing Czar Nicholas (the first) criminalizing of a homosexuality. The communist parties of western Europe all campaigned for sexual liberation and many a western homosexual saw the Soviet Union as the utopia of their future. And yet in the heart of Moscow where amongst the socialist homosexuals, the androgyne soviet females, the celebration of abortions, the legislation enabling an immediate divorce for unhappy couples, and so on and so forth, where in all this do we see trans? It was not there.

So from this, how on Earth can we arrive at a population level of persons in 2019 who would be trans if not supposedly supressed/oppressed of 0.5%, let alone 1.2% to 3.7% of an earlier mentioned New Zealand study? I can scarcely imagine the rate being 0.00001%. Or are we to believe that trans was more persecuted still than the homosexual and consequently driven almost universally underground? Are we seriously perhaps expected then to believe that the L, B and G have also been keeping the T down all along?

Digressions aside and returning to the matter of desistence, sadly stories of changing one's mind (or formations of one's mind) are not restricted to children and adolescence. The trans lobby also seeks to supress growing reports of adults who reach the approx. 10 year mark, regret having transitioned and wish to return to their natal sex. Although the secular reader will recognize the ideological bias of his Pentecostal Christianity and perhaps be uncomfortable with it, I commend the reader to visit the website (sexchangeregret.com) of Walt Heyer, an anatomical/natal male become female become male again. He is contacted regularly by adults with trans regret. Heyers case is an illustration of many things, two of which being that his trans dysphoria, like many others, commenced in childhood and was unequivocally related to small "t" traumatic events of childhood. The second is that if a trans critic happens to have a religious affiliation, the trans lobby will seize upon it to ignore any argument made, no matter how sound it is. The trans lobby also seeks to ad hominem the trans critical American College of Paediatricians (not to be confused with the official American Academy of Paediatricians) as being fringe Christian lunatics, rather than engage with their conservative argument.

There can be one final possible rebuttal to Zucker. There is the work for example of deVries et al in 2011, who looked at desistance rates in those who have transitioned socially in childhood and with puberty suppression to continue onto cross sex hormones. None of the 70 subjects desisted. All 70 continued on into cross sex hormones, this provided as proof of anything the translobby wishes to argue (though with a follow up interval that, like a horse race half run, is too short to answer the question if any will have trans regret in future). We ought to be cautious about these and other similar results. This debate is best not evaluated as a competition between success of outcome rates, the likes of which a physician might look for in comparing two different medications with equal side effects. Such data are certainly not proof of the validity of the claim of the child to have been born into the wrong body. That question is asked and answered definitively by Zucker and others in studying the natural history of the condition, and in the fact that desistance is then very high in the minimally manipulated child. It really ought not to matter to anyone if in the years to come each and every 4 or 6 year old trans child who is placed on an intensive and immersive path results in adults who universally persist in their claim to be opposite the natal sex (i.e. zero desistence). This would only be proof of the power of an ideology to take a Herculean grip on nature and engineer humanity to their own ends. This is conceptually no different to taking the child who claims not be able to run, maiming them for life and then claiming to have proven them to be congenitally crippled. As any neuroscientist familiar with the works of Hubel and Wiesel can say, you can take a kitten, suture up one of its eyes for the first few months of life, this rendering the kitten more or less permanently blind in that eye for life, when it would have otherwise had normal vision. The outcome of bio-political experiments fails to inform the default ontology of the person, except in the mind of the philosophical pragmatist whose idea of truth is whatever works.

How Did We Get This Far? The Makings of Genderosis

Hopefully by now the reader will be sympathetic with my argument that those promoting transgenderism in children (and perhaps adults also) suffer a psychopathology we might call "genderosis", though seeing it as a dangerous groupthink Munchausen by Proxy Disorder will do just as well. The question arises just how did this madness arise? I don't suppose to know the answer to this question, though I will venture some speculation as to its source and direction beyond that that might be found in the implied motivations of the early trans activists outlined earlier.

The Role of Psychiatry and Psychology; The business model of a profession is the advancement of guild power, this being a currency as good as money, both currencies to be maximized in the stock of its psychiatrist and psychologist shareholders. Psychiatry's strategy is to in turn maximize diagnoses in the populace for as long as it is politically possible without tarnishing the brand. Once upon a time to be a political dissident in Soviet Russia or a freedom loving slave in the USA might have provoked psychiatric diagnosis and treatment. Once upon a time to be an emotional woman was to be a hysteric to be locked up and even lobotomized. Even those residing in the modern Camelot were not immune from danger, the case in point being Rosemary Kennedy's lobotomy. More recently there was homosexuality, taken off the psychiatric table back in 1980 with the issuing of the DSM III (in practice it was de-pathologized many years earlier). And once it was a psychopathology to be transgender, though the tide has also has turned in trans favour. The caring professions in their pragmatism have made a deft move in doublethink and doublespeak, retaining the diagnosis of gender dysphoria qua being troubled by gender incongruence, as a means to both legitimize trans ideology and transitioning as a diversity to be celebrated, whilst retaining the authority to declare it so as secular priests who are to bless and anoint the trans individual as having passed the test of normality, and by extension placing upon the path of punishment those who disagree and "stigmatize" (a word itself laden with religious symbolism). The guilds have deftly managed to ride the tide of political correctness and understand the powerless ones are actually the trans critics who are to be educated out of their perceived ignorance and prejudice. This transphobic prejudice and the patient's own conflict (introjected prejudice) are considered the object of treatment. And so psychiatry can breed another disorder and another treatment and bask in the light of being the saviours of the people, that is until the suffering that is their product runs its life cycle and they invest themselves in another. If ever the current trans hysteria falls out of favour, the guilds and clinics would quietly pull back and a generation later sell the story that they never believed the nonsense in the first place. I'm not suggesting it's all power politics however. The psychiatric impulse is, and fair enough, one of compassion and care. Yet much infractions upon liberty can be cloaked in the language of care, as can absolving the person of personal responsibility. Other chapters address the same issue. And the language of compassion can be as aggressively weaponised just as suicidality can be weaponised, and both employed in the trans issue to silence the arguments of the trans critics. Something I did also predict and unfortunately did not publish before the fact was that trans persons would be taught that their suicidality lay in their introjected stigma, i.e. other prejudiced persons drive them to suicide, and transitioning in childhood is necessary to save young lives. By extension the message would be it is the trans critic who kills the child. Never mind the buried secrets of the trans person as someone who just might have had small or large "t" traumatic experiences of childhood and that their neurosis extends far beyond the trans question, just as David Reimers suicide (see section on John Money) was more than this also. Never mind that excellent data exist to suggest that transitioning is not the panacea for neurosis and suicidality and that indeed transitioning is far from a cure. For example in the often considered ultra-liberal Sweden, Dhejne and colleagues show even post operative transgender persons have suicidality far above age matched others. Most alarmingly, sex-reassigned individuals remained 4.9 times more likely to attempt suicide and 19.1 times more likely to die by suicide compared to controls in the normal population. Is it not possible that the perceived persecutions by bigots is a red herring? The question of suicidality however is provoking a pragmatic question. Let us say that the experiment was rerun in an alternate universe and Dhejnes cohort not had sex reassignment and the suicide rate been even higher still (i.e. higher than 19 fold the population norm). This would suggest that suicide rates are lowered by transitioning, though not cured. It would also suggest a co-morbid neurosis perhaps driving the transgenderism, or at least be congruent with such a hypothesis. It would not be evidence of the trans construct nor the basis for a political demand on the world any more than stating "I will kill myself if not recognised as being a house cat and allowed sit on any lap I choose" proves I am a cat and that you must acquiesce to my threats. The tragic consequence of a fact does not a posteriori create a different fact entirely. It only does this if one is a philosophical pragmatist. A free person ought never be bullied into assenting to another's fantasy.

The Overextension of Radical Feminism; When Simone de Beauvoir famously wrote that "one is not born, but becomes a woman." she was not referring to the obvious temporal playing out of a person's development such that "a woman does not start off as a baby girl". No she was obviously referring to what she perceived is the oppression placed upon the girl by a patriarchal world to be what men want the woman's role to be. Nonetheless the seeds were sown. Radical feminism continued down the radical rabbit hole, with Judith Butler describing gender as "a free floating artifice, with the consequence that man and masculine might just as easily signify a female body as a male one, and woman and feminine a male body as easily as a female one." And so when feminists wanted the right to be treated like men, and a want to openness for men to be like women (e.g. in assuming the role of what might have been called a housewife), for some the next step would be that the woman might actually be a man, and the man actually be a woman. And when applied to childhood, where early feminists saw (rightly) that a girl can be interested in "boy play", the trans-activists take the liberation further into positing that that girl might be a boy, and vice versa.

The Overextension of Radical Individuality; The trans movement had its start largely on the European mainland, and the Netherlands played a key role in this, as it has in other novel medical practices such as doctors murdering people under the euphemism of physician assisted suicide. Yet there is no denying the United States is a thought leader and focus of cultural shift affecting its own citizenry along with that of other Anglo (and many non Anglo) speaking nations alike. These are often the nations who mock America whilst wilfully becoming her all the same. And part of the American dream in general and especially in following the popular self-psychology movement that prevails to this day is the notion that you can be anything and anyone you want. Indeed, you deserve to be whatever you desire. We have all been exposed to the tropes of the adult who needs go "find", "reinvent" or "discover" themselves when previous generations might have considered these statements evidence of arrested immaturity. There is also the libertarian non-aggression principal that shines on in all those not tainted by psychiatry's diagnostic stains and the overuse of involuntary treatment (i.e. even in hard libertarianism all is permitted if it does not harm others). The social rewards of being seen as tolerant and liberal can become a call for those of the Pharisaic mood who wish to be publically praised to invent new categories of persons to become tolerant about. What necessarily follows is the creation of phantom enemies against which a liberating nation or individual might virtuously fight to save the downtrodden. And these aspirations for liberation and liberating can reach dizzying heights from which bombs of many a kind are dropped, and ironically many liberties are seized upon. The problem is that someone who can sit back and dream of becoming anything at all in the future, is in danger of being simultaneously diffused or limited of knowing and being anything in the present. Every little boy and girl can one day be president the American child is told, being asked to close their eyes to the reality that life does not actually work that way. And so a culture that aspires to radical freedom and lofty aspirations might well be ripe to become a culture radically unanchored to the biological and other givens of the world, and all sorts of experiments in ways of living that John Stuart Mill might have underwritten follow from it. In a country where any little boy (or girl) can become president, any little boy can become a girl. And don't you dare disagree or I'll kill myself, the blood being on your hands.

False Certainty and Radical Insecurity; To anyone honest with themselves and who works as psychiatrist and psychologist, if they are old enough they will come to the illuminated though disenchanted view that people are becoming more insecure and infantilized, and that we now have a society of adults less able to be adults to their children. It is part of the purpose of this book to say that psychiatry and the helping professions, far from curing personality disorders, are actually breeding them on an industrial scale. Now on the matter of personal identity there are two kinds of persons who are strident, dogmatic and insist the world be made in their image or none at all. One kind are those with hyper surety. The jihadi who straps a bomb to his body must be fastened by great faith in the cause and the hereafter to counter the drive to protect their body and life in this world. The other kind of militant individual who cries out to be recognised are those whose identity formation is anything but sure. There is something in the shrill tenor of the trans activists and many of the trans individuals themselves, in frantically wanting children transitioned as soon as possible and in attempting to silence and "de-platform" trans critics that collectively suggest these individuals are anything but sure in their identity and fight against those who fail to recognize it. Quite the contrary. They are, in a classical psychodynamic sense, persons and organizations with borderline personality structures whose identities are diffused and frantically clawing together a sense of solidity when stating they are solidly something they are biologically most certainly are not. Their identity is as fragile as a butterflies wing. The finger that points towards my claim being the truth of their psyche lay in the fact that the trans movement as a whole includes and embraces as valid the gender fluid, the pan gender, and many others crying out for validity. It includes those who say also that their gender depends on the weather, the colour surround and so on. This is an attempt to make solid what is not solid, as if saying it is so makes it so, and screaming it makes it more so. And I'll venture to speculate that part of their psyche is aware of their own terrifying fragility, making the screams even louder and the demands to censor more insistent. The transactivists running the show of asserting identity are persons without identity, and in their strident demands they doth protest too much.

The Death of God and the Atomization of Woman and Man; This book is not an apologetic for any faith, and so the faith of the author (or lack of it as the case may be) is something not relevant to the argument. What is vital to consider is whether Nietzsche's obituary was correct re the death of (the belief in) God. Nowadays Orthodox Christianity does not at all figure in any formulation of humanity and its problems in government, science, medicine and the humanities. All are detached from the faith of old, this fact untouched by whatever attendance the American mega churches gather within and whatever people purport to believe in the various census that fails to measure how people really live their lives. The only echo of a dead God might be certain principles of ethics that form the basis of what remain of our moral givens, yet these too are formulated as if God were never alive to have set the co-ordinates of moral compass to begin with. Instead the appeal is to neuro-ethics, humanist dialectic or a neo-Darwinian utility, with the deity not given his due credit. And with Gods passing passes also the sacred separations and the binaries he announced through the author/s of the book of Genesis. Chapter one is all about separations, and chapter two extends on this to the fundamental variable of the human person in becoming separate from God on one hand, and separated into man and woman on the other. Now in the post-postmodern world man (ironically for lack of a better term to reflect the new potentiality in a trans world of "persons"), is alone. And man is the sole measure and maker of man. And so man will be woman and woman will be man, and both will be animal now and more animal in future. And this diffused trans-human will seek to integrate itself into biological and inorganic technologies that may emerge in time and attempt to make man into man's image of God. Atheist humanists and Orthodox theists alike will see the end of man in the decades and centuries to come. Trans-children are just another step on the road to the tower of Babel inhabited by variations of Baphomet.

Related to the above point is man as a free consumer and unit of consumption. The trading in others (i.e. slavery) was abolished in the west, and racist oppressive separations with it. And this is rightly so. Certain oppressive separations between woman and men had also been removed, taking for example the victories of the suffragette movement. This too is rightly so, with a righteousness such that who am I to even affirm it just as if my opinion matters a damn. And now the trans movement wants its freedoms too, or so goes the narrative. The problem with this ever greater demand of freedom for an ever greater range of identities is not simply that some identities are illegitimate. The problem is the context of the times within which freedom is exercised, this one being consumption and selfish individualism. Some would say a recognition of an ever greater fractionation of identities must lead to an affirmation of the individual after seven billion fractionations are complete. This is philosophically sound as you are not me and I am not you, and a comprehensive description of each other cannot leave any two individuals exactly the same. This too is fair enough and might be a favourable direction to a point insomuch as radical individualism breaks the divide and competition for victimhood between cis vs trans, man vs woman, left vs right, black vs white and so on. My prognosis is more pessimistic, though I think it might be historically borne out in stages and seem a fantastic fiction to the reader now. The current trans movement might simply be a step in a punctuated march towards this bleak future of atomized units where a person once stood. Were I to imagine myself as the marketeer to consumers or a statist agent with power over the person I too would sell trans and many other freedoms and choices besides, targeting a market as young as possible and guilt tripping adults who might run contra the product. And

I too would sell a diverse mix and match product line, where the individual can "discover themselves", be "gender creative" and engineer themselves with biological attributes that in all of human history was labelled as male or female, yet even now is increasingly divorced from sexuality and named on purely anatomical lines, i.e. breast, vagina, penis etc. And another marketed item off the shelf would be gender as self-identity, be that male, female, both, neither or any one of the innumerable other possibilities of infinite alethic fluidity. The manufactured choice would be marketed as the exercise of a freedom of choice or a discovered immutable state of being, each depending upon the political tide of what the consumer wants to hear. And then independent still would be sexual appetites; to have sexual congress with the woman with the penis, the man with the vagina, the gender fluid, the pansexual, the one endowed with both genitalia or whatever. And will the individual choose the wallet or the clutch purse, the dress or the suit or all of the above? All of these freedoms or discoveries would be made by the consumer whilst being steered by myself as marketeer or the state agent with its own agenda as to what it wants the consumer to be in their consumption. Nothing in the person would be solid in time or over time. And so the individual would be a unit of production by the state for state purposes, or a unit of production of the market to be consumed by itself. Forget about the nonsense of the left eating itself in wars between groups in so called identity politics. Even the individual would coil itself up like some pathetic ouroboros and individual identity would eat individual identity. This aided by transhumanist technology marketed to us by our betters would be the final blowing out of the person. What remains in this eschatology would be a being with consciousness and qualia, with drives, emotional states and verbalizations. But we would not recognize this being as something free, individual and human as we know it. It just might think it is. And this is not a leftist or postmodernist conspiracy. It is the inevitable outcome of the enlightenment and modernity.

And so what to do about it?

The answer to the trans question is simple. Any adult who claims to be a man/woman trapped in a woman/mans body arrives at the claim as an adult having reached the age of majority. The trial by which they must pass is a childhood of affirming the sex of their birth, this being part of a child's education into the reality of the world. All efforts to convert the child to a gender incongruent with the biological givens ought to be challenged and prosecuted as acts of child abuse, however well intentioned. That having been said, all bullying of all persons ought to be likewise challenged by the village as aggressive and uncivil acts. In this endeavour we might ironically actually consult those more conservative and transphobic in the art of good manners. Yet bullying against one who holds a belief does not in dint of being bullied prove the belief they hold is true, this being the realization of the most basic logic imaginable. I'm amazed how often it escapes us that perceived victimhood cannot assail truth, only the appearance of it can be overcome. I am further proposing that we consign gender back to the world of language studies and that sex be the sole descriptor applied to the human as something discovered as fact, not assigned as a social construction. Should it come to pass that the child emerges as an adult who wishes change the public face of their identity to that of identifying with the other sex, like any adult they ought to be free to make their own way in the world unto their own "pursuit of happiness", taking sole responsibility for the outcome that they wrought on themselves and paying their own way in the process. They ought to place no expectation upon any other to address them as she or he, or to either perform surgeries upon them or finance the same by the public purse. Amendments to these transactions ought to be completed only on the basis of a contract between free persons, all else being a tyranny. Threats of suicide, however much they might be held as sincere at the time and however tragic if acted upon, also cannot be allowed to be functionally coerce anyone to action about anything. Disagreement is not an act of aggression, and suicide is a choice.

RESPONSIBILITY. AKRASIA AND ENKRATEIA.

"For the good that I would do, I do not; but the evil which I would not, that I do."
St Paul

"But to manipulate men, to propel them towards goals which you-the social reformers-see, but they may not, is to deny their human essence, to treat them as objects without wills of their own, and therefore to degrade them."
Isaiah Berlin

Scarcely a day goes by when I am not confronted with some desperate family member demanding I lock up their drug using loved one and force them into a state of abstinence (I say using and not abusing as one cannot abuse an inanimate substance). To say these family members are well intentioned souls tortured by seeing their significant other destroy their lives at the end of a needle, pipe or bottle is quite obviously the case. They have my sincere sympathies and this chapter is not to trivialize their emotional pain. Nor is it directed at the equally obvious fact that were I to grant the wish and psychiatrically incarcerate the consumer of drugs, that abstinence would endure for only as long as the incarceration persists, along with perhaps an additional few hours or days until they source their drug of choice again. No the question is why drug use, even repeated drug use, is a matter for psychiatry specifically or medicine in general? Why is use per se seen as a health problem? Why will the family member scream down the phone at me that their loved one has a disease and cannot control of their own behaviour, replacing mere implication with the certainty that I must control the consumer's behaviour for them. Why is criminality never mentioned, though throughout my career criminality has almost always been the case (i.e. cannabis for the most part has always been notionally subject to some legal sanction, as has public drunkenness to say nothing of methamphetamine and other "illicit" substances). Why then are police nowhere to be found unless the patient threatens suicide?

Not surprisingly, I place the blame at the feet of psychiatry. Long before Leshner wrote in the journal Science in October 1997 the non sequitur "that addiction is tied to changes in brain structure and function is what makes it, fundamentally, a brain disease," psychiatry viewed it in the same way. And to this day one will be hard pressed to find an article by the psychiatric intelligentsia that does not refer to drug use as a public health problem, repeated use as "addiction", a "chronic relapsing disorder", a "brain disease" or many other medicalized and materialistic permutations of the same.

The Reward Pathway

Almost every review article of addiction will mention the so called 'reward pathway" and "neuro-circuitry" of addiction. I'll hazard to say that the whole reward and addiction pathway story philosophically revolves around not a circuit (which is circular) or a pathway (which is a metaphor involving something material by which a person with agency may move from point A to point B). Instead the "pathway" is, at its most basic, the physical extension of nerves fibres from an area deep in the brain (the ventral tegmental area, or VTA), to another area deep in the brain (the nucleus accumbens, or NA). This single extension constitutes part of the "mesolimbic pathway", a pathway which psychiatric trainees and medical students will also invoke if they are asked what pathway in its excess is involved with some of the expressive symptoms of psychosis. The chemical substance released from the former (VTA) onto the latter (NA) is called dopamine, and many a lay reader will have heard of it. A hedonic mental experience correlates with pleasure seeking behaviour externally and correlates also biologically with an activation of the mesolimbic pathway and dopamine release. From this basic splay of neurons we can elaborate many other inputs and outputs, from which circular feedback loops can be said to truly occur. There are bidirectional connections between the mesolimbic pathway and the frontal cortex, the amygdala, the hippocampus and other centres, like fractals within fractals each of these areas contains sub-centres and sub-circuits also. Let us not do an injustice to the complexity of the brain, which is gargantuan. In fact, given that the whole array of "circuits" include sensory perception apparatus (of cues) and the motor outputs towards behaviour, anyone with a modicum of imagination and an undergraduate knowledge of neuroscience can construct a model of addiction and circuitry involving the whole brain without exception of any part. And why stop at the brain when the circuit extends out into the world, as it does in any system of input and output. Feedback and prima facie causal circuits reach back tens of thousands of years and outwards thousands of kilometres of space. This is not a biological model extended to absurdity, though it does reveal something of the silliness and arbitrary nature of the neuroscientist who, when examining a complex social behaviour, points to a part of the brain and says "there it is", "there begins and ends the circuit". By the same token neither is it absurd to say that the materialist philosophy behind the biology all boils down to doing something that gives you pleasure and that little squirt of dopamine you get from it. Whatever other brain centres are required, and however the consciousness is thought to be an emergent distributed property, the binding together of more than one brain module, in some way the materialists ultimately think that little spurt of dopamine is you. As was made clear in chapter 3, does it really add anything to the metaphysics of the mind brain / body problem to say that the mesolimbic pathway is further connected to area X of the brain which correlates or thought to be involved with impulsive inhibition, or area Y thought to be involved in anticipation and expectation, or area Z with anxiety as a driving force to use? As was also made clear in chapter 3, between mind and matter is a metaphysical divide that I contend will never be bridged. And a knowledge of biological connectedness does not advance us one jot or tittle towards the answer of phenomenological binding in consciousness.

Many more facts besides make the brain disease story problematic. Firstly, the same mesolimbic reward pathway is involved in any hedonic experience. It is not pathognomonic of addiction and does not make of it a different category to habitual pleasure seeking in work, love and play. Nor do elaborations outwards from the basic mesolimbic core constitute the coming into being of addiction, for they too are common. Take for example the cues to nostalgia and romance from a sight not seen for years. Or an anxiety provoking day at work associated with the want to get to the car and listen to favourite relaxing music for the drive home, or simply to "get pissed". All pleasures and pains and hedonic seeking involve more than the mesolimbic pathway, without a categorical divide within the brain. And plasticity of these pathways is a response to use, not the cause of use, even repeated use, which is choice.

Secondly, this biological reduction is predicated on what the brain is seen as being, either something we are or a tool we use. People use pathways vs people are pathways is the basic philosophical point of division, also as partially addressed in chapter 3.

Thirdly there is the non sequitur of a change in structure and function in the balance of power between pathways somehow being the argument of the change in the brain being a disease. A change in structure and function is often a consequent of use, lack of use or misuse as the case may be. Learn a musical instrument or a martial art. Change in structure and function of the brain. Become a cabbie and learn the knowledge of the London streets. Change in structure and function of the brain. Decide to languish in a haze of cannabis smoke. Change in structure and function of the brain. Switching from the lifestyle of the latter to that of the former, or the former to the latter will involve a change in structure and function of the brain. Even a materialist must of necessity admit this is the case, as their whole metaphysics is dependent on this basic fact. Now some changes in behaviour and consequent structural and functional changes are harder won (or lost) than others. This is a microcosm for life writ large where the good, the beautiful and the true takes effort and sacrifice. And there are horizons of potentiality beyond which no human can pass, whether that be their brains or themselves. Anyone involved in recovery from stroke or anyone wishing to add to any skill base knows this well. But in the absence of a stronger argument of why change is disease, I will continue to insist that the behaviour and what one does with the will is the dysfunction and it is only in metaphorical terms a disease. That drug use is often maladaptive and repeated compulsive use to the exclusion of more fruitful behaviour is harmful to the user and society alike is a common sense truism. We also ought to grant that certain connections (impulsiveness inhibition pathways for example) become weaker in the addict and maladaptive behaviour promoting pathways said to be become stronger, just as an unused muscle may atrophy. But a pathway and its weakening/strengthening is a correlate to the self, not a determinant of the self, and not a definition of what the self in its being is. No one has found the self in the brain. The brain is the canvas upon which the addict paints their will. No one can paint too far outside the lines, though everyone can choose where they apply colour and shade and when they paint over what has been done before.

But the Addict is Robbed of Free Will. They Are Special.

Nonsense. Beyond this desk where I write this chapter is a door. And beyond the door are hospital patients. And I read from the patient presentation list that one is a child with an allergic rash, one is a pregnant woman with problematic vomiting, another is an elderly gent with hip pain and possible fracture, another child has asthma, another is "post ictal" (i.e. has had an epileptic seizure). There are several "chest pains", and it's more than likely at least one of these is having a heart attack, soon to vanish downstairs to the cardiac lab. The list continues on and on. Now I ask the reader to engage in a simple exercise of calibrating their common sense intuitions with the reality of the world.

I invite the reader to imagine something brutal to be sure, an experiment I'm not ever suggesting be done in fact. Yet here is our gedanken experiment.

Imagine yourself holding a gun to the head of the pregnant woman. She is informed that if she vomits you pull the trigger. Or toward the elderly man with the busted hip you point the gun. As Christ told the cripple to up and walk, you say the same. Or the asthmatic turning blue you tell them they get the bullet if they do not under sheer force of will open up and re-oxygenate their bronchiolar tree. Or the patient infected with the virus they must will a billion viral particles dead. Or the epileptic will face our little firing squad if they don't hold themselves back from the seizure. Or tell the skin not to rash at point of a gun. On and on the list goes. These are disease over which the person has limited to no control. Now we might say that the heart attack is informed by poor diet and such or the hyperemesis is informed by the choice to do what one necessaries in order to become pregnant. This is not the point. Nor is it the point that the mind can do amazing things all on its own to modulate pain and to soldier on in the face of injury and disability. With some Herculean effort people can even hold back an insistent diarrhoea for a little while, or hold back a cough until with tears in their eyes they can hold back no longer. Psyche and the soma are linked for sure. Yet common sense often defines the limits of mind over matter, and we need not call upon the doctor to instruct us. Even those yogis who are said to be able levitate (though no one ever seems to film them) seem ironically unable alter the shape of their lens. Consequently, even they put on their spectacles in the morning. Returning to our diabolical little experiment, the odds all would be shot would be high indeed. Their disease will have its way with them and there is little they can directly do against it.

Now let's imagine the same experiment, only this time replacing the above subjects with the alleged disease of addiction. Now the trigger is pulled if they reach for the bottle or the pipe, the bong or the needle. And our subjects know we are serious as they have seen us execute the previous cohort of innocent women and children. Try not allow our common sense intuition be contaminated with what we think may happen as per our indoctrination by psychiatry. This is not a psychiatric guild exam. This is reality we are appealing to now. What say the reader? Will they reach for the drug? Will the trigger be pulled or not?

I have not the slightest doubt that if such an experiment were performed that the survival rate would be enormously high, proof positive and beyond dispute that drug use is neither seizure nor rash, stroke nor vomiting. It is pure and simple choice. Will power, as terribly unfashionable as it is, exists!

As it so happens, the experiment has been run by a real monster. Mao Tse-Tung and the Communist party of China took power in the 1949 revolution and set about reforming the country. Part of the problem that Mao faced were anywhere from ten to dozens of millions were addicted to opiates (mostly opium itself). That they were addicted, I will argue, was a matter of choice though it didn't help that the British had forced the opium trade upon them and even fought two wars to this end in 1839 and 1856 respectively. You see in those day we did not fight the war on drugs so much as fought a war for drugs or the war with drugs. Mao wasn't about to waste tens of millions of bullets, and people means productivity for a new power on the march. Later with the great leap forward these tens of millions would kill off literally billions of rats, insects and small birds in order to fix several other real public health crises of the times (but that's another story). And so Mao staged some very real yet very symbolic brutal public executions of drug barons and simply told the addicted masses to give up the poppy for the good of the people or die as an enemy of the state. And give up they did. Now I'll grant the story is not as simple as that. Mao was not driven by principle as from political pragmatics. An earlier Mao himself traded opium out of Yanan to finance the revolutionary effort. A later Mao killed many more tens of millions than he sought to save. And for the teeming mass of comrades he saved to then kill, ceasing opium took effort and a mobilizing of mass social pressures also, a drive to a new state of belonging part of the people by seeing opiates as the enemy, not in toto a bad thing. And whilst he decimated opium use he did not eliminate it completely. Forever and always there will be an underground drug trade and organized crime. Still, no one can deny that Mao ran the world's largest and by far most successful drug rehab facility, putting to shame the best rehab clinic you will ever find in the western world. If the incentives are perceived as being high enough, people can and do exercise choice.

The next political figure to do even a remotely similar thing was Richard Nixon and his "Operation Golden Flow". In the closing days of the Vietnam war many thousands of American serviceman were "addicted" to heroin, which I'd speculate was readily available in the golden triangle after Mao pushed the centre of production south. American serviceman also used copious amounts of military sanctioned stimulants, cannabis and psychedelics, though this too is another story and the balance shifted more towards heroin by 1971. Nixon was concerned that returning serviceman would remain addicts and join the ranks of the urban black underclass. His solution was a simple one. A seat on the plane stateside was contingent on them being clean from heroin. Those who did not take him seriously were turned away at the tarmac until they proved themselves clean. Lo and behold these soldiers terribly afflicted with the disease of addiction, with supposedly reorganized and "hijacked" reward pathways stopped use and got on the plane. Even more surprising to disease mongers, only a minority continued a life of heroin state side, and only a minority of addicts even sought replacement of heroin with cannabis and alcohol, the latter of which has always been a problem. Back in the land of the free and the home of the brave they no longer faced intermittent cycles of monsoon and mosquitoes, of boredom and bullets and blood or any of the usual sights and smells of Vietnam. They had different connections and different meanings. All of this was the connective tissue upon which a change in choices was made. But it would be as much a nonsense to say that a Saigon Monsoon bio-mechanistically caused them to use heroin as it would be to say the sight of the statue of liberty bio-mechanistically caused them to stop. Indeed, it cannot even be easily argued that drug use was fuelled by psychological trauma of war. Just as much use was had by those who never approached the front line. It was part of the counterculture of the 60's and 70's to use drugs. People used drugs because they wanted to and enjoyed the altered mental state more than they disliked the consequences. It has always been thus.

Incidentally, punishment has a flip side, that being reward. There is abundant evidence that addicts given cash incentives can modify behaviour. Scale it up and imagine our patient with atopy who will get a luxury holiday if their skin does not rash, vs the addict who will get the same if they refrain from substances. Do we seriously think both are diseases equally beyond personal control? Would we seriously place our bets symmetrically across both groups?

Why do we see some people as powerless to addiction?

Part of the problem is the overreach of medicalized thought, of genetic determination, of brain pathways etcetera (vide supra). Part of the problem is also phenomenological and philosophical, something I'll call the cannot/do not fallacy. The addict might be described as someone who desires not to use and might be painfully aware of the negative consequence to use, both in their lives and that of loved ones. But they use anyway. (Or they might be described as someone who denies the painful obvious fact of their misuse. That said, even those disinclined to believe a psychodynamic psychology of "psychotic denial" will see in the addict who says they don't have a problem the want to deny the obvious, an implicit acknowledgement that even they know the truth). And yet despite the desire not to use they find themselves compulsively using, where compulsivity is a technical term of art to mean they have a powerful internal drive within them that results in the behaviour (the compulsion), a drive which is discharged for a time after use only then for it to gather force again. And so the addict might pass through all of life saying they are doing something they do not wish to do, yet do anyway. Surely they are moulded into an automaton with their conscious awareness of the events only going along for the ride? Here is the point where we ought not to lose our phenomenological, or logical, nerve. For it does not follow that from what one does do, that one cannot do differently.

To begin, people have mixed motives. By exercising choice, the user may be advised start their road to abstinence by forcing their will into the moment of clarity in seeing just how they lie to themselves. There is a part of the addict who derives satisfaction from use. One hears all the time from psychiatry ever greater procrustean reasons why the addict might want use, almost always at some point allowing the user absolve themselves of responsibility. Absolution from responsibility is the zeitgeist. I can and have lived literally years without ever hearing from a psychiatric colleague that being drunk or high simply feels good, and desiring what feels good is as human as being human can get. And this part of the addict dislikes the discomfort of the come down, withdrawal or the boredom of returning back to a world of abstinence. This part of the addict would rather we stop badgering them and allow them have their high. And this part of the addict will pay lip service to the impact of their use, as a means to garner sympathy or simply have the complainant shut up for a time. We cannot discount the place of subtle agency in choosing this part of ourselves and wanting to be an addict even when other parts of ourselves wish we were not. It is not fashionable to press this fact upon the user as psychiatry is full of soft caring minds in socialist health care, that or small business people who do not wish to irritate a consumer out of using their services. Nor would psychiatrists like to admit that to declare the patient bereft of free will is in proportion with elevating the intensity of the problem and themselves as the intelligentsia with the expertise to stop something beyond the patients control. Viewing addiction as a brain disease is also an excellent strategy to gather funding for the research industry. When the reality of an alleged medical illness is brought under question, follow the chain of whose egos benefit from the medicalization. And follow the money to the thought leaders in the field, and to the regulatory and research agencies for profit from it. And remember the psychiatric ethos as per previous chapters. The epistemology is pragmatic. The truth is what is useful. Nothing is more useful than money and power.

Secondly, we must not medicalise too much this moral weakness in the will of the addict as if it is a unique and reified phenomenological category. Take the following examples. Someone wants dearly to apologize for that offence made years earlier. But they never pick up the phone. Or they want to learn that foreign language and never pick up the book. Or they want to correct their diet and never give the dessert spoon a rest. Or they always say they will take out the garbage. Sure enough they feel guilty if they don't, yet never take it out anyway. Or they want to exercise more and yet never buy the running shoes. Or they wish to overcome their fear of flight. Or they find themselves each week writing a list to write to that old friend and the list carries over weekly in the diary for years (something I'm guilty of). Or they fly off the handle and become irritable, regretting their anger later and vowing to change. The list is endless. I do what I do not want to do they say, and from it they say (not altogether erroneously) I am what I do not wish to be. Yet would we say they too are addicts of a kind? Would we say they are automatons to their faulty brain circuits? Not at all. We would say they are human. Most humans, nay all humans on some level, never gain a victory over themselves. They are akrasia versus enkrateia, score 1:0. The addict simply sits upon a spectrum upon which we all, without exception, stand. We might all say we love to gaze on the beauty of nature and we all care about the environment, But the smart phone and automobile has brought to the fore just how "addicted" we all are. In fact, rather than my banal examples arguing against the medicalization of addiction, in our age the banal has been swept into it. Think of the aggressive and adulterous celebrity who sheds crocodile tears as they speak of their "sex addiction" and their "anger disorder". Some psychologists seriously lobbied to include compulsive shopping disorder in DSM 5. People want to lie to themselves and in psychiatry they have a secular priest only too willing to give them the demon addiction they are possessed with, absolve them of responsibility and then enter into an exorcism not likely to end.

This is where we come closer to approaching the cannot/ do not fallacy. Imagine any one of these individuals manage to escape the gravity of habit and inner conflict, the drug user included. This will surely be a proof not just of the exercise of free will in general as it also be a proof the requisite quanta of free will, the moral strength, the will power, exists in them as individuals. We might say (though this would be silly), that they have the lucky gene of free will or their frontal lobes luckily managed to seize the balance of power that fateful day the tide against addiction turned. And there will be much rejoicing. Yet what of those who pass through life and draw their final breath always dipping their toe into the pool of a life better lived (i.e. abstinence), yet never to take the plunge. It will be concluded as an empirical fact that they lacked the constitutional strength to make that change, the proof being the outcome come the end of the trial, our natural experiment. And this will be inductively taken to be proof that there are a class of people who truly are compulsive automatons, who cannot change and so need either saving or excuse mongering. From this will come ever greater elaborations towards hijacked brains and overpowered and reorganized brain circuits, of fMRI results and all manner of nonsense and psychiatric industry. But pray tell how can anyone conclude from an unrealised outcome that the person lacked the potential? How are they seers of souls in order to reach this conclusion? It is as if to say that if they see me die having never purchased that item on the shelf what follows is to conclude I never had the funds in my wallet? How do they know that? How can they know that? The assumptions made are logical fallacies of the highest stupidity.

Besides, saying that some people cannot ever control themselves irresistibly attracts many others who wish to be included in the leagues of the powerless to excuse themselves of their misbehaviour. Absolution of large responsibilities is the gateway drug to absolution from all. There is abundant experimental evidence in the psychological literature showing that if subjects are lead to have their belief in free will challenged, they tend towards more selfish and immoral behaviour. Perhaps addiction disease mongers come close to actually breeding the very thing they think is a fact of the world, the disease they wish to cure.

Driving in the Wedge of Choice

Before becoming as jaded as I am, I spent a great deal of time diving deep into the phenomenology of my patients, far more than I can speak of most of my colleagues as ever doing. Where they would spend 45 minutes in psychiatric assessment and the standard interview, I may spend another 90 minutes in conversation exploring the mind of the addict who chose to admit they had a problem. In my own practice I have never ever met the addict who did not have those times, even a fleeting daily moment, when their consciousness and conscience did not exist at a mental crossroads. On one side of the crossroads was the drive to use. On the other the call to the duty not to, all that they said they wanted to do and be, or all they wanted not to do and not to be. And in the middle they stood, unable to deny that however weak and feeble they were, however much the product of habit had them pointing their feet in the direction of use, that weak and feeble person went by one name and that name was choice. My primary psychotherapy for addicts is to take those times, stand within that moment, choose to rip it open ever wider and choose to stand within that time as an ongoing moment. So as not to find oneself mindlessly walking left at the crossroads, make each moment a moment of choice. Opening up this moment to a state of permanent choice creates a tension one will wish to escape. But hold the tension all the same, for the tension is choice and emotional discomfort an exposure to how weakly we have exercised it. Always be aware of the temptation to collapse the choice into habit and always be aware how wily the will to use can be in presenting the mind with a lie. The house needs milk. I am going to buy milk. Is my dealer loitering near the grocery store? Is the liquor store next door to the grocery store? Will that step towards the much needed milk bring me closer to using or further away? If so then say no to milk or go purchase milk with each moment a meditation not on the goal of the milk as opposed to the goal not to use. Never let the guard down until a change in behaviour creates a new armour and many chapters are written into a life of different habits. Addiction is that part of yourself that will tell the little lies you want to believe, in order to keep you bound.

For some the fight against addiction means going a step further and changing ones set and setting. Like Odysseus resisting the sirens call, if not attending parties will sustain sobriety then bind yourself and don't attend. Or go further, question the very value of parties. If it means changing work to a lower paying less tempting job, then do that also. If it means leaving the sweetheart who keeps you in the gutter with the bottle that is a choice also. Odysseus chose to be bound to the mast and his sailors chose for their ears be filled with beeswax. The sirens call is more addictive to any drug. I am Hermes to your Circe, and can only offer the advice you already know to be true. The rest is up to you.

A note on Liberty and Decriminalization

Hopefully I have convinced the reader that addiction is not a medical disease, and that it ought to be uncoupled from psychiatric industry and ideology. Is this to imply it is not a social ill either, or that the user ought to be left in the gutter to rot? Not at all. There are medications that can assist the addict in the utilization of their choices to the life better lived. These are currently the province of doctors to prescribe, though often ought to be prescribed far less than they are, as addicts can easily just exchange one drug for another. I've known people who spent five years on heroin and then the rest of their lives on methadone (which is similarly dangerous) or buprenorphine, making of the psychiatrist someone no different than an alternate drug dealer failing to act on the principle that a drug that is not medically required ought not to be prescribed, except as a transitional object towards no drug at all. And for those wishing to escape the gutter any healthy society would naturally foster the power of family and benevolent institutions to help them, of greater connectedness to their fellow man (and woman). Part of the thesis of Johann Hari's bestseller "Chasing the Scream", was the revelation that drug use often correlates with lack of social connectedness and is remedied by the same? This is evidenced both in observation of humans and the "rat park" work of Bruce Alexander. I wish not to scorn Hari's valuable book, and encourage the reader towards it. Yet only a world made sick from self interest and excess medicalization would be surprised at a fact so obvious. Social connectedness a salve for the addict? Who would have thought? Astonishing!

But what of the law? In this I am with a different author, that being Peter Hitchens in his brilliant book "The War We Never Fought", another I can commend to the reader. In my own psychiatric practice, I've never seen the war on drugs as seriously being fought. Certainly the western world has never done as Singapore does and never did as Mao did. And so our governments may wish not to fight the war if they wish, though it would be disingenuous to say it was fought and lost. Unless a police officer takes a particular disliking to a person or there are multiple or repeated other charges I've never seen drug laws seriously prosecuted. Most of the time all a drug possessor or petty dealer need do to avoid going down the road of any minor prosecution is claim to be suicidal. They will be dumped off at the hospital and that will be the end of it, the police thanking their lucky stars they dodged some extra paperwork. To such a person I ask them please quid quo pro. Be kind to the psychiatrist and recant the insincere threat when the police leave the emergency department. Should the user happen to face the magistrate for drug offences there may be a fine they have no intention of paying and the state will not pursue, or a claim to a history of mental illness will be made. They will then be leaving the dock to enter not a prison cell, but the sunshine outside, if not the rooms of a psychiatrist. And so the cycle will repeat. And the street will know that apart from some fancy seizures of supply and arrests of middle and top tier dealers and distributors, that there is no real risk to the user from state, regardless of what the law might say.

Does this imply I suggest the war on drugs ought to be fought? Not necessarily. My own inclination is towards a radical liberty and to remind the reader of Mills axiom

"The only purpose for which power may be rightfully exercised over any member of a civilized community, against his will, is to prevent harm to others. His own good, either physical or moral, is not a sufficient warrant."

Of course it is possible to argue that the addict has left the civilized community and so is in forfeit of liberty. However, that would open us towards the slippery slope of a state which could arbitrarily divide the citizen from the barbarian, and so enslave or tyrannize the populace on mass if they fail to make the grade.

The problem is not entirely resolved however, neither by cherry picking statistics from the pro drug Portuguese statistics favourable to the libertarian cause, or by the principal of carte blanche libertarianism itself. For the libertarian, a mereological problem arises with the accretion of liberties within the one person, when each liberty can be argued to be valid on its own. Might there not arise problems from combinatorial freedoms? And moreover the problem is the effect this necessarily has upon others in the liberal society simply from the exercising of these multiple liberties. Let us imagine the case of the cannabis addict who fritters away their day in an unmotivated haze, this mixed with occasional paranoia. Now we might be able bring ourselves to the callousness of turning our back on them, especially if they wish us to. But they will break their families heart and purse. Are we to be callous to this also? Are we expecting that their family enter into that nirvana state of liberal individualism, to harden their own hearts, to "look after number 1" and simply cease to be attached to kin? And what if the product of the users liberty is to burden the tax payer with the cost of a disability pension they have obtained on account of the psychiatrist who described them as having exercised choices masquerading as "a brain disease"? Ought the liberty to become stoned entail a loss of liberty to the tax payer in having the fruits of their labour taken from them, even if this fiscal injury is just one slice in the death by a thousand cuts? And what if stoner, in or out of their paranoia, becomes violent? Cannabis alone can add to the disconnect between the potentially moral actor and the immoral act, though methamphetamine or alcohol can also clinch the deal or do perfectly well on their own. It is all well and good to speak of persons as having liberties up to the point of the fist actually hitting the face, though this is of little comfort to the neighbour of the ice addict waving their fist in the air. Let's take it a step further. You might own a gun for protection and I might own the same. The American reader might see this as a constitutional right, and the state having no right to obstruct one who might bear the firearm to the ends of their own protection within the boundaries of their own property. I am sympathetic to the sentiment. Yet back we are to the question of combinatorial liberties. Do we defend the right of the methamphetamine user to patrol their cannabis farm in the wee hours of the morning with shotgun and machete at their side? The shot is not fired yet the menace is hardly trivial. Does it really make any difference if we take the shotgun from them if they have the machete, or more lethal still the automobile? Or what are the elderly to do in a yet to be gentrified part of town when they do not feel safe to go outside and into the howls of drunken and drug addled masses, though no violence has yet been done? These are very difficult questions, questions in which all libertarians must imagine themselves to be the elderly neighbour of one who is intoxicated and unpredictable, or the parent of children living on the other side of the fence. Yet these are neither medical or public health questions. These are moral, social and political questions. A civil society cannot endlessly sustain a mismatch between liberty and responsibility. We cannot allow liberty to do anything and everything one wishes within the non-aggression principle without the calculus of risks increasing beyond the braking strain.

Some Small Steps Within Liberty

I do not pretend to yet have the answer to the question of what to do in law when individual liberties collide with one another. But as one experienced doctor committed to the fact that drug use a matter of choice, I think that I and any citizen ought to have the liberty to make clear what is clear; that is that addiction almost certainly always results in one or another kind of harm to others. The current treatment paradigm in addiction psychotherapy is the cycle of change model of Prochaska and DiClemente, this asking us to identify how prepared the user is to change (pre-contemplation/not interested, contemplating change, preparation for change, action within change, maintaining abstinence) and tailor our psychotherapeutic approach accordingly. Actually I'm quite sympathetic to the model in itself. Providing it not be dogmatized, it has much merit. As practiced, it unfortunately very often also asks us also to imagine the addict like approaching a fragile and flighty animal of the wild (my analogy, not theirs). Approach too fast or with too great a spirit of confrontation and it will turn tail and dart off into the forest. Or put another way, if the addict is not ready or putting up psychological "resistance" we are to simply invite them for a conversation when they are ready. To do otherwise is to risk frightening them off for good. And heaven forbid us being "judgmental"! Even when they are ready for change we are told to help them identify their own reasons, as if to prescribe additional reasons would be to scare them once again into the dreaded state of being "pre-contemplative to change". Rarely if ever are moral duties part of the picture presented to them. It's always about the pros and cons as the patient sees them, this being more pragmatism, more atomized "me, myself and I" ism in this case. Pragmatism be damned. I'll submit it ought to be part of every therapeutic encounter that the addict is given a healthy dose of Burkian thought, a dose of reality that their use is a failure to return on the investment made by their forbearers and a failure to attend to the needs of those in the present and future. And regular users of intoxicants ought to be assumed incapable of holding a firearms or driving licence at all, not simply at times of confirmed intoxication. They ought to be told at each encounter that intoxication will not save them from the full force of the law for whatever sins of violence and mischief when drunk or stoned or high.

So an exchange might go something like this, and for the materialist I'll include some of what they are wishing to be included also. Let's imagine the conversation is with a crack cocaine or methamphetamine addict. We might say, as is patently obvious, that cessation is a matter of choice towards being a better version of themselves. We might warn them that their mesolimbic pathway has become a tad lazy in the excesses of its exposures and downregulated its dopaminergic apparatus, though only by about 10-15% so says the data (a similar thing occurs in medicated ADHD kids, so parents be warned). These neurological changes may persist for many many months and in abstinence correlate with lower mood, craving and a lack of hedonic response to what other people experience as healthy simple pleasures (though I'm not at all sold on the notion the biology is the whole story). Not a very enticing prognosis in the short to mid-term. But they can nobly bear it if they choose, and gain existential (though not hedonic) satisfaction that in abstinence they are not participating in a sequence of transactions that has vicious biker thugs acquiring luxury real estate and people being fed to dogs in some Mexican cartel town. I will tell them that without drug use they can study. They can get a job. They can be someone worthy of a worthy cause if they wish, they can love and be loved.

Or what of person in their late teens or early twenties who "self medicates" their anxiety with cannabis and spends all day either playing video games, getting stoned and amotivated and occasionally loitering in the nearby skateboard park.

They are, needless to say, unemployed and not in study. They are, needless to say, each day moving closer to a future of becoming unemployable altogether, if not chronically psychotic. To grant them the radical liberty to use ought we not also to grant them the radical responsibility of their actions? We can offer them the psychotherapy to help with the underlying anxiety, it being an article of faith on our part that the anxiety is anything more than an excuse and to be formulated as a want to "self medicate". To take the offer is up to them. If they don't, surely the tax payer ought not to be burdened with a lifetime of paying for the sequelae from their habit. But these users know they exist within liberal democracies with social security safety nets (even the United States has a robust safety net). And so across the world the user in the fact of their using chooses to make their fellow citizens suffer. We might inform the user that every day they get stoned that their parents (if they have parents or anything approaching an intact family) suffer on account of their choices. And if they, or we, cannot bring ourselves to be sympathetic to their parent's plight in virtue of the parents being abusive, neglectful and failing terribly in their own duties, there is that ten year old neighbour on one side who deserves an adequate older role model. There is the octogenarian on the other side who deserves the caring visit of someone from time to time. We should not be shy of telling this young person that the sins of their own omissions lead to the sufferings of both neighbours and the world at large. The world at large need repeat the same to them, for large scale social shaming does work and has value of its own. The user sits as a nexus between generations. To both neighbours they have responsibility, in addition to themselves.

It makes little difference to drug addiction if the drugs are either decriminalized or legalized. Granted white collar entrepreneurs are less savage than organized drug criminals, though being able to operate and profit above or within the law does not save one from the core sociopathy of greed and callous exploitation of another. It merely tempers the manifestation of it and diffuses it such that the harms are less graphic. The user might choose to make the entrepreneur rich, just as they have the cartel or meth lab. More fool them. Likewise, decriminalization will almost certainly result in a larger government bloated with layers of regulatory and taxation apparatus, with bloated social security needs and with the taxation revenue going wherever the government wishes, including military excursions that make feeding a Mexican villager to a dog look like a minor misdemeanour. Yet the problem is this, the problem being one which the state is just all too willing to collude with the polis to bring about. Our crack addict or alcoholic or cannabis stoner cannot be an informed and rational actor. The state finds itself in the midst of optimizing the outcome of two intersecting functions. The first to keep the polis productive enough to maximize taxation and state income as a corporate entity whilst retaining political power. The second to render the polis too distracted and intoxicated to exercise free thought. The addict contributes to these problems, much like the populace soaked up the drug SOMA in Huxleys Brave New World. This, along with the failure of the addict to live up to the potential within themselves and their potential to their kin and the village is what makes even legalized addiction a moral wrong and a depreciation of the rational actor part of the equation the libertarian wishes to strengthen. A libertarian political realist would see that the road to legalized carte blanche drug use is likely the road towards a larger government, this also being contra the libertarian mission. The problem with uncompromising libertarians is that, like those who do not read Kants ethics carefully, they fail to see that liberty and certain categorical imperatives exists within a civil society, not without. And why promote a change that can only result in greater barbarism?

SANITY. ON AGREEING TO DISAGREE

"What would have happened if they [new methods of physical and chemical psychiatric treatments] had been available for the last five hundred years?... John Wesley who had years of depressive torment before accepting the idea of salvation by faith rather than good works, might have avoided this, and simply gone back to help his father as curate of Epworth following treatment. Wilberforce, too, might have gone back to being a man about town, and avoided his long fight to abolish slavery and his addiction to laudanum. Loyola and St Francis might also have continued with their military careers. Perhaps, even earlier, Jesus Christ might simply have returned to his carpentry following the use of modern [psychiatric] treatments"

William Sargent (psychiatrist)

"All are lunatics, but he who can analyze his delusions is called a philosopher."
Ambrose Bierce

Whatever science is, is debatable. However, in what is arguably the world's most prestigious and aptly, if unimaginatively titled, scientific journal, "Science", its January 1973 issue published what was arguably more a piece of investigative journalism than a representation of the journals namesake. Whatever it was, I commend you all to read and read again the aptly titled "On Being Sane in Insane Places". The cast were 8 in number, including the articles author himself, Professor of Psychology David Rosenhan. Each presented to various psychiatric admissions departments, from east to west coast of the USA. Disguising their real identity (except at some level for Rosenhan, informing the hospital executive who ostensibly kept the matter secret from the treating staff), they all reported hearing a voice say notionally enigmatic things, "dull", thud", "empty" and also all reported a non-descript sense of existential disquiet, what Jaspers may, at a stretch, have considered a primary delusion. Apart from this, in every other way they behaved normally. Every one of them was diagnosed with a serious mental illness. All were hospitalized. All were medicated with powerful major tranquilizers (aka antipsychotics), though almost all the medications were pocketed or water closeted.

Several conclusions of this study were obvious, chiefly that psychiatrists cannot distinguish the real from the fake, and from this we might be tempted to question what is, or if there is, real psychosis is at all. Or to put another way, all diagnosis in psychiatry can be said to be couched on an implicit act of faith in one's fellow man to be as they say they are. Additionally, the study demonstrated the irresistible pull of diagnosis. Psychiatrists simply cannot live without it. They lose all moorings without the labels they ascribe to people, and a history of the silliness of psychiatric taxonomy is not far from being equivalent to the history of psychiatry in toto.

Apart from the devastating core finding, several more observations or conclusions can be drawn, some of which I observe to persist across time and space to my own career.

Firstly, American psychiatry may not have needed the DSM to achieve inter-rater reliability (i.e. consistency in agreement between different diagnosticians as to the diagnosis in like kinds of presentations). As stated, all patients were diagnosed with mental illness. Seven of eight of the patients were diagnosed on admission with schizophrenia, these same seven being diagnosed with "schizophrenia in remission" on discharge. Rosenhans study illustrates that prior to DSM III, psychiatrists were perhaps more reliable than they are now. The only problem is they were reliably wrong at the outset, and reliably too arrogant to simply revise their diagnosis to the admission they got it wrong. The most reliable of diagnosticians are those who practice the zodiac. Just ask the person their date of birth. The rest is easy. And so what?

Secondly, were these same patients to live in an age with rapid electronic communication and integrated hospital databases, they would be on record as having a history of schizophrenia, and any future unusual behaviour would be interpreted with this past in full view. The next admission may well be longer still, for a patient can be in remission from an illness, but remission is not synonymous with cure. It should not be lost on the reader that this forever binds the patient to psychiatry even when they walk out beyond the threshold of the hospital gate. On re-entry more would need be done the second time around, possibly a long acting injectable antipsychotic (though this was not available in the early 70's), especially were it to be discovered they threw the pills in the loo as this is historical evidence of "lack of insight" and "non-compliance" with oral agents. Schizophrenia is one of many diagnoses that is for life, a stain that can never be washed away. The only cure is a complete revision of history for the patient him/herself, or better yet for the whole of psychiatry. And Rosenhan himself also chillingly writes "eventually, the patient himself accepts the diagnosis, with all the surplus meanings and expectations, and behaves accordingly". Or as every good torturer knows, they all break eventually.

Thirdly, the average length of (involuntary) stay in the experiment was 19 days. Putting aside the moral aspect of this extended deprivation of liberty (more than some criminals face in the penal system for serious offences), and putting aside the cost of the medications that pollute whatever ecology the sewer pipes drain into, the real cost of the study in today's dollar terms was enormous. (average 19 days/pseudo-patient X 8 pseudo-patients X at least $1000/day is >$150,000). It is remarkable that these hospitals or the state did not file suit for fraud. My suspicion they did not do this was on account of the publicity that would have surely resulted, and the many weaknesses in the psychiatric art that would surely have come to light was the greater liability.

Fourthly, "real" patients often detected that the pseudo-patient was a fake, though this was not the case with staff. Moreover, Rosenhan himself observed that most of the time the allegedly authentically insane co-patients were as normal as him.

Fifth, Rosenhans pseudo-patients quantified the numbers or time of encounters between staff and patient and he writes "those with the most power have the least to do with patients, and those with the least power are most involved with them". I've observed this myself. Psychiatrists will in the abstract say they like and wish to help people (don't we all?). In private practice they do just that, as a person seen is money earned (and from more of the former flows more of the latter, as with any small business). But my observation is that most psychiatrists, however much they may say they like people, don't like that subspecies of person we might call the patient. In public practice it is not unusual for those higher up the totem pole to delegate to the juniors the time spent with people, under the self-serving guise of granting the junior doctor the experience they need. The junior doctor will see perhaps at least five patients per day for every one or two the consultant sees, the remainder of the day the psychiatrist talking about the patients, and pottering around the endless pathological proliferation of paperwork that keeps most the hospital machine spinning, chairing meetings etcetera. Most public system psychiatrists are happier as managers than clinicians and suffer no unhappiness if they go the whole day without seeing a patient. As Rosenhan also observed, they often had the time to engage in more than the bare minimum with the patient. They simply chose not to.

Sixth, though it would seem the hospital staff were duped, the pseudo-patient subjects/malingerers themselves were duped in perhaps a much more pervasive and embarrassing way. These pseudo-patients are said to have been unanimously surprised to the point of shock it was so easy, almost certain before the fact that the psychiatrists would see through the sham. How might this speak to a zeitgeist of misplaced confidence in the probing mind and intuitions of psychiatrists as if they can see into the soul of the person? And how much this might speak to societies misplaced confidence in authority figures in general? My own psychiatry professors spoke to the medical student with amusement about a public seeing psychiatry as a fraternity of seers who could almost "read minds". Why just amusement? The very fact they were not as horrified as I was at even the countenancing of such nonsense suggests more than a little comfort with the idea. The psychiatrist is then inclined to imply "A seer I'm not. A prophet I'm not. But a sage? Of course!"

Finally, after the findings were informally distributed on the psychology/psychiatry grapevine, yet before they were published as such, one particular institution took umbrage at the prospect of being scammed. In their hubris they believed they would not be fooled a second time round. They were, well, psychiatrists after all. Rosenhan took up the challenge and announced that sometime within the subsequent 3 months an undefined number of pseudo-patients would present to their admissions department. Of 193 patients admitted, 41 were thought to be pseudo-patients by a member of staff, 23 by a psychiatrist, and 19 patients were thought to be fake by both a psychiatrist and one other staff member. These proportions would be much higher if excluding the patients already known to the hospital. Every hospital is familiar with several, or many, patients who are so called frequent flyers. These would not have been suspected due to their chronicity with the service over months or years, and so would effectively reduce the number of potential suspect malingerer/pseudo-patients somewhere below the number actually admitted within the 3 month interval. But this adjustment needn't be necessary, as the joke was on them. Rosenhan did not send a single patient their way. How many fake patients slip through the system when such arrogance doesn't have its guard raised? Of this we can only speculate. However much we may have sympathy with those who believe in psychosis, once again it is an article of faith to believe there are authentic psychotic patients at all.

But of course that is the issue is it not? Rosenhan's study can easily, though not as easy as some may think, be rebutted given its artificiality. Most people who say they hear voices are justifiably assumed to be sincere. Parenthetically, another population of those who may not be so sincere are those evaluated by forensic psychiatric services. Forensic psychiatrists cannot as a matter of manifest fact discern if an individual's social mischief is driven by a complete break with reality in the general sense, and a break so great as to have rendered them ignorant of the law. All they have is the patient's narrative and their own hubris to see through a con. Though not a forensic psychiatrist myself, I have seen many a patient to whom was given what was essentially an insanity defence. From my own conversations, what incidentally emerges when the rapport is up and the guard down is that they did the crime for no other reason than self gratification or the passions of emotions, in full awareness of the law and often with steps taken to evade it. They may or may not believe they are the queen of Sheeba. But that is not why they committed the crime.

Pseudopatients aside, in the remainder of those we encounter we might ask not if they are lying to us, but if they are lying to themselves. And we might wish to ask just what is so special about the symptoms of hearing a voice or believing unusual things as to make ostensive sincerity meaningful, especially when freedom is at stake?

What is psychosis?

The so called psychotic illnesses are many and divided by different nosological systems (all such systems being arbitrary and constructed by a group of elites, these are not equivalent to a taxonomy of physical disease as might be found in a textbook of pathology).

Taking the criteria of schizophrenia as per DSM 5, the psychosis of psychiatric concern can be defined as one or more of the following, pervasive over time, correlated with social/occupational dysfunction (always easily able to argue this criteria when one wishes), not explainable by drug intoxication (but convenient for psychiatry, recurrent drug induced psychosis will be treated "pragmatically" as the same psychosis anyway) and not part of an illness that is explainable by illnesses as diagnosed by physicians (such as brain tumours etc, i.e. real medicine)

Delusions; broadly speaking a delusion is believing something that the politically incorrect might say are crazy, and tenaciously holding to these beliefs despite evidence to the contrary.

Hallucinations; considering the five basic senses, an hallucination is experiencing the perception of a sensory stimulus without any such stimulus as objectively having been made, most commonly auditory phenomena, so called "hearing voices"

Disorganized thinking; insomuch as speech reflects thought, the speech does not make sense and by implication the thoughts also are muddled. Talking nonsense in other words, hopefully this book not being an example.

Disorganized behaviour; the behavioural accompaniment or analogue of disorganized thinking, the actions are not goal directed and do not make sense.

Negative symptoms; the absence of flourishing and expressive behaviour and thought, examples being amotivation and laying around all day, not showering and having withdrawn from engagement in the world and perhaps even lacking animation in dialogue with oneself.

Here I'll focus just on delusions, auditory hallucinations and disorganized thinking, to argue just how fragile is the concept of psychosis.

What is disorganized thought?

In ordinary human life, thought is expressed semantically and syntactically in speech acts, with words articulated into clauses, these further articulated into sentences which might be further elaborated to form larger chunks of the speech act that is the equivalent of paragraphs of written text. We expect that responses from the interlocutor address the theme or question asked, and that the response is intelligible and directed to the goal of the conversation. "How is the weather?" one might ask. An intelligible response might be "it is raining. Do you want to borrow my umbrella?". Problems arise when the architecture of the speech act, and by inference the thought, lose architectural integrity. Milder examples of this might include a simple lapse of logic as might be expected in common discourse. Or it might include highly intelligible responses that nonetheless have absolutely no relevance to the question asked, leaving the listener wondering where on earth the response came from. Broadly speaking these responses might be called "tangential", by way of invoking a geometrical metaphor, or knights move thinking in reference to the non linear jump of the chess piece. The irrelevant responses may continue to trail off and never find their way back to the point. There are gradually greater manifestations of thought disintegration down to what has been described as word salad, where even the words within a clause have nothing connecting them together, as if one if hearing randomly generated selections from the dictionary. One may speculate that in some cases mutism may represent the severest form of thought disorder, where thought is so degraded or muddled that it cannot find its way into any act of speech at all, perhaps from the crowding together of whatever preverbal chaotic soup lay in the mind of the patient who might be psychotic. Now it must be said that pure word salad is rarely seen by psychiatrists, with the vast majority of utterances containing at least something intelligible. Even an example of severe thought disorder such as Question "How is the weather? Answer ""well I went and saw a show and the chair is over there today, horray and good day" is not common in the patient diagnosed as psychotic.

Whilst at first blush these and other examples of so called thought disorder might be considered psychotic, the crucial question is if this easily separates the mad from the rest, the them from the us i.e. if ostensive thought disorder is necessarily psychotic and what the justification might be to draw the line here and not there or nowhere at all. And if not, then ought we avoid overplay the significance of the phenomena, for it is remarkable just how common thought disorder is when one looks for it, or rather listens to it. Take for example the audition, the first date, the anxious talk with a powerful other (common in dialogues between junior and senior doctors), and many other situations besides, especially had between anxious poorly educated ineloquent often drug addled patients of marginal intelligence who have their liberty threatened and the pressure of stating their case for freedom before an authority figure who has the power of the state behind them. What we normally pass over in virtue of the context, empathizing with the person and filing in the gaps where we can, we miss just how thought disordered we have all been in the past. A cancer is a cancer is a cancer, whereas thought disorder is not necessarily anything to do with medicine, and rarely so severe and enduring over time as for the physician to conclude that the person cannot function without assumed loss of responsibility and deprivation of liberty.

What is a delusion?

The DSM III- through to DSM IV TR defined delusions as "false beliefs due to incorrect inference about external reality" whilst the DSM 5 defined delusion in much the same way and pulling in the buzzword "evidence". It's definition; "fixed beliefs that are not amenable to change in light of conflicting evidence".

The DSM 5 also defines a subtype of delusion as bizarre ""clearly implausible, not understandable to same-culture peers and not derived from ordinary life experiences". Pray tell what is "clearly" the case without elucidation?

Kaplan and Saddock, in their text commonly used by psychiatric residents defines delusion as a "false fixed idea not shared by others"

The Oxford handbook of Clinical Psychiatry is more detailed, stating a delusion is a

"pathological belief which has the following characteristics

-is held with absolute subjective certainty and cannot be rationalized way

-it requires no external proof and may be held in the face of contradictory evidence

-it has personal significance and importance

-it is not a belief which can be understood as part of the subjects religious and cultural background"

Let us examine these elements of the definition.

Falsity

"What is truth" asked Pilate of Christ. This was Pilates jaded response to Christ for the latter stating that he was, in a sense, the manifest personification of truth. Despite this being at odds with what Pilate the pagan no doubt believed, he washed his hands of the matter and the rest is, as they say, history. Nevertheless, what was perhaps a rhetorical question for Pilate becomes one about which we might demand an answer. And not just a question of what truth is. The crux of the issue when subjective truths collide is when, nay if, we ever have licence to label some beliefs as normal/acceptable and others as "pathological". Embedded within this question is the assumption there is and ought to be a "we", as opposed to a collection of "I"'s. Let's see if this is the case

So an atheist, Jew, Christian, Muslim, Pagan and a schizophrenic walk into a bar. The Pagan says there are many Gods, the "Abrahamists" they there's one, the atheist says there are none, and the schizophrenic says he is God. He knows this as the devil told him so. None of the other believers however can agree on the substance of the deity, or the metaphysics of his/her/its/their extension into creation. Before a ruckus arises the party are distracted by a debate between another who says the Earth is flat and yet another who says the Earth is spherical, and this splinters off into a debate between the atheist and the Christian who, as it turns out, is in the fundamentalist tradition of Archbishop Ussher and believes the age of the Earth is more or less six thousand years and the Vedic who believes people have walked about the Earth for an aeon. Another eavesdropping pair then are triggered into a debate over the fate of the Earth, whether the weathers will change towards the heralding of a new ice age or the polar caps will melt and the Himalayas become beach front property. In every exchange the protagonists have one fist shaking while the other contains the papers or website addresses in accord with their evidence and the anecdotes of personal experience. And then things get really nasty over the subject of the current US president and Brexit as the bar patrons start tearing the place apart. This upsets or amuses the schizophrenic. He may either believe he is the president or is maliciously followed by CIA agents of the same. The bar is very large and echoes of other arguments can be heard, clauses and fragments where we can barely make out the words abortion, vaccination, proper parenting, gender, veganism and more. Promptly we depart into the cooler night air.

A moments reflection will grant us the obvious, that every adult human being on the planet (or disc as the case may be) has multiple beliefs that others ardently consider are false. Some believe a leader is a proto fascist. Some believe he is saviour from fascism. Some believe the Earth is doomed whilst others consider such a proposition scaremongering. The atheist steps out of the materialist manifold of space and time into metaphysical space to proclaim there to be nothing present save for transcendent nothingness where even the semantics of nothingness itself loses meaningful sense, as does his materialism in taking the transcendent step in the first place. And we are all familiar with the potpourri of the other religious traditions that do not define themselves through radical negation. Return we do to Pilate, only now we are he. "What is truth" we now ask, yet this time with a twist. Instead we ask who has the political right to discriminate between all possible falsities? Whether you have had the misfortune of having been labelled schizophrenic or not, somewhere someone on some matter will think you are wrong about something. They will think you are very very wrong. In fact they will think you are so wrong that they will conclude you are crazy. Moreover, not just someone will think this, but everyone. Fractionate each and every belief that you hold and seek another who disagrees with you. Sooner or later the group who unanimously agrees on all matters will collapse to n=1, i.e. you yourself, the individual. And this is if you are fortunate (or boring), as persons within themselves change their views over the course of a lifetime or even a day. Falsity thus must give way to liberty within a rule of law or we all becomes tyrants whilst simultaneously all becoming delusional. Or as Christ might have told Pilate, if one does not agree then go in peace and shake the dust off one's sandals on the road out of town. In this sense Christ and Pilate might have been in agreement.

Fixedness

The notion of fixedness and imperviousness to contrary evidence is somewhat of a tautology. After all, why would one wish to unfix a belief if not the resultant from conflicting evidence, whether this evidence be from reason, empirical observation or some other kind of revelation (with an upper or lower case "r"). The feature of fixedness (of belief) is too close for comfort to the meaning of falsity as both are intimately informed by, and dependent upon, changes in what one takes to be the calculus of evidence, not sitting in parallel to it. Are the psychiatric intelligentsia sure of what they are saying when they throw out words which blend and weave into one another without a coherent explication of the sense in which the words are used in relation to one another? I'm sure they are not. Is this not a kind of higher order thought disorder? A philosophical psychosis even? But never mind.

One way we could conceive of fixedness is in terms of fervour, an intensity with which the belief is held irrespective of the evidence base. Yet fervour is something more of the passions is it not? Fervour does not relate to the dispassionate deliberation over a proposition in rational and empirical terms and the certainty of its truth. Even this is an artificial separation as belief is usually held with some kind of attachment, some affect, some passion and fire within the vector of intentionality towards the proposition. Are we proposing that every human being ought to be a kind of hyper autistic rationalist? Is passion to be made the enemy? This is patently monstrous! Or are we to medicalise the individual for how far they behaviourally go with the belief dearly held? Surely this behaviour is a different matter to fixedness of the belief as such, though the same in a different sense as one informs the other.

This so called "delusional intensity" calls to mind the patient who was once admitted against their will as psychotic for the beliefs he held against tattoos. He believed they were ugly, representative often of satanic, violent and anti-virtuous symbology (especially in men) and stood like bad architecture to mar the aesthetic landscape and damage the spirit of the community, surely leading to the corruption of morals now and down the track. This belief was not held with any greater elaboration than that that of a social critic. It was not lost on me that the referring private practice psychiatrist was, under the expensive suit, an aficionado of, and personally stained by, much tattooists ink. On the other hand, I personally could sympathize with the patient, recalling a time when only bikers, convicts and sailors sought out the tattoo parlours that were always in the seedy back alleys of town. Now it's a rite of passage for almost every young man and (especially) young lady to have a skull, sword, six pointed star, flower, narcissistic quote or an epitaph somewhere on their person. But you see this belief was strangely passionately held in this particular young man, and the patient took it upon himself to evangelize against ink, chastising those he passed in the street, occasionally preaching it on the corner. This will not do. And so he was described as delusional in virtue of holding the belief with "delusional intensity" on one hand and given the attendant "risks of misadventure" on the other. For, or so the argument went, if he annoys someone he might be assaulted, and must be protected against the misadventure that his illness might bring upon him. Psychiatry would not advance the idea that perhaps he ought to be free to speak his mind and those who assault him face the police and the judiciary. Such is the erosion of responsibility in the age of hard neuroscience that no one is accountable for what they do, the victim is the criminal and the criminal the victim. This patient was accordingly detained and treated against his will, without the slightest engagement with his ideas. Neither did psychiatry engage with the idea that behavioural fervour is the stuff of many adolescents and all revolutionaries of all religious/irreligious and political stripes. It is the stuff of those who are true to their beliefs. To crudely paraphrase Vaniegem, a revolutionary without action speaks as with a corpse in his mouth. There was no formal difference between he (our patient) and they (the revolutionary). And if a patient were not true to his/her beliefs might it be argued that he has negative symptoms, depressive amotivation or some other symptom of mental illness. Damned if one does and damned if one doesn't to a system who wishes you damned.

Or in talking about fixedness are we speaking of lack of openness to change, which is synonymous with stubbornness and as much a passion as the fervour to persuade. Take any case of ones professed faith in who they are, who they were, who they will be, what they will do and how they will evaluate the world, including significant others within it. What are your cherished beliefs? Would you, as a fundamentalist Christian, when presented with fossil evidence and geological dating not just conclude that six thousand years ago God created a shabby chic Earth that just happened to look old? Or that the science has been corrupted by the father of all lies, i.e. Lucifer? Or would you, the atheist, if waved at by a statue of the virgin not conclude that against almost infinite probability all the vibrational states of the atoms of the marble moved in the same direction at the same time, and more than one would expect. Or that the quantum probabilistic field within which the atoms may lay synchronized into what may be thought of as movement? In such a case the miracle could be interpreted as little more than the playing out of Clarkes first law, that any sufficiently advanced technology (or scientific knowledge perhaps) would be indistinguishable from magic, or in this case miracle being scientistically explainable. What would the blessed virgin then need to do to get your attention? Or maybe nothing would convince you otherwise that Lee Harvey Oswald was a patsy, or that the Apollo 11 really did, or did not, land on the moon. Would any of you betray your Marxism, despite it not yet creating the utopia each time it is tried. Would you ever rape your own child, or believe such an act to ever be morally justified? How can you be so sure in your fixedness of what you won't do tomorrow, when asked questions about moral givens? Why are you so fixed in what I assume your answers to be? Would you give up believing in the fidelity of your husband even after seeing his strange phone records and he tells you that man in the singles bar just looked like him? Just as is the case with falsity, we each hold beliefs that we will doggedly hold to the end. Damn what the so called evidence shows, whether that be science or material evidence or journalism or the well intentioned friend states who says we're "crazy" and attempts to knock their sense into us. So what?

The criteria of fixedness also calls to mind the patient who recalled vividly (and I would say symbolically), a time when "military police" took him in the night, anaesthetised him and replaced his liver with a mechanical version. Now the party line in psychiatry is that we ought not entertain such delusional ideas as his by hypothesis testing such as X-raying for metal livers. For such would, as it were, play into the hands of the patients psychosis. Strangely though this kind of hypothesis testing is just what the doctor orders in the methodology of cognitive behavioural therapy for the neurosis such as anxiety and obsessive compulsive disorder. But such hypothesis testing is discouraged in psychosis. As luck would have it, for some reason we had medical cause to perform an abdominal CT scan (essentially a glorified Xray) on our cyborg patient. Lo and behold no mechanical liver was visible and we accordingly challenged him on his belief. Our latter day Prometheus accepted without protest our "evidence". Without skipping a beat he immediately concluded that at some time the buggers must have taken him in his sleep again, replacing the mechanical liver with a real one of flesh and blood. Well that flexibility puts paid to fixedness of belief. Or does it? Is he truly delusional then? We can always shift gears ourselves, and crucify him on the cross of psychosis for what he did believe occurred in the past, or for what he even countenances as possible. Yet what have we proven save for our own guile to nail someone and keep them nailed if we are so inclined, to keep them in the clutches of psychiatry.

So let us drop the word fixedness altogether and simply approach the issue of belief held in the absence of confirming evidence or in spite disconfirming evidence. Does this not return us to where we started, with the matter of falsity and what constitutes evidence? What right ought the state have to interrogate anyone on how they arrive at the beliefs they hold? How might the state and the guilds of psychiatry themselves have arrived at the final answers to the deepest questions of epistemology and the assumed value of truth, when the philosophers haven't managed the same?

Cultural Context

The Oxford Handbook of Psychiatry (and all psychiatric guilds also) makes a most curious qualification that a belief can be appropriate (i.e. non pathological) if it is held as flowing from the subjects own cultural background. Putting aside the subjectification of the individual by use of the very word "subject", it's a very traditional British formulation, quite at odds with the current state of affairs in a multicultural post EU UK, and at odds also with the individualistic spirit of the Americans. How many who court beliefs fully developed in another culture may be captured into the net of satisfying such a criterion, and thus be on their way towards being diagnosed with, as the Handbook states, a "pathological belief"? The situation calls to mind all the stories of the westerners who becomes disenchanted with traditional Christianity (or probably just bored and looking for novelty). And run away they do to join the Ashram, only for the Guru to state that they cannot be Hindu and are best back in the Anglican Communion where their karma intended them to be, with the Father, the Son and the Holy Spirit rather than Sat, Chit and Ananda. Would psychiatry also seriously entertain the possibility that someone was delusional if embracing a cultural belief incongruent with their own background? Would the white upper middle class suburban youth meet the criteria of incongruence with their own cultural beliefs and practices if they adopted the persona of the urban black rapper? The list is endless, tacitly suggesting to us that we ought to know our place and ride in our lane. The subtle hints of identity politics lay everywhere, hiding in plain sight.

Let us then be more individualistic and say that someone cannot be delusional if the belief is part of any cultural and religious background, giving them freedom to escape their own cultural backyard. Then the question of background itself comes into view. Is this not a war against the individual and against progress that they must attach themselves to an identified state approved antecedent and cannot formulate their own culture? How far can the thread to the past be stretched before a belief becomes, sui generis, unique and accordingly vulnerable to being declared pathological? Was Christ or the Buddha sane in forming a religion out of an existing one (Judaism plus/minus Platonism in the case of the former, Hinduism in the case of the latter), i.e. both being culturally congruent with something that came before? Or insomuch as the new religions they founded were radical departures to all that came before, were their beliefs pathological, i.e. psychotic? Surely this is a case that can be made, the same for the founding fathers of many a paradigm shift in science, the turn towards classical liberalism in the modern era and so on. We can easily imagine a counterfactual history where Christianity sat side by side with a psychiatry, moving from the schizophrenic megalomaniac madness of Christ himself to that of a mass delusion and gradually onto Constantine ordering its removal from whatever could have been the DSM of antiquity. For by that time it had become culturally established, the belief of the many making the belief no longer pathological. From Copernicus to Darwin we can imagine other original thinkers and doers similarly stigmatized. Perhaps the better proposition is that delusion itself in a sense did not exist prior to its invention as a construct by psychiatry, just as law created crime which can only otherwise be universalized over time and place by appeal to transcendent moralities.

Yet this does not drive home the central point. Ultimately such a clause appealing to cultural congruence so as to give licence to a belief as non pathological is not just word play. It's a sinister and evil war against the individual. And more contemptuously it the act of the coward bullying the weak. For what it proposes is that the beliefs of one prophet or avant-garde thinker can be pathological in virtue of the novelty. Perhaps two or three believers would suffer the same diagnosis of a shared psychosis. Yet when the movement reaches an undefined critical mass, where the people can assemble and take up pitchforks or form a voting bloc, then they are dangerous to power. And then they are no longer deluded. Then they are a culture, a religion (or negation of) and so on. The notion of the voting bloc is important insomuch as the institutions of psychiatry are thoroughly in bed with the state, having displaced the church and so giving the illusion of church/state separation in the secular western world. Still the form of such an arrangement remains. Psychiatry would do better to admit it's cowardice. Either that or declare in a coherent way what is a pathological belief and what is not, take the ideological stage with the other religions and act (and fight) consistently come what may against larger and smaller opponents alike. If then the legitimacy of every culture and ideology is up for grabs then psychiatry, qua a culture amongst others, itself enters the arena of vulnerability. Thus it's cowardice is not simply a war against the individual, yet also a want to grant immunity to itself from prosecution as deluded.

Belief as such

Much is predicated on the idea that beliefs need to reflect the world. Yet where is the evidence this need be the case? This idea is itself ironically a belief, and one which sits outside the material world as it is. Rather it is a statement of what beliefs ought to be. And a belief of what a belief ought to be, insomuch as it might better reflect the world, might also have greater survival value, yet maybe not. Take the case of confidence in oneself against insurmountable odds, the hope of a miracle when life is at its bleakest. Often this is enough to survive through great adversity. Or take for example the basic thread of the atheistic existentialists, that life is ultimately meaningless and absurd, and so the only meaning is found in the construction of meaning, which is to say lying to oneself. Why a lie? For this reason; This subjective meaning may feel itself to be a victory whilst being subsumed within the greater metaphysics which is cut through and though with inescapable nihilism. One can never escape a transcendent nihilism that reflects back upon, suffuses, and defines, the meaning we think we have constructed for ourselves. In any case, the belief about what a belief ought to be contains within itself a moral argument as how we ought to live. And a belief of what a belief ought to be writ large by powerful persons and applied to other persons against their will becomes a political act of the moral tyrant. And moral propositions, however much they may be held as truths, are outside of a basis of evidence the likes of which are the standard criteria of delusion. They are experienced as faith. A belief is a propositional attitude. Hume thought they could be differentiated from fears and desires. I'm not so sure. Where is medicine and psychiatry in all this, except as some entitled child who thinks it has already mastered the content of the philosophical conversation and deserves a place at the head of the table whilst not being able tie it's dialectical shoes. My suggestion, itself a belief, is primum non nocere, "first do no harm". If the individual is aggressing against others this is the job of the minimal state to police and prosecute. If not, leave the person alone.

Beyond the Phenomenological horizon of Jaspers

Is there anywhere or anyone else to which or to whom we could turn to know what delusion is as opposed to just another variant belief about which we might say "live and let live"? Well from the frankly silly little unconvincing aquarelle that is the definition of delusion we have discussed, we come to the thickly obscured canvas of phenomenology, obscure as from Lambert to Brentano to Husserl to Jaspers et al, philosophy cannot seem to agree what phenomenology is. Nonetheless I'll try my best. Broadly speaking, it is the study and taxonomy of mental phenomena with the goal of establishing the basic elements of experience and the vectors of relationship of one experience to another, the ultimate in omphaloskepsis. For example, I may have a fear. The fear is directed towards something (the directedness or aboutness being an intentionality), where the fear contains within itself a representation of the feared object. This object need not be an object in the world. It can be an idea or something in the abstract. What are the qualities of the feared object as experienced in the mental state? How does fear stand in relation to belief, sensation, desire, planning etcetera? When did it arrive in my consciousness and what were its antecedents, if any? This sort of thing is phenomenology. So far this is simple to grasp, though matters get trickier if we are to consider ourselves, our identity and selfhood, themselves as objects of descriptive introspection. To do this is to stand apart from phenomena. But what is the self standing apart from the self? Arguably this degree of separation obstructs from knowing as a true phenomenologist ought, i.e. in purely unadulterated subjective terms, where being and self are one. Only then can we know what it is to be. But then what can we say about this raw "beingness", without holding oneself out at arms length, in so doing losing grasp of what it is to be? Is the reader confused? Good! It is these more metaphysical speculations that takes phenomenology from the realm of banal descriptivism to existentialism and even the outer suburbs of the mystical city. But such sojourns off the clear and simple path fortunately or unfortunately were never used to evaluate and contextualise how phenomenology might be appropriate for psychiatry. They should have, for the banal is subsumed within the higher metaphysical orders which either validates the former or repudiates it. A pity as these are the very questions crucial before engaging with Jaspers. Ergo my engagement with Jaspers will be the Jaspers as taught to psychiatrists, not an expansive review of the man and evolution of his thought.

Karl Jaspers, the prodigious and morally upstanding psychiatrist turned psychologist turned philosopher more than any other allied (his version of) phenomenology to psychiatry. Most psychiatrists would not know how to pronounce his name let alone anything more about his thought. What they might know however is the notion of "empathic understandability". Jaspers project was to engage the patient with radical empathy, though I would say not radical enough (vide infra). To place oneself within the mental shoes, as it were, of the patient, without ostensive judgment and to listen to all the inner experiences of the patient, their relationship with one another (i.e. the experiences) and with the temporal chain of events in the patient's narrative of his or her inner world. This was the method, with the goal being deep intersubjective understanding. And so you might encounter the patient who believes their spouse to be unfaithful. How and when did they come to arrive at this belief? Do they believe their spouse is unfaithful as the latter has been coming home late at night, they were seen in town with an ex girl/boyfriend, they smell of a unfamiliar perfume etc? This Bayesian line of reasoning is something with which anyone could say they empathize, though the infidelity still might not be the case in truth. Or did the belief arrive in consciousness like a sudden migraine one morning, in blazing certainty and in the absence of any antecedent experience that could constitute "evidence", where evidence is a chain of thought and experience with which the psychiatrist could empathise or fail to empathise as the case may be? For how could such a certain belief reasonably arise de novo? Or did the belief arrive in consciousness as a result of thoughts and experiences the likes of which the psychiatrist, try as he or she might, fails to empathise as logical or common sense entailment, say for example if a letter arrived in the mail with a stamp askew or upside down on the envelope. "Then I knew he was cheating on me" the patient says. "How this event (the askew stamp) entails or leads to the belief in the other (the infidelity) is beyond me" the psychiatrist will think. This is the psychiatrists unsettling experience, making impossible the act of empathy. Such empathic un-understandability need not appeal to a definition of delusion as earlier described, the belief instead being formulated and understood as the product of a process. The un-understandable belief passes beyond the horizon of phenomenology. And so the experience is considered delusional, and the person is considered psychotic.

So far so good, but is it? Take the matter of the beginnings of the delusional journey, before or perhaps instead of the askew stamp used as a reasoning for the belief (spousal infidelity in this case). As stated above, the phenomenological journey between psychiatrist and patient may reveal an initial phase before the formed system of beliefs that are the alleged delusions, a sense that things are not quite right. This is the so called delusional mood. Or the belief may arise as stated in a flash, without reasoning, an autochthonous delusion, which as in Chekhov's Ivan Dmitritch" of Ward 6.

Coming upon a revelation or sudden awakening, insomuch as one cannot identify readily an antecedent thought, is un-understandable. But is it? If we permit the possibility of the existence of the unconscious how can we say what is primary and what is autochthonous? Think of the times your conscious mind worked on a problem, say a math equation. It may take you thirty minutes from first encountering it to the final solution. If you are interrupted mid way through, the answer may come along in a flash some minutes, or hours later while riding the subway or sitting on the toilet. The total conscious time taken to solution was in the latter case substantially less than thirty minutes. Obviously the unconscious in its mysterious machinations was working on the problem all along, though we know precisely nothing more than the output as to the existence of the unconscious, and nothing at all of its architecture. Think also of what other problems the individual faces and "works on" all the time. Someone one day experiences a sudden sense that things are not quite right, and looks upon the world as something alien, a vast instrument laid out before them that has suddenly fallen out of tune, with all the movements of the persons and machines around no longer melodious. Now there is just cacophony, metaphorically speaking. Between their slumber in normality and this allegedly psychotic first moment has been an interim in which their psyche has been exposed to the banal, the kitsch, the consumerism, the media, the rising sin, the fading virtue, the bucket list that just keeps getting fuller, the loss of youthful innocence, the unwelcome arrival at adult responsibility, the growing middle aged crisis, the unwelcome arrival of old age, the realisation of mortality, the looming seven year itch, the base drives seeking justification, the crowds and changes and so on and so forth. The list is limited only by one's imagination. One day something starts to crack from all this, the scales fall from their eyes. Something is not quite right. Now we may debate what the allegedly psychotic may conclude from and following this first move into alienation, whether the investigations (i.e. the thoughts) that come after the delusional mood and first autochthonous shift are psychotic or not. Yet how on Earth can we medicalise the shift itself? It has no predictive validity in advance. We must de-pathologize the idea of delusional mood as it (technically speaking) also lacks discriminative validity. I've lost count of the number of persons I've encountered who woke one day, realized pre-rationally (or arguably trans-rationally) that something was wrong in the world or at least their world. And this disquiet rumbled within them towards great changes in their lives, perhaps even by that afternoon they had found religion, a divorce lawyer, a resignation letter or a caravan out of town.

Another problem is holding these patients to an account of justifying their basic (i.e. autochthonous) beliefs. This too is quite unfair.

Even persons who work in mathematical and so called scientific investigations must rely on assumptions so basic, so sui generis, that they can only be operated with, yet cannot be explained in more atomic terms. Vastly complicated technologies rest upon mathematics. 2 add 2 equals 4. But where is 2 and where is 4 and why is the latter the square of the former? It just is in some way that is either a matter of faith or radically ontologically true, whatever its utilitarian value. One can operate on these assumptions as knowledge yet one cannot justify the assumptions as knowledge. For in what sense can I claim to know? I can walk forward in knowledge, operating with tautologies and basic assumptions. Yet what have I added to say "I know" what I believe when it comes to basic beliefs themselves. Or what of the friend who can describe their ideal mate, yet when he/she comes along they feel nothing or might say they know (i.e. believe) the person is not right for them, and instead can only feel something for someone less ideal, often far less ideal? Will we not fail in empathizing with our friend, lest we subscribe to a belief in man's fundamental drive to self-destruction? Or what of the friend who, despite evidence to the contrary, says they intuit "I just knew he/she was/wasn't right for me. I don't know why I know". Why are these individuals also not psychotic? Is it because we empathize with the metaphor of "the chemistry was/wasn't right"? Is it because we accept the place of intuition, even if we question its application? Have we shared in their psychosis?

However strange, it is most unfair to look for the patient's basic experiences and beliefs, the hinges upon which other beliefs and behaviours may turn, and then to expect them to justify these basic beliefs when no one alive can do the same on every thought that forms the basis for action. It would be a trickery were the psychiatrist not so ignorant.

Another problem arises how we may accomplish this when embarking on the empathic journey with at least one preconceived goal, that of empathic understandability itself. This is a goal which smuggles along with it all the prejudices Jaspers sought to avoid, or ought to have avoided. In his writings he speaks of the pathological belief as if it is a priori something that exists as separate from the non pathological, just waiting to be understood, or rather I should say identified by its un-understandability. The very notion that one may in principle reach a point of empathic un-understandability and that this somehow fleshes out an objective psychotic state of affairs is only one such prejudice, as is many other covert notions, such as the limitation of symbolism as explanation, the limitation of symbolism as permissible when projected out as concrete belief and a mode of life, that a lie to others is not pathological whilst a lie to oneself is, that I may have already decided the patient is delusional and I am using Jaspers method to justify what I have already adjudicated and so on. Now surely to engage with the phenomenology of the patient entails an identification with the patient in all their psychic experience, perhaps even unto an entering into the alleged madness itself. To truly stare into the abyss is to look headlong, with the unavoidable result being that the abyss stares back at you. Only now you are the one staring out. And when one achieves this ultimate act of empathy, then where is the madness? Perhaps back in the world of the accusers, back in the world of the allegedly "normal". Might Jaspers horizon say more about him than about the patient, and how un-intrepid psychiatrists are in making the effort to empathize as the Jaspers known to psychiatry might have suggested to us? Or worse it is a show trial leading to the justification of the charge of madness by the judge who is also first the prosecutor? Who is empathically watching the one with authority to judge by empathy?

Let's take the following examples of patients who would, and indeed were, surely diagnosed as psychotic and who were treated forcibly against their will with domesticating medications and involuntary hospitalization.

There is the case of the young lady, more or less typical of many female patients I've seen over the years, who come to believe she is being followed by some powerful presence and persecuted by all and sundry. She believed that her body was literally behaving as a marionette, with her abusive ex-boyfriend pulling the strings and controlling her every move. Sometimes she would move her lips and tongue to speak, her ego cut off from identifying herself as the agent behind the voice who spoke. It sounded like a womans voice she would admit, and indeed sounded identical to how she imagined and remembered her voice to be. Nonetheless the voice was that of others she would say, and the speaker was a male. And this belief was held literally. Her thoughts also were not her own. Her own were taken from her. Occasionally when her identity emerged she would just become what was once termed "hysterical", and scream violently about her rights as a woman (her words), surely a clue to any with even a modicum of curiosity to ask the deeper questions. Now let us break this all down. No psychiatrist I know would let her go free, let alone tolerate her beliefs as another kind of normal, a damaged normal I'll grant you. Her beliefs were unfounded in ordinary terms of what might be considered evidence. Technically they were considered "bizarre" delusions. People do not possess other people and cannot control them as one would control the movements of a puppet. When my arm raises it is I who raise it, unless another holds it and moves it and is observed to be doing so. Who can empathise with the impossible? But let's look at her from a different angle, one not wedded to psychiatry at all as to what psychosis and schizophrenia is. What if she had been used and abused, perhaps even prostituted out by men (plural) in the past? This indeed was the case. What if her opinion came to naught and her body was not, in a sense, bio-politically her own? And the man or men whom she loved and towards whom her ego was diffused were using her as the object she once allowed herself to become. I say "allowed" for at one point she did have responsibility over the maladaptive steps she took and the drugs she imbibed, and this book is a defence of personal responsibility. To my mind her alleged psychosis was her existential pain writ large to a malignant degree. It was quite easily something with which I could empathise, all considering. True her beliefs were not materially and efficiently true. So what? How might we answer such cases, especially when the individual rails against being hospitalised against their will, medicated against their will, and inevitably with a force that unavoidably must on some level recapitulate the sense of powerlessness against powerful others, in this case me? With such patients I would rather grant them radical freedom, ideally coupled with radical unfreedom for the vermin men (and/or women) who preyed upon them. And I would rather do this even with the risk that they may never recover as any well intentioned person would wish them to, as in the vast majority of cases psychiatry never can effect such recovery as one would wish. But alas it was never so. Never were similar patients not diagnosed with schizophrenia or bipolar disorder. They are brought to the hospital, by police more often than not. They are forcibly treated. And the pimp walks free.

Or what of more systematized persecution. I've lost count of the number of patients who have some variant of a belief that they are in a kind of Truman Show like experiment, observed by others for some greater amusement in a large cage with them the only exhibit. Often the observers are said to be government or family. Unlike the character in the film, they have never seen a lighting prop fall from the "sky", and never ferreted out the hidden camera in their home, though not for want of trying. And nothing will convince them otherwise at just how canny the observers can be at covering their tracks. Even I might be an actor they wonder, though most of the time I'm able to avoid involvement, that is unless I'm punitive towards them myself. I'll let the reader analyse the implications of this shift in their beliefs with the shift in our mode of relations, from interested other to punitive other. Examples of these cases take on many forms, some coming into closer approximation with the film, especially in the immediate years following its release. This should also serve as a hint to mainstream psychiatry that so-called delusions are not likely brain diseases as opposed to psychological creations for which the brain is an indispensable tool for sure, yet not the architect as such. Cancer is cancer is cancer down the millennia. It's form and content change not. Its incidence can change with the emergence of environmental carcinogens (e.g. as in lung cancer and mesothelioma). But delusions are infinitely more plastic. They can be one generation the demons and the next generation big media (is there really a difference?). And another generation in another person along comes the Illuminati, paedophiles and the biker gangs, whatever is the cultural material or boogie man of the times, bearing in mind that sometimes the boogie man is real and the biker gang really is out to get you. After all, there is more than enough paranoia to go around. Sometimes these Truman Show like experiences tread far from analogy to the plot of the film, and become these other things and many more, with the warfare even waged on the spiritual plain. But, and this is crucial observation, all of them have one thing in common. It is a feature with which we all can empathize. In each and every case the sufferer is a person of interest. They are important even as they are caged or hated, hunted or abused. They are the centre of a kind of an attention the intensity and breadth of which few ever "enjoy". And I use the word "enjoy" deliberately, though with qualification as their suffering is certainly neither denied or discounted. Nevertheless, a life of persecuted importance may be perversely preferable to that of bland dissolution into the meaninglessness of the masses. And not just the masses, but often to a lower rung than all those on the ladder. It is better for some to be Jeanne d'Arc and risk being burned at the stake, than be that nothing little village boy or girl who few knew, fewer cared for, and none at all will remember. If this drive to significance is the primary pathology, this is something about which one may readily empathize. And so is not pathological at all, by the standard of those who set the standard (i.e. psychiatry) and yet who cannot robustly defend it.

Here are some additional cases that this maladaptive drive to preserve narcissism informs many of the cases of what we call psychosis in general, or delusion in particular. The first is also from popular culture, which derives its power in part from our capacity to identify with the protagonist. Consider the film Total Recall. In it the main hero is a garden variety construction worker who chooses a virtual holiday in a dream state. Things go awry and he discovers himself to be a previously amnestic secret agent, never a humble construction worker at all. Part of the plot concerns the question if this discovery is authentic and the product was never purchased, or part of the dream, i.e. the product the ordinary man purchased. For what a vacation it must be to relish in high adventure, and moreover to believe it is true, even though death lay in wait at every turn. The second example is from the life of many persons who thankfully evaded psychiatry. I can recall the world of the 1970's through to early 1990's, when huge swathes of subculture were under the spell premillennial terror. I knew dozens of persons who believed the world was coming to an end, the beast of revelation would soon rise and famine, pestilence and all manner of Satanic and/or secular Communist persecutions would creep over the land, and indeed into their very lives and homes. Some sold their homes as, well, why not when the end is nigh? Were these people facing persecution the likes of which any sane person would prefer avoid? Arguably yes. But oh what a glorious drama, as I can tell you from first hand experience these people were, more often than not, happy and enlivened with meaning. Needless to say none required medications and most settled in with the rest of the sheeple in suburban insignificance, wage slavery and reality TV addiction come the other side of the millennium. And then and only then in suburbia they became depressed and were psychiatrically drugged. Perhaps Satan won after all.

The third is an example of a specific patient in real life, who failed to escape the clutches of psychiatry. He believed himself to be a Van Helsing like character. All around him are vampires, including the clinic receptionist. He was not so sure about me, and gave me the benefit of the doubt. The risks were real for him too, for these vampires were not likely to grant him immortality and the key to the vampire executive bathroom. Instead if he failed to maintain moral strength and a strangely described sense of psychic fortitude, they would turn him to mince in a glorified meat grinder he was sure literally existed yet could not confirm ever sighting. He thought it was kept out the back of the hospital. This patient came my way when the vampire film genre was all the rage, and he was of the vintage whose unconscious may have remembered the human meat grinder of Pink Floyds music video "Another Brick in the Wall Part 2". Now I ask the reader, who would this man be if not the bane of vampires, themselves a metaphor for the selfishness of the world and their meat grinder arguably the call to conform?

The answer is he would hold a menial job and stand in peril of a confrontation with the fact that his youth was gone, his wallet was always near empty and he had nothing and no one. In saving him from the vampires, psychiatry aspired to grant him just that kind of terrible mediocrity with the drug it forcibly injected into his backside every 2 weeks. The question psychiatry never asked itself is why they would prefer him to be a victim of the state's metaphorical meat grinder and not the one of his own psyches creation, most especially when he looked me in the eye and told me that were he not forced to, he would never ever take the medication, even if the medication seemed to correlate with the vampires losing interest in him. Inject him is precisely what we did, as we always do. We bit him where the vampires didn't.

Finally, every psychiatrist can easily identify the many patients who react in response to the so called delusions, often to their detriment. Take for example the patient who in looking for hidden cameras comes perilously close to being electrocuted. Or the one who drowns from swimming out too far to avoid aqua-phobic aliens. Or the manic who buys up useless old items and travels to the other side of the world in the fervent belief that he can market them at Christies and make a killing, wiping out his life savings in the process. That acknowledgement of risk being given its due (and more on it anon), neither can any psychiatrist deny the substantial fraction of patients who much of the time or all of the time do not behave as if what they (supposedly) believe is true. Just this morning I had a patient who would say he is fixed upon the belief that people are waiting outside to kill him. And by his side is his wife whom he claims is part of the nefarious conspiracy. The strange thing was his warmth towards her, and the grin whilst he conveyed this story. Why was he not frightened of her or why not gaze upon her with the hatred such a conspirator would deserve? Psychiatry has long written off such incongruences as part of the irrational split, the "schizein", within the thinking, the "phren", the incongruent affect etc. Psychiatry has long assumed this incongruence to be a symptom itself of the disease. I'm not so sure. Likewise, psychiatry ignores the fact that most of the time our schizophrenic can be flexible to changing other beliefs apart from the core delusion, and so clearly do not have a global impairment or cognitive inflexibility per se. Could it be that at some level all of those whom we might call delusional have created a lie for themselves to live by, the degree of attachment to the lie being what we equate with lacking insight? Take a thought experiment, a village of the so called sane. They are told the barbarians are coming down from the hills to rape and plunder. Some freeze, some prepare to fight, some take flight. But all to a man, woman or child would surely react and fly up the Yerkes Dodson curve. And all would settle if no barbarians were there. Were these villagers medicated schizophrenics some would do the same. Yet they may just lull about in anergic languor as the "antipsychotic" ablate their drives. A village of unmedicated schizophrenics or those refractory to treatment however, under the deluded belief that the barbarians were at the gate would, in a sizable minority of cases, also just tell you so and nonetheless go about their daily business, occasionally peering over the pickets to see what was, in fact, not there. We ought to ask ourselves a difficult question. Is it not conceivable in what is betrayed by the (lack of) behaviour of this subset of schizophrenics, that there are layers of belief? Is it not possible that they are lying to themselves, and part of their psyche knows it's being lied to?

What's with the voices?

The psychiatrist enters the room and engages the patient in conversation, only to find they are somewhat distracted, their head inclined at key moments within the conversation as if the room is occupied by patient, psychiatrist and a third interlocutor the psychiatrist cannot see. That mild distractibility is the subtle hint to an intuitive psychiatrist, though the cat may be out of the proverbial bag when the patient abruptly turns sideways to face empty air and talks as if to respond to a voice telling them this or that, often a derogatory comment, a commentary or even a rebuke against the psychiatrist and a warning not to trust them. Needless to say this is a voice only the patient can hear as no one is actually there by their side. As with so called delusions, one will probably be tempted to conclude this strange behaviour not simply the mark of a garden variety eccentric. Is it not surely a marker of the insane?

An important point to raise at the outset is that auditory (or other sensory) hallucinations are in practice a phenomenological composite of more than the raw qualia of the percept of the sound itself.

To begin with, hallucinations are not entirely separate to the case of delusions. In ordinary cases the only power an hallucination can have is the patients belief about the hallucination. A patient may be distressed by a recurrent voice telling them to kill themselves. Yet there is a world of difference between this experience known to be emanating from their own mind and the belief that the voice is from another external agency, perhaps human with whom they live, perhaps some supernatural entity. Perhaps they did not know who or what is talking to them and have not thought to consider the question beyond the commitment to the belief the voice is not a product of their own mind (this is in turn confounded with the concept of insight. See how psychiatry is an intricate web of begging the question). The list of possible external agents is endless. Insomuch as this "belief about" component of the phenomenological whole is notionally delusional, we have dealt with it already in principle and found it problematic. Can it not be formulated that the delusion is simply a stubbornness to refuse the obvious, and so a delusion is a difference of opinion between persons as to what is the case.

What is the obvious? It is, as said, that the patient is the architect of the message they are "receiving". Yet it is a message they audibly hear you may say, this is what defines the auditory hallucination as psychotic. Not so fast. I might tell you that a little voice inside my head told me not to gamble on a car park close to the hospital entrance and under that beautiful tree this morning, as this little piece of blue chip real estate would surely be taken by another. That same little voice told me that I'd better cut my prospective losses and park in that other street. Having made the gamble and failed to get the carpark, that little voice may tell me I'm an idiot and ought to have known better. That little voice can be very punitive. Such a narrative you would listen to without raising an eyebrow, all because my turn of phrase "little voice" is metaphorical. I know it. You know it. And you know I know it. So at worst what is pathological about the hallucination of hearing voices is the conversion of the metaphorical (and perhaps also the symbolic) into the literal hearing of an inner speech act, where inner speech is a metaphor for thought. Abundant evidence, even neuroscientific evidence, can at least be said to support the model that the auditory hallucination is disavowed inner speech, that little voice in the heads of all reflective persons. There is even some evidence of, on at least some occasions, excursions of vocal musculature during the hearing of the voice. But why hear it as opposed to think it? Why not? Can this not be conceptualized as a normal variant of human experience, that thought be heard? Remember we have already dealt with the matter of the patients belief about the voice (qua a quasi amplified inner speech act). Nonetheless it behoves me to explain how such a conversion may occur, and how it may make sense in adopting a more broader empathic approach to so called hallucinations.

When Esquirol first coined the term hallucination in the middle of the 19th century, he saw it as a form of madness (delire), yet saw the core feature of a hallucination as an involuntary creative act of memory and relatedness the person has with themselves and the world. Falret thought the same. This is not far from conceptualizing it as an inner speech act held stubbornly to come from an external agency. Now the matter of it being involuntary renders the hallucination no different to bone fide stimuli on one hand (I cannot easily filter out the sounds of those ambient noises that involuntarily enter my ears), and bone fide thoughts on the other (no one can claim to be the deliberate interior generator of all thoughts that enters one's mind. The best most of us can ever hope to manage is what to do with the thoughts having arrived, this being the outcome of choice and a dialectic within the self and between the self and others). It is the inescapability from our own thoughts that finds its analogue in the inescapability of the auditory hallucinations. It is the fact that none of us is truly the first maker of our own thoughts that finds its analogue in the voice as being heard as the "other".

Let us imagine the following three cases, each of which I'll argue are a continuance upon a spectrum.

Let us imagine I were raped, neglected and otherwise mistreated. From this and for various psychodynamic reasons about which we can only speculate I come to believe I am worthless, unloved and unlovable, and have temptation to kill myself. I might look upon the world and believe it to be a human jungle, to quote Tennyson "red in tooth and claw". I am always on edge that someone may target me for exploitation. Is my lot an unhappy one? Surely yes. Yet is this the stuff of medicine? Ought this be the stuff of the state in demanding I be reengineered towards normality and forcing its normative demands upon me? Surely not.

Now let's imagine that sometimes when especially distressed, I hear a voice telling me I'm worthless or to kill myself. All the memories of what happened or might have happened flood in at once, along with my relatedness to them. That is to say all those metaphorical voices from my present and all the memories of what others might have told me in the past, or what I may have concluded they were telling me as an interpretation of their behaviour, that is to say what they told me with words and also "told me" with deeds, all this is pulled within the present interpretation of experience. All the angst and the anxiety of the time approaches a crescendo of phenomenological alchemy where affect and content of thought transmutes into the form of a voice. Transiently I may even have the thought enter my mind that someone is out to get me (a persecutory delusion). At such times the psychiatrist, in their ever present drive to classify first and ask deep questions later, may say I am experiencing a pseudo-hallucination, a most incoherent term of art as what I am experiencing, qua a percept in lack of an objective material source of stimulus is by definition a hallucination as such.

We can forgive the psychiatrist, as the term pseudo-hallucination is goal based
to differentiate a particular class of patient from another (vide infra), and the
whole political exercise of classification and management need hang together to
a pragmatic end. We might be especially forgiving of the psychiatrist if at the
time or soon after I the hypothetical patient has the capacity to recognize the
voice is a product of their own mind. Once again we smuggle into our evaluation
of the voice the sine qua non of a delusion (i.e. belief about a proposition) and
with it also is conflated the concept of insight (a euphemism for submission
to psychiatric opinion, i.e. if you fail to agree with me you lack insight). The
reader will see all these terms of art are different facets of the same thing. To
the reader I might additionally ask the same questions. Beyond folk prejudice and
your affective response to the patient to which is entangled notions of care, what
are your a priori's, your "before the fact" premises from which to argue that this
alchemy ought to be either the stuff of medicine or is necessarily pathological?
Why is this alchemy not permitted, as a political act, to fall within the bounds of
what a human is permitted to be without molestations upon liberty and labelling
as "mentally ill" by agents of the state?

Let us imagine you see me months or years later, only now the voice is
with me often regardless of my affective state. Now my pseudo-hallucination is
a so called chronic auditory hallucination and I have been rebranded a chronic
schizophrenic. Now I always refuse to countenance the notion that the voice is
a product of my own mind, and may converse with the "voices" often, being
observed to "respond to non-apparent stimuli". I refuse to admit that I am the
alchemist in the transmutation of thought, of memory and of affect charged
inner speech into auditory perception. And so what of it? Once again, in what
sense is this disavowal of responsibility necessarily pathological? Why does it
demand a response by the state? If I ask you to think of a number between one
and ten and the number six enters your mind did you choose that particular
number before it's arrival? Insomuch as no one can claim to be the architect of
each and every one of their own experiences in the world, and no one can claim
to be the architect of each and every thought that enters their mind, no one can
claim that at least some disavowal of being the architect of mental phenomena
is necessarily corresponding to a fact of the world and human experience. Some
may externalize responsibility further up the spectrum of what one does with
mental phenomena after having so entered the mind. This is the stuff of all the
psychotherapies. Do you feel angry and say someone "made" you angry? Might
you not conclude from the lack of warmth and false politeness from that officious

bureaucrat that the state is at least indifferent to you or at most hostile, which is to say they are metaphorically "telling" you that you are grist for the mill, that they are "out to get you"? And what if this interpretation of social experience is, as an act of alchemy, heard audibly as coming from the other? And what if the presence, politically speaking, of the other is always there in a sense as a valid symbolic interpretation of the modern world. Though no one particular agent of the world is standing before you at the time you hear the world speak, the world still spins. Its aggression never rests. It and agents within it are always there as a perceived spirit of intention, a mood, a symbolic representation of deeper themes and agendas. Once again so what? Why is this alchemy to congeal meaning into voice not be permitted, as a political act, to fall within the bounds of what a human is permitted to be without molestations upon liberty and labelling as "the other" by agents of the state? What monster might you be to try save me from myself and my eccentricities, and so murder me as I am?

Finally, hearing voices is not normative in the dry statistical sense of the term. Yet looking cross culturally and across the lifespan (especially the youth), voices are much more common than one may think at first blush. Before Esquirols medicalization and the slow turn towards what Szasz called the therapeutic state, hearing voices was not always and universally accepted as demonic possession as those pejorative of the pre-enlightenment would allege in their attempt to argue they (i.e. psychiatry as an alleged science) saved us from the cruel iniquities and folk superstition of the previous age. Often visions and voices were interpreted as eccentric, benign, of symbolic worth and even theological value, or perhaps all of these. I'm thinking here for example of father Ferropont visions in the Brothers Karamazov. It is simply a myth of historiography and a propaganda of psychiatry that the disease symptom/sign of the hallucination was discovered. It was and is instead a normal variant of human experience reformulated as disease. Even today in many parts of the world the hearing of voices is often very common and perfectly appropriate when protected from the clutches of psychiatry by cultural context. Pick any group of what we may dare say are pre-modern peoples and try take from them their voices and visions, go try build a hospital large enough to accommodate those who have them. Even in our English speaking post industrial neck of the woods, take yourself into a state of sleep deprivation and even you might begin to see things or hear things. As a doctor I've been there. Or take yourself into a state of existential alienation or loss of connectedness to others and the same may occur, even in a city or sea of people, for we are beings seeking connectedness and will invent it if we are starving in the midst of plenty. Similarly it is extremely common for otherwise sane mountaineers, shipwreck survivors and the like to have the so called extracampine experiences of another person nearby, even to see or hear them at their side. The one cries out in its solitude even by those whose conscious mind claims to prefer being alone. And then there is bereavement and the patently obvious psychological motivations to seeing or hearing the afterglow of the departed loved one. Some may be tempted to believe these are legitimate visitations of the departed. Would any reader claim to be able prove this belief false, let alone force the experiencer to heel and disbelieve what their psyche, albeit the unconscious, has chosen to be true to them?

Risk

We have come to the point where those wishing to medicalize beliefs and behaviours invoke the matter of risk, this being essentially much of what much of psychiatric practice is about anyway, principally risk to the society in having a deviant roaming about and secondly reducing risk of medico-legal sequelae to the psychiatrist in not properly controlling them. What if the allegedly deluded individual performs an action that harms themselves or others, this action informed by the belief (or "belief about" in the case of voices). Note I did not use the turns of phrase "driven by belief" or "caused by the belief" or "stimulated by the belief" or "made to do" as such would be to presuppose the absence of free will and deny a capacity for deliberation that ought to be assumed the default state of the adult unless and until proven otherwise. We must labour very hard to escape the language of the ideologies within which we have become (only partially I hope) indoctrinated and use language consonant with having made the escape. I have discussed the matter of risk above in the chapter on drug use and in the chapters to follow also. For now it is enough to repeat, or at least to consider, that what one does as a behavioural response to a belief ought not necessarily provoke in others any behavioural response at all, especially not necessarily an aggressive or coercive response underwritten by the state. Much less ought the behaviour of the one who would be patient ever deductively (albeit a posteriori) be the basis of a medical diagnosis. That is to say, the behaviour does not retroactively make of the belief a pathology.

Hopefully in the sections above I have convinced the reader that the boundary between the normal and delusional belief is not so easily made, and moreover this may reflect that such a taxonomy of belief, i.e. normal vs pathological, is simply not the case in ontological fact. That is to say, beliefs are beliefs, and that is that. To be sure some are truth based and some not.

So what? Apparent falsity as judged by you, me, us, so called science or more often as adjudicated by an appointed agent into which state power is invested is not enough to medicalize anyone without medicalizing all sooner or later. We simply have no robust argument of what a delusion is outside of our use of the word to control a kind of deviancy, and as a euphemism for a critical mass of shared prejudice. Let's look at a couple concrete examples of risk. Someone believes that aqua-phobic aliens are out there and have designs to kill him. Sometimes they even control his movements, and have performed nasty sexual acts upon him, as aliens are often allegedly apt to do. Needless to say there is no material evidence of any of their visitations. And try as one might, arriving at empathic understandability is hard to come by without deeply diving into the symbolic realm. In any case our world be patient views their phenomena as literal. Now it is a matter of manifest fact that there are many free persons in the world who will express a belief in the existence of aliens, of having seen them, of even having been abused by them. So what? Where do we draw the proverbial line at which point we may dare medicalize such a spectrum of beliefs about the universe, those who may or may not dwell within it and our experience with them? I've never met a psychiatrist who can successfully debate this against me without condemning sooner or later half the schizotypicals, pagans, hippies, artists, ascetics, eccentrics, conspiracy theorists, malcontents and misfits down all of human history. Many psychiatrists retrospectively do just that to the extent it seems only those who did not leave any biography can be free from being diagnosed. Every famous person seems to have had some mental illness or another so says one psychiatrist or another. Fortunately, I know several psychiatrists from whom such an alien molested patient may be allowed escape unmolested by medication and forced hospitalization should they end their narrative at that, though this is sadly a minority of the whole sample of psychiatrists I've known. But what if the person of our example, a rational actor, decides one especially persecuted night to risk his life to escape the aliens by swimming out into the centre of the lake. Recall the aliens are aquaphobic. To be sure it's a desperate act, perhaps to escape, perhaps retaliative, perhaps out of spite. And naturally it engenders some risk and our patient might almost drown, or drown for sure, and such might even be their intent (just as the ascetic or dissident might self-immolate or starve from hunger for example). But there is no denying rationality in the behaviour from the system of their belief. Yet I do not know a single psychiatrist who would not see this, as a behaviour in virtue of it being a "risk of harm to self or others", as somehow recasting the whole belief and phenomenological picture as pathological and using it to justify saving the patient from the freedom to act according to the belief they have. This is a logically very weak move to make. It appeals only to the drama of the situation to invalidate the acceptability of another's belief. It is the political control over anothers body and freedom, which is very human. But it is not any more rational than our patient taking the fatal swim.

We may compare the above with crime. Criminal belief is only actionable if the consequent is a criminal act, a concrete behaviour. Of course one can imagine an omniscient celestial judge damning us for our silent rages and that which we covet without fair and moral acquisition. Yet in the fallen world of fallen man one cannot be charged with the crime of a mental representation of a crime, such as fantasizing about robbing a bank. Only from the behavioural act of conspiracy to rob the bank from which is present material evidence of conspiracy (not claims of intent or disclosure of fantasy), or only in the act of robbing of the bank as such, might we be able limit an individual's liberty. And the prior fantasizing is not made criminal after the fact as an additional charge. Even my positing such a word play of an un-actioned "criminal belief" is to illustrate a point, criminality in this case being a metaphor for the thoughts of one with a poor character (or rich and very human imagination), for thought is not crime. More of this in the penultimate chapter. But at least when we say that the person carries a thought that if carried out would be a crime, there is some conceptual homology between thought and behaviour, the picture in the mind (the fantasy of the criminal act) being the immoral representation of the immoral act (the crime itself). It is worse for psychosis than with crime, and the trap is bipartite. The first horn is the intolerance we might have of the thought itself. Often simply holding the suspect belief can be fertile grounds for being placed under state control, given such control flows from diagnosis and the risk of what they might do, along with the notion that the patient ought to be saved from the deleterious state of having the aberrant belief itself, the psychotic illness. But we have argued above that the psychotic thought cannot be distinguished from any other as pathological. We can only say it is the thought held by a non-criminal social deviant. And so what? The second horn upon which the individual might have their liberty impaled is the behaviour. Yet how does behaviour placing self or others at risk somehow alter the picture in one's mind to something else? There is no thought behaviour homology as there is with the criminal fantasy. In what sense can it be argued that belief in aliens is permissible only up to the point at which attendant behaviours incur a risk of harm to self or others? And having passed the threshold we say "ah, you can be permitted your belief in aliens only if you do not take the belief so seriously as to live it. You can believe in these aliens and not those aliens. It can be you in this relationship to aliens and not that relationship to aliens". You see if belief is not pathological and suicide is not pathological, placing the two together cannot be pathological.

As I once regrettably and to my shame told the loved ones of so called delusional patients, "we are saving them from the prison of false beliefs, a prison far more insidious than the deprivation of liberty in a psychiatric hospital" (I'm paraphrasing). Is this so different from the Orwellian idea of thought crime and all the horrors of the worst totalitarian ideology, all the more so as carried within the mind of the totalitarian agent is a sincere spirit of benevolence. For me then, as it is now in mainstream psychiatry, the matter of risk of harm to self or others is merely a tool of argument in favour of control, playing upon the language of care and fear. It does not somehow breathe life into lifeless arguments seeking the medicalize beliefs as pathological.

What I am proposing is to drop the sham and pretence of psychiatry as medicine and science. Any intervention to deprive the individual of liberty, to stop them from harming themselves or others, and intervene after such attempts have been made ought to appeal to either acts of criminal legislation (harm to others) or an entirely unscientific un-medicalized state of human affairs with attendant language such as is found in morality, philosophy, religion and the basic folk prejudices of the family and the village. I would neither blame the loved one or concerned citizen who drags the self-described alien abductee from the lake than I would blame the alien abductee themselves for taking the fatal swim. What is to be blamed is the agent or agencies who repeatedly ignore the call of the individual to have their liberty restored come what may, be it jail or the grave. From concerned citizen or loved one does not (or ought not) a police state make. Psychiatry continuously and egoistically denies the hue and cry of patients who say they prefer to risk death at the hands of aliens, vampires and the CIA rather than life involving psychiatric hospitals and psychiatric drugs. Such love is hatred in disguise.

Again, what is psychosis?
Very early in my career I came to see the only way psychosis could be defined was either in terms of an unjustified undefined common-sense prejudice, i.e. "of course he's insane", or alternatively in an observation of the use of the word, with criteria and ostensive definitions just props in a ritual. This was when the

penny dropped, that the definition of psychosis is entirely bound up in the use of the word. I was a junior doctor then. No one understood me, nor wanted to, and I quickly fell into a troubled silence. Only later did I discover other philosophic voices who might have been sympathetic to my own. Empathic un-understandability may seem like a wonderful tool when we cherry pick unusual or concocted examples such as misplaced postage stamps as nonsense evidence of infidelity, and allow ourselves be seduced by an argument after we have already settled on the conclusion. Here we have designed our own seduction, and in seducing others are being sophists in the worse sense of the term. Here all we are appealing to is motivated consensus. It is not at all clear if we are in a place of consensus the likes of which we may be when making logical inference or agreeing on the material solidity of the world by dashing our collective feet on a stone. It gets worse though for logic, and infinitely worse for psychiatric rules and surveying the phenomenological landscape looking for psychotic signposts. Stones will be stones, though the nature of their solidity of these too were questioned in the formulations of Berkley as made in the third chapter.

Wittgenstein spoke of the use of words in language as not having any definite meaning in themselves, the meaning only becoming manifest in the use of the words in a custom of human activity. Were someone to yell "duck" we know what to do, not as a conscious act of interpreting the word, as opposed to an act generated by the hearing of the word and embedded within the context of the event itself. Often the action we take upon hearing the word has no connection with thought at all. Perhaps in language acquisition thought never did sit "meta" to action and context, as the primary driver of language itself was learned custom. Upon hearing the word "duck", do we look for a duck as an ornithologist might? Or raise the rifle to shoot as a hunter might? Or take it as a message that the companion has found something delectable whilst passing a Chinese restaurant? Or do we lower our head to miss the swinging boom as a sailor might when the captain yells "duck"? The word/sentence "duck" is an observation, a command or a celebration and much more and nothing in and of itself divorced from context. It is the simplest of what can become far more complicated examples of what Wittgenstein called language games. We might add to this vast list the custom and terms of art in psychiatric diagnosis in general, and the rituals of constructing the patient as psychotic in particular. But this is a devilishly complex language game, and one that can take years of synchronising language use between masters and apprentice (not only for reason that the psychiatric masters are often inconsistent within and between themselves, technically speaking lacking reliability even with the DSM 5, and incoherent also if forced into real argument), and between masters and their masters within the greater hierarchies of power or the history of psychiatry. This formulation of psychosis as language based and contextual also "reframes" emergency department physician's tendency to label any disruptive and disorganised behaviour as psychotic, and why internal medicine physicians seem not to be able to diagnose idiopathic delirium, having the talent to confuse it with psychotic illness at almost every opportunity. These species of laudably authentic physicians are simply playing a different language game, with different goals (i.e. to dump the patient into the arms of psychiatry). It is not that they misdiagnose delirium or psychosis. They are defining it differently in practice, and only acquiescing to psychiatric opinion out of professional courtesy, not as an act of being corrected to the truth.

Allow me to restate the case to follow in various admittedly pleonastic ways, to further liberate the reader from being trapped in a false idea of what psychosis is, for we have seen what it cannot be. This repetition is necessary and ought to be forgivable as tiny drops of unlearning against the ocean of the standard view into which one has been indoctrinated. The standard definition of delusion in particular we have seen is not worth the paper it's printed on. The Jasperian reading is also deeply problematic. He was thinking some sophisticated empathic encounter with the phenomenology would bring us to the essence of psychosis in the patient. He was thinking you require some expertise in reaching into the patient with a penetrating phenomenological gaze and finding something there corresponding to the word psychosis, a word object denotation, a something being there and pointing to it the way we might do with a physical pathology, a cancer or thrombus for instance. (or the collection of physical evidence pointing towards a specific behaviour such as a crime).

But you see there is no systematic answer to the question of what is psychosis, no coherent definition that is a priori to what we do with the word, no pointing through the person, as it were, at the essence within them of something we call psychosis.

Psychosis is the word ascribed to a broad range of psychological phenomena and psychologically informed behaviours of, usually, non-criminal deviancy, not as an actual concrete object that the word denotes, but the words meaning is diffused out over the whole process of the diagnosis as a goal based practice. Psychosis is not some essentiality in the patient. Nor is it in the point when the psychiatrist arrives at diagnosis, as if it becomes the case in the grasping or understanding.

The diagnosis is often in the "dyadic" interaction of patient and psychiatrist both. It is their diagnosis, and more so the whole ritual or ceremony, it is also what becomes of the person so diagnosed, its function in the world.

Being psychotic is this and it is this in toto; there is a manifold upon which the construct might have its meaning, i.e. the historical pattern of the use of the word before the current encounter between psychiatrist and patient and how that is shifted and shaped over time. This encounter might be with a different set of players, yet it is similar to the diagnostic ritual of the past, i.e. it's shifts are not rapid. There is a technique or custom passed down. There was simple psychosis, Soviet style psychosis (political deviancy), Morel's degenerate démence précoce, Kraepelin's dementia praecox, Bleuler's schizophrenia, ED physician's psychosis (dramatic behaviour), internists psychosis (overlaps with delirium if not dementia), DSM schizophrenia (neither equivalent with that of Bleuler or Kraepelin) etc. All of these were or are "true". They are just the settings for different language games. Then in the encounter at hand, the current game at play, it is what the patient says, what the psychiatrist asks, what the psychiatrist proclaims is the case and how the patient is treated, fitting the present encounter to those of the past use of custom. Or it is like a secular marriage (I say secular as the analogy only succeeds if removing the sacramental mystery). The celebrant does not discover the couple to be married. Neither are they married simply by the proclamation of the celebrant, or in the celebrant coming to a point of knowing they are married. They are married by partaking in the ritual and it's meaning to the wider world. The meaning of a word is in its use.

In summary, the rule or definition comes as an explanation for what we do, which is in practice to medicalize a social deviancy of this particular kind. It is as if we are saying we agree about delusions when we encounter them, and now find need to discover the essence of them by the invention of a definition/rule to justify what we do. We all agree you are crazy. Now let us decide why we agree. When combined with the question of liberty, this is the very definition of a show trial, far removed from a phenomenological study. And this a posteriori definition is ultimately empty without recourse to explaining it by way of the examples which are the very custom of its use. It is then made circular, the arc of the circle with the thinnest edge being the definition, as the definition or rule doesn't have any strength of its own despite its formal pretentions. Furthermore, having been divested of the logical strength of the definition/rule, we needn't have any faith in our grasp of it as pointing us towards something. We think we have a mental hold on something in our definition. But not only is the definition obviously lacking, it can never be proven true. It cannot be shown to point towards itself, let alone something beyond itself to which it is said to represent. And neither can the phenomenological enterprise. What if we all agree 100 patients are delusional (or not) according to our ostensibly shared use of the Jasperian process of empathic understandability. And then we start disagreeing on the next patient. What if you start saying you can empathise with the patient and I say I cannot? Curiously we both think we have been using the same process all along. We both swear we have been following the same rule. Now our disagreement at the one hundredth and xth case might prove that one of us has lost our way, that one of our phenomenological powers have dulled. Yet in the fact of our certainty to have both all along been following the same process, and the now emergent fact of our disagreement, we find instead that we were not following the same rule all along, or any rule at all. What we were following was not as solid as we thought. It was a dance upon air, where we each stood on one another's feet. We just had mutual adherence to a custom, the mutuality of which has been revealed to be imperfect. Now the mutuality is gone. So just who of our one hundred patients were delusional? Were any? What does it even mean? To the young and budding psychiatrist who might ask me what psychosis is I cannot give them the psychiatric definition and keep a straight face. All I could say is go and sit in the interview room. See the ritual. Calibrate yourself to the ritual. And one day you can take the interviewers seat and partake in the ritual yourself. And then you will see that psychiatric diagnosis is not something you do as in discovering. It is something that is doing itself. A psychiatric diagnosis is a "mastery of technique" as to its use. It is pragmatism rearing its ugly head again. But we continue dancing upon air, convinced it is solid. Idolatry!

Don't misunderstand me. I do believe in objective truths. Neither am I denying the reality of "madness". I'm anti-pragmatist, anti-relativist and a realist of a certain qualified kind. People with certain deviant behaviours and thoughts certainly do exist. They will say mad things and do mad things. And this might annoy people, embarrass family and even place themselves in grave danger. They might not flourish in life, and usually don't without a substantial buttressing from the family or the state, where the latter sadly very often comes to replace the former in the states relentless war against marriage, family and community. Nevertheless these mad persons do not easily or at all fit into the infractions upon sections of criminal code legislation, begging for some other options for micro/macro social engineering and control. And so they will find themselves sitting across from the psychiatrist, our secular shaman invested with the power of the upscaled village, a village which seems to want to lose its collective liberty. The psychiatrist/shaman will tell the village if the patient is possessed by the demon psychosis, or not. The psychiatrist certainly exists too. As has been made clear the diagnosis ontologically depends on their participation. The language game has already commenced before the patient arrives at the interview room, in the suspicions of the laity, how they seek a place to alienate the individual, to find some other prison in which to place them, in wishing to find someone to explain them, to solve them, the decode them, to change them, to help them, save them, absolve them of responsibility, treat them, restore them to being a comfortably normative object for the state and its various subjects. The complainant laity certainly exist also. How the complainant recognises the customs not to play and whom to call, (e.g. the white coats and not the boys in blue, except the latter as adjuncts), and the ends they seek...all is part of the custom. And when sitting across from the psychiatrist he/she will ask x, the patient will answer y, and the word psychosis or schizophrenia will come to be invoked. And the attempt to return the person to normative function will begin, with force, with domesticating medications, and with periodic confinement if necessary. And that is all psychosis is. No more fruitlessly looking for aberrant chemical imbalances or brain shrinkage (these will come after the psychiatric drugs). Just the playing out of the consequences of whatever special deviancy is a la mode by the psychiatric orthodoxy of the time and place. Whether it be hearing voices, believing you are the queen of Sheba, believing you ought to be freed from slavery or having the cognitive dysfunction not to recognise the self-evident correctness of Soviet Socialism, it doesn't matter. All can be psychosis. So if you wish to enter into the church of psychiatry, then please untie yourselves of the knots your professors have bound into your mind. Please do what you will do shamelessly and with clarity. Be honest to all involved, starting with thyself. You are an agent of the state, a political actor, a complement to the police in minimizing social deviancy. The patient is mad because we agree they are. That sentence is both the beginning and the end of the dialectical show. But should this chapter lead you to feel a sense of doubt with your erstwhile cherished power of discernment of the mad from the normal and what it all means, hallelujah. Let the doubt be like acid dripping onto the untruths of a troubled mind. Doubt and doubt some more. Spread it amongst friends.

THANATOLOGY. ON PRIVATE PROPERTY.

"They tell us that Suicide is the greatest piece of Cowardice... That Suicide is wrong; when it is quite obvious that there is nothing in this world to which every man has a more unassailable title than to his own life and person."
    Arthur Schopenhauer

"When suicide is out of fashion we conclude that none but madmen destroy themselves; and all the efforts of courage appear chimerical to dastardly minds ... Nevertheless, how many instances are there, well attested, of men, in every other respect perfectly discreet, who, without remorse, rage, or despair, have quitted life for no other reason than because it was a burden to them, and have died with more composure than they lived?"
    David Hume

Camus is credited with having first said of suicide that it is the "only one really serious philosophical problem" Well he would say that, wouldn't he. So convinced he was that existence was absurd, that the question was whether to take flight into superstition and myth, or let go of existence altogether. I'm not sure I agree it is the philosophical problem apart from the consequence of the projecting his "mood of absurdity" out into the world. Perhaps as an atheist he wanted the world be absurd so he could cast off the shackles of religion and its attendant moral injunctions and conduct his affairs with moral impunity. But who knows. If absurdity is transcendent, then how can he escape it? All of his analytical reasoning towards what is meaningful and the conceptualization of absurdity must also be absurd, making the whole thesis an exercise in self-contradiction. And hence I would say his project was moral, political and necessarily theological as opposed to a work of a dispassionate metaphysics. Nonetheless I'll pause from criticizing Camus too much, for in fairness there is much to the man and his thought that is commendable. Moreover, when one looks at psychiatry's conception of suicide, it evidences a kind of absurdity that may lead one to despair and a want to exit if not from the existence, at least then to exit from psychiatry. Why? Well, for all the critique we may level at Camus, credit is his due. For it ought not be lost on us that he placed suicide in the correct category, i.e. a philosophical problem, not biological, not medical, not social even, but existential and individual. To the extent the state it it's appendages become involved it is also legal and political. To the extent to which it is a moral act, it is also subsumed back into philosophy at least, if not theology also and as stated above.

But a younger version of myself should have known better in the naïve assumption psychiatry would see suicide for what it is, or at least for what it isn't. Or at least to care to ask deeply the questions Camus asked. Back many moons ago, before entering the church of psychiatry and when fishing around for a PhD project, I happened upon a conversation with someone who was working on the "genetic basis of suicide". "How strange" I thought, though politely did not say, as they fervently described their project with the enthusiasm of one who had just begun a PhD, as opposed to labouring to write the doctoral thesis at the end when each word is panful and hated. I had a background in genetics and none at the time in psychology and the humanities. Like many a science major, I erroneously heaped scorn on philosophy. But even then it seemed immediately obvious, a priori obvious, that a suicide is a behaviour of one living in a web of psychological relationships with self and the world, a choice made by a free agent, however hastily and ill considered, and however for or against the grain of surrounding opinion. It had never crossed my mind that had Sophocles lived in the genetic age he might have figured into the plot the Oedipus family having a faulty gene or that a counterfactual history might have seen the samurai or religious martyrs recruit on the basis of genetic testing as to their proclivity towards their own death. Or perhaps Sophocles would have ceded to scientism, with humanity all the worse for it. Sure, what might possibly be found is a genetic proclivity towards alcoholism as a very common contextual factor in suicide, though this is a far cry from determinism. Or what might be found is a genetic proclivity to impulsively or other features of personality that may be correlated with an increased risk of suicide. Yet these variables seemed many degrees of diluted separation from the act itself, and thoroughly divorced from the context of say, the suicide from unrequited love, the act made poignantly sweet from sad songs and made warm from the liquor before the blood runs warm and the body goes cold. All this is to say, the old nature and nurture

ledger within scientism simply won't do in any case I've ever seen of threatened/
accomplished suicide, and I have seen countless attempts after working on the
front line in emergency department psychiatry for longer than almost any other
psychiatric doctor I know. I might as well have asked this scientistic geneticist
what gene (or second order epigenetic mechanism, for genes aren't the whole
story), as a meaningful explanatory datum, determined their choice of career
as a geneticist? And not just a geneticist, but which gene determined her gross
reductive medicalization of suicide, the interest in this specific project? Or what
gene determined the band she listened to on the radio in the lab today or the
postcard of that tropical island she placed above the PCR machine? All this too
would have been absurd, were it not also horrifying. For at the ends of every
attempt at genetic over-determinism is, if not eugenics, a drive towards social
engineering, a want to "save" people from their genes, the genes of others,
and from any notion of free will and personal responsibility. Such appeals to
compassion and saving people drive the funding for the gene hunt in the first
place, for money creates the thoughts that attract it, and thought creates money
in turn. This kind of reductionist ground is also revealed in psychiatric practice
in the belief that lithium salts and the medication known as clozapine have, in
addition to manifold other effects, a specific and independent anti-suicidal effect.
Why? Do these medications act upon the suicide receptor or suicide brain circuit?
What nonsense! However much orthodox psychiatry might speak of the so called
biopsychosocial model or person centred care, make no mistake it is driven
to consider suicide a medical illness, the act being an epiphenomena of events
occurring in the brain. The whole language game is geared in that direction with
"triggers" to suicide, "what made you take the overdose" etc. Such reductive
nonsense is lubricated by metaphor also, for the cells that comprise the body can
commit "cell suicide", otherwise known as apoptosis (for those of the academic
lineage of Sir John Kerr the second "p" is silent, apoptosis being, etymologically
a metaphor for the falling leaves of Autumn). For example, at certain stages of
development cells may involute and die, the resultant being that we can have
separated fingers as opposed to a webbed paddle of a hand. Or a cancerous cell
may "commit suicide" after damage from radiotherapy, providing the cell has
retained the "program" and capacity to "decide" and effect its suicide as an act
of cellular civic consciousness, much like the character in the zombie film who
kills themselves while they still can and before they turn into the walking dead.
The reader will see in one cellular phenomena I've made appeal to multiple
metaphors, of conscious deliberation and decision, of computation in the cell

having the program, of telos in the ends to development, of sacrifice for the common good in cancer, of changes in the weather in the name, and so on. I once made a joke, unfortunately seriously taken, about writing a paper arguing that suicide of the person was just an evolutionarily upscaling of cellular suicide. Yet cells do not commit suicide. This is a metaphor. People do.

If we bookend my career from that conversation to the present day, we now have a "Camusian" despair at the absurdity of the zero-suicide movement sweeping the Anglo speaking psychiatric world. Very much framed in corporate newspeak, if one peruses the website of the likes of zerosuicide.org as the largest of several international organizations, one will see it populated psychiatric doctors and psychologists rebranding themselves as "thought leaders", "re-designers" (pray tell of what?), "educators", "movers", "top influencers" and (my favourite) "full scalers". Whilst it's organization and language are nauseatingly corporate (without the tax burden of course, why not add "monetizers" to the list?), it's lofty goal is totalitarian, hence the aspirational name to drop the suicide body count to zero. The only way to even countenance such an aspiration is either to be open to bio-political totalitarian control and abolition of individual autonomy, falling into the Foucaltian trap (more on this anon), and/or a drive to change the very substance of the human condition on a crypto-Orwellian scale (fullscaling?), and/or to have an absolute wanton ignorance of human history. The movement also seeks to craft the way in which the mental health clinician and populace speaks of suicide, in turn to craft the way the both think about suicide. For it seeks to abolish language such as "killing yourself", "successful suicide", "committing suicide" or "taking your life" for fear that this makes a statement about personal agency, or moral judgment or value or goal directedness. Suicide is like a seizure, something that happens to someone unless saved by the hero psychiatrist.

Its 2015 International declaration opens with the statement that, on average, there is a death from suicide every 40 seconds. This is reminiscent of a distant past when I could recall the preacher standing aside the pulpit clicking his fingers at the rate at which souls enter hell. He wanted to save souls also, and what horrors he could have done with a slick website and the powers of the state at his side to deprive liberty of those who might decide their own fate. Yet another example that the powers are not separated. The state replaced the church with psychiatry and forced the church to the margins.

It continues, this being current at the time of writing this draft

"Suicide is a complex, multifaceted biological, sociological, psychological, and societal problem with few resources for prevention. As a major global health problem, it is estimated that it will contribute more than 2% to the global burden of disease by 2020. Suicide imposes a huge unrecognized and unmeasured economic global hardship in terms of potential years of life lost (YPLL), medical costs incurred, and work time lost by mourners."

They had to mention the money didn't they, as economic concerns drive the funding for burgeoning industry. There is no model offered to integrate and give meaning to the four contributors to complexity, two of which sound so similar as to be arguably synonymous (perhaps we could say sociological, societal and social just to increase the word count and appear more erudite. We then ought to add the word "socialist" also). Reading a book is also all these four things in being biological (requiring vision and the biomechanics of page turning), psychological (motivation to read etc), social (the economics, supply and marketing of the book within the social milieu) and so much more. These words are empty of explanation of what it is for you to read this particular book and this particular time. Reading a book can be simple or complex depending on one's point of view, as can everything else for that matter. And so complexity can be everything and nothing, and in praxis becomes code for the claims made by an elite intelligentsia that they are the only ones to understand the phenomena to which the word "complexity" is attached. Putting that aside for now, the zero-suicide movement (and yes in places it explicitly invokes the word "movement") also explicitly makes of suicide a disease, hence I imagine the need in turn for the social "redesigners" of this suicide industry to counter those naysayers who might seek to dissolve it back to the individual with liberty making their own choices in the world.

I ask the reader to keep in mind those three things, i.e. a) zero aspiration, b) the power of psychiatry underwritten by the state to deprive suicidal persons of their liberty and c) viewing suicide as a complex "disease" the likes that only the psychiatric intelligentsia can understand (or if not a disease all its own, the manifestation of a psychopathology or mental illness all the same). Against this apogee of the new psychiatry, let's look at some typical cases from history and my own experience, and what psychiatry might have done, or did indeed do. Of each historical/mythological case I can assure the reader that if any psychiatrist is even aware of them, that this was most certainly not the result of psychiatric training, though it should be. To each case I challenge the reader to formulate the goodness of fit between the zero suicide ideology and the reality of the human condition. Hopefully I can start to dislodge the reader from what might be the conviction that suicide is a dreadful epidemic that must be stopped at all costs, as opposed to a tragedy to be grieved. We shall see.

Suicidality in the mythology of antiquity was, as presumed fiction, not a representation of historical events in time. Nevertheless, mythology is a reflection of human concerns, the way they are managed and the way the author might have suggested they are to be managed. Though we be neither Gods or kings, mythology is, in its way, stories about us in a time before it was contaminated by psychiatry. One can look back at the works attributed to Hypocrites and find mention of mania and melancholia not as descriptors of so called psychiatric mood disorders a la DSM so much as instead descriptors of noisy and quiet delirium in severe physical illness. That small piece of trivia is a digression, but an important one corrosive to the notion that psychiatry looks back and discovers unconstructed disease. Similarly, if one looks at, for example, the latinized Fabularum Liber (Book of Fables), by Hyginus one will find suicides aplenty in the literature of ancient Greece. Yet within these plots will not be placed anything that can be easily equated with alleged major depressive disorder, bipolar disorder, schizophrenia or any other so called mental illness for that matter. No, those protagonists, some few dozen in number, took their lives for reasons of great pathos, not pathology. From Antigone to Themisto and everyone in between (including in Sophocles renditions most of the house of Laius), they killed themselves out of pride, shame, lost or unrequited love, vanity, social disconnectedness, all the well worn themes of human drama in literature as in life.

The list is hardly restricted to the mythological. Here is but a tiny elaboration on our already tiny sample. Cato suicided as a political protest, as have countless others up to the current age (I'm thinking for example of self- immolating monks of south east Asia). Antony and Cleopatra suicided in a drama that presages and partially resembles the tale of Romeo and Juliet. Kalanos suicided rather than live as an elderly invalid, as has countless others for the same reason down to the present day. Of how I have lost count of the number of times I have been called to the bedside of an old person who wishes to die for no other reason but age and infirmary or on account of intractable pain. "But they are suicidal...", says the physician as if this one terrifying word dissolves all humanity and good sense into the inhuman void of psychiatry. The savy physician might appeal to a gnostic argument, that they might have "masked depression" and this drive their suicidality. To the one who insists a mask is being worn, no pulling at the face will convince them it is not there. Needless to say when a patient states "but for the fact I'm in pain I would not be suicidal.." this is a call first, second and third for the psychiatrist. When I politely suggest to the physician they may wish look at the analgesics, I'm met with a dumb look of perplexity.

Returning to the history lesson, Judas suicided after a radical confrontation with his sin. How many Samurai suicided out of honour, indeed even as a natural expression of their commitment to Zen and an ever readiness for death that could only ever be fully actualized by meeting death at the hand of their own blade, if not also the blade of a comrade. Even the enemy is their comrade in bringing them into a confrontation with their meaning in death. And we have all heard of Socrates, who accepted the hemlock for no other reason than to be true to himself to the end. Insomuch as he might have been allowed to escape Athens and his death sentence yet chose not to, his was a case that places martyrdom within a conceptual spectrum where homicide and suicide become blurred (though in my opinion this would be an error). Then there are group suicides, as in Masada and a couple millennia later in Russian/Ukrainian villages as the Reich closed in, and some German villages suiciding a few years later as a red army sought vengeance for some twenty million of their own dead. Then there are terrorist murder suicides, perhaps with Samson being the first. The list is so long as to paint psychiatry thick with embarrassment, were they not either ignorant of history or hell bent to interpret all these cases as undiagnosed mental illness… if only they could. Dilettante or philistine. That is the differential diagnosis we might give to the case of psychiatry. Ancient sources also put paid to the notion that limiting access to means can limit the behaviour. Ajax had his sword and so fell on it. Females usually didn't have a sword handy. So a cliff, a river or a rope was used instead. Making loved ones the custodians of the medication and putting the kitchen knives up high might limit the access to means for the one who might impulsively reach for an aid to self killing making a scene. This is common sense. But for those determined to do it, antiquity proved that where the spirit is willing, the flesh shall follow. This is a truism that the suicidologists will say is a myth.

An emblematic case from my own experience

There I was sitting amongst colleagues discussing the suicide of the patient of a colleague. As usual and if pressed all would admit that suicide is nigh on impossible to predict, and the tenor of the meeting was the usual political babble of a working "culture of no blame". All the same the purpose of the meeting was to transport ourselves back in time, and discuss what we might have done differently to see the suicide coming and prevent it. If the reader is confused at such self-contradictory lack of logic, then so was I. The case was of a man who killed himself. His tale of woe began after moving from a war torn almost lawless place where gun attacks were common, to a place where they were exceedingly rare. And here he moved, in part to the furtherance of his safety, only to suffer severe injury at the hands of an idiot with a gun, a reckless act though not intentional attack. He would have many painful surgeries. The shooter evaded justice on a technicality, and so the patient took to drinking and arming himself, not with a plan of revenge as opposed to simply feeling safe. Unfortunately, his gun was not legally owned and so he was the one facing charges, along with multiple surgeries. Now one way to formulate the case is in terms of "major depressive disorder", "medication" required, the suggestion of "house calls to review his mental state" and "psychiatric admissions". This was the talk of psychiatry. This was all they could, and did, say. What was obvious however was that here was a man made a victim of fate and the blackly ironic humour of the world. Moved from a place of war. Shot in a place of safety. Prosecuted when the real criminal walks free, and his body was injured, and injured badly. He could not say there was a certain quantum of good in the world, and life was painful. And so he ended it. Where is the place of medicine here, or the state except as a further source of taking the man's freedom away and saying there was something wrong with him? Would psychiatry have the gall to prevent him to choose his end as he did? They would if they could.

Or take the case of the young woman brought into hospital by police (plural) after threatening to throw herself on the railroad tracks. That's three police policing suicide, and three less police policing crime, and not her crime either, for such patients are mentally ill don't you know, and so no charges are laid for public nuisance etcetera (laying charges incurs paperwork and ought to be avoided as a strained judiciary will do nothing anyway). Her behavior was very dramatic and potentially lethal, yet she had been assessed only hours before in the same emergency department for the same behavior and discharged. And now with me and within ear shot of one of the police officers she clearly stated, inter alia, that she made the threats with the express intent of worrying her mother and not to end her life (her intent to worry succeeding in spades). And so not wanting to reward bad behavior, I discharged her also, and kindly requested of the police that they not return her thrice. "But she's suicidal" came the reply, as they spoke as if the word evokes in them an animalistic reflex to act, completely divesting themselves of their common sense. We agreed to disagree, that should she repeat her threats they may conceivably return her for assessment every six hours for the term of her natural life, and every 6 hours I would discharge her. There are countless other patients besides in similar situations. Patient number one is brought into the emergency department with threat to suicide, and engages in argument with another already there for the same reason. The first threatens to kill the second. I ask the police if they will prosecute the threat that their own ears have born witness to, the answer being they cannot as no crime is committed. A threat to kill another incurs no penalty. A threat to kill oneself involves a deprivation of liberty and takes at least two to four police officers off the beat.

How did suicide become medicalized? I would not be so bold as to suggest that 17th and 18th century England was the first place and time, yet it certainly was an early place and time, and one of the nuclei around which the anlage of Anglo psychiatry could collect and construct itself. If one reads, for example, Blackstones "Commentaries on the Laws of England", suicide was correctly seen as a crime against the self, a felo de se. In the case of completed suicide, the indictment hardly can be met with any defence against the charge, for the accused is there hanging by the noose (though I have in my career encountered three clear homicides that were unfortunately written off as suicide). In England of Blackstones time a suicide, qua a crime was met often by harsh fines and asset seizures that the estate of the departed were forced to pay. And so the poor family was left to foot the bill. This is to say the poor family were effectively the ones punished by the crime of the suist, and with no recourse to escape from the fine. And the penalty was not just with coin and assets. The loved one also faced an ignoble burial and the family face social shame. How does one escape all this miscarriage of justice where the family is punished for the crime of the departed? The escape was the construction of the insanity defence, defended by family with the accused in absentia. If the departed could be posthumously proven to be insane, certain forgiveness may be possible, both in terms of debt and social stigma. It made no sense of course, for the family cannot of necessity be guilty for anothers crime against themselves (and God). Much harm to truth could have been averted had the government not been as greedy. Nothing much has changed.

But enough of mythology, history and personal experience of what might be called rational suicidality, though more on this anon. After all, what lessons from a few thousand years of humanity have to bestow upon us of today? The reader might be of the belief that emergency psychiatric departments are nowadays filled with persons who have taken leave of reason and their senses, the ostensive insanity being from no fault of their own of course, and which may carry them into the arms of death, in extensio, as part of the disease itself. This, or it may be thought the emergency department is filled with suicidal persons who are involuntarily driven to wanting death on account of some gravely melancholic illness, some depressive "disease" that takes over their person and renders them unable to see the sunshine and rainbows that others "objectively" see is part of their world. To encounter such a rare melancholic patient is to encounter a psycho-physiological abyss. Such cases are far from being the norm however, and I have long witnessed in colleagues the paradoxically pleasant surprise they experience when encountering a truly depressed person to whom their heart reaches out spontaneously, a person for whom they need not make a deliberate attempt to quell the "negative counter-transference", where counter-transference is now nothing more than a euphemism for disliking the patient and failing to sympathize with their plight. We must not take too harsh a view of what is often (self) ascribed to be negative counter-transference, as it is often an aide to diagnosis. Moreover, when one points the finger at others, as the saying goes, one points a few fingers back at oneself. This is to say that the one who passes judgment on the negative counter-transference of the mental health practitioner are themselves exercising a negative countertransference of a kind, this time against the practitioner, and guilty of the same judgmental sin they see in the other. The splinter in my brothers eye, the forest growing out of my own....

In any case, the assumption as stated above is incorrect. Apart from the procession of psychotic and dysphoric methamphetamine and cannabis users, emergency psychiatric departments fill on a daily basis with individuals who profess to be suicidal on account of the passions and problems of daily living (which they often opaquely acknowledge) and often an infantilism in personality (about which they are often determined to be unaware). Their plight is often the likes of which a friend of mine once remarked "we in the developing world have real problems whereas you in your world need invent problems for entertainment"

Take for example the adolescent girl who passionately hated her stepfather. He had been banished for a time by the mother, though soon to return full time as mother and stepfather were involved in talks to reconcile (unsurprising to the psychoanalyst reader this hate was held with a tinge of love and a want not to be abandoned again, and the love for mother was with a measure of hate, for she drove him away the first time). For the reader who would be latter day witch hunters the answer is no, there was not an inkling of a suggestion that he had sexually abused the girl as an attribution for her suicidality, to a hammer everything need not be a nail. Her mother wanted the father figure restored front and centre in the family circle, and demanded she bend her knee so to speak, and respect the man who would be king. This was a demand to which the daughter responded, in a sense literally, that such an acquiescence would be over her dead body. And so she threatened suicide and was brought to me. She had of course the set criterion for diagnosis of a major depressive disorder, for such criteria are exceedingly easy to meet. She was "depressed", sullen and not engaged with her usual hobbies, as frivolity and leisure are seldom befitting the occasion in times of war. She was excessively sleeping, a behaviour for which she had excellent insight to be an act of escape, and not interested so much in eating with the family either. Why would she? Then there were the suicidal threats, another criterion in the checklist towards the diagnosis a la DSM 5 of a major depressive episode, and a doubt that she would win her war and her future to be a happy one (i.e. hopelessness, another criterion). The whole pseudo-depressive symptomatic set cried "protest" and she fought with what was her only weapon, instilling fear in her mother, making of her suicidality a sado-masochistic act. Yet to those around me, from the mother aghast at my formulation to the emergency staff and the psychiatric machine, this was illness that demanded treatment, and none would heed my simple anti-prescription that there is not a pill in the world that will change the situation. Apart from the stepfather exiting the stage, the only remedy was for the mothers stubborn will to break, or the daughters. And my strategically feigned perplexity that they would even have an expectation otherwise fell on deaf ears. Certainly an SSRI was prescribed by the psychiatrist who came after.

Or take the almost endless march of young men, often burley, muscled, with tattoos often up to (and sometimes now sometimes unfortunately within) their eye balls. These are the kind that one might pass in the street and think them to be intimidating, not only given that some of them actually are bullies. But when their sweetheart ends the affair these alpha males are reduced to a blubbering suicidal mess. On occasion the now ex sweetheart attends the scene with him, delivering a mixed message in the very fact of her presence. And yet both will then look doe eyed awaiting the magic of the psychiatrist, as she will tell the blubbering mess that he is here to "get the help" he needs. Once again all and sundry assume a medication will be involved and that I will, nay I should, have an answer in the form of a diagnosis and so on. Once again I am the secular priest who sanctifies them as diseased. But why and what is this help about which she speaks and he assents? What is the diagnosis? She has left him, for the moment anyway as she oscillates between love object and mother object, for the moment in the phase of the latter. Either she changes her mind and takes him back, or he reconciles with the reality of her choice (or current disposition) and moves on. It really is that simple. I could dull the anxieties in his mind with drugs probably more safely than the illicit drug dealer or bartender down the street. I could give him some words from Epictetus, with psychiatry not to thank for the stoic wisdom they have only partially plagiarized (and not the better part at that). But psychiatry doesn't have anything special to offer outside of ritual, authority and a rebranding of much that has come before, including the pangs of lost or unrequited love.

Suicidality often also mirrors the case of the misuse of domestic violence or restraining orders, a sadomasochistic weapon in the battles between (and within) the sexes, between parent and child or between neighbour and neighbour. If you report me to the police for assault I'll report you to the police because, after all, false allegations like many sins and indeed many crimes attract no consequences. If you proclaim your emotional pain and seek to distress me by crying suicide then I will do the same, with psychiatry serving to sanctify both claims, as the "mental illness" of each wrought upon the other. We in psychiatry can make of the boy who cried wolf a boy facing a real wolf with real teeth. That is our authority in the village. We can easily be accomplices to bad behaviour en route to breeding personality disorders. Thankfully I never started counting what would become innumerable cases of revenge suicidality in threat or gesture. And then there are the variant consequents of other bad behaviour. e.g. of the suicidal older adolescent girl who sent risqué photos to a male she barely knew, only to have him circulate the files amongst the peer group. The following evening that same male was in the emergency department, suicidal out of fear that the girl's older brothers would teach him a lesson out of school. The whole kindergarten circus keeps playing on. Or there is the observation that the best way to start an epidemic of suicidality in a school is to parachute in a charismatic little wuthering heights dying swan of a young lady espousing the virtue of suicide as she cuts herself. Then stir the social pot and wait for others to start cutting in turn, all catching "mental illness" and leading teachers to fetishize the same. Make no mistake. Suicidality is a social idiom and a contagious one at that. Yet not every contagion is a disease, and no social idiom is the stuff of medicine unless the doctor steps across the social and political divide and makes it so.

Or take the alcohol abusers. This cohort probably dwarfs all others. They are brought into the emergency department drunk and suicidal, often not remembering anything of the previous evening when they reach sobriety in the cold light of the next morning, amnesia to suicidal ideation inclusive. Yet still the spectre of suicide hangs in the air. They made the threat or performed the gesture. Once again the expectation is often placed on the psychiatrist that he/she cure the patient and that they be followed up for days with laborious safety plans, especially if the presentations are recurrent of the suicide attempts are near misses. Yet the answer to pseudo-complexity is once again simple. When beer is in, brains are out. To drink is to court a suicidal drive again, and to depress the mood over the longer term. To drink or not to drink. That is the question when applied to suicidality in this case. The patient knows it. The psychiatrist knows it. Everyone knows it. It has always been thus.

Or take the borderline personality cohort. These women (and very often hysterical young men, the over diagnosis in women being a form of soft chauvinism) often have had very unpleasant upbringings and not so pleasant current life circumstances also. I spoke something of these patients in the second chapter, in asserting the non-existence of type II bipolar disorder except as a model within which the psychiatrist may work to medicalize dramatic personality disorders, and from which to justify the prescription of domesticating medications. In the embodied mind of the borderline patient is an emptiness, a parent or other who is missing and a void that never enduringly filled, and usually is never temporarily filled but by distress. For these patients their lives are in perpetual chaos and the suicidal ideation is often never far from their mind. It is not unusual they come to see the hospital as a kind of giant mother object, each nurse another muscle or sinew who holds them in a warm embrace for as long as the admission lasts. The problem is of course that no admission lasts forever. And there is no evidence, not in my experience nor in that of the literature, that hospital admission does more good than harm, failing to put the slightest dent in the psychopathology whilst indeed infantilising the patient even further. And so at the stroke of midnight they appear, in crisis and in undeniable psychological pain, with an addiction to admission made stronger from each admission they receive. Often a well meaning psychologist or family member has told them they simply must present to the hospital, that they need admission and it will surely be granted. Promises made can always be made by those who have no part in the delivery. The vehicle by which the patient gets what they want, undeniably a drive often sincerely felt, is nonetheless amplified by what they know will be others response to it. And that vehicle is largely culturally specific. In some non western countries the embodied distress and emptiness may be somatic aches and pains with barely a mention of the want to die. In my world, and probably the readers also, the vehicle by which the distress is communicated is suicidality. With the "S" word comes the inevitable battle of wills between an emotionally dysregulated and psychologically damaged child trapped in an adults body, and that of the mental health clinician who wishes either to preserve the resource of the hospital against the interests of the patient, or admit them as quick as possible so as to call the interaction to a prompt close. One protagonist is playing the game to be admitted and the other (the psychiatrist) to avoid granting the same, while the first might deny the desire whilst advertising the very thing that will effect it, a lie to themselves and to others "I hate hospital but if you don't admit me I'll kill myself, and no other option will suffice". The situation is like the proverbial child who, in wishing a piece of candy and the parent denying them the wish, the child may threaten the hold their breath. A most rare and resolute child may even make good with the threat, hold their breath and pass out (or so I'm told as I've never observed this myself). Now no child is Palemon and neither parent or child is Ondine. Before long the physiological drives inevitably overcome to restore breathing, for no child would ever come to grief from such a strategy of breath holding. And just as well. For it enables the parent who would be a true parent to stand their ground, refuse the child the candy and win both the day and, more to the point, the wellbeing of the child, a demonstration of resoluteness to principle paving the way to the crafting of a better adult from forcing a development of delayed gratification and so much more. Scale up the stakes and we have a similar situation in the emergency department. "If you do not give me this cherished admission I will kill myself" is often the explicit statement, and almost always the subtext. Only this time the patient is liable to mean business, or at least to be more serious if not granted what they demand. When the game is in play, this move to externalize blame and responsibility is as much if not more a punishment to the clinician than a threat to escape from the pain of the world. From this change in dynamic one may ask where does narcissism and anti-sociality end and the borderline personality begin, when the threats is made that the blood will be on the psychiatrists hands, not as a statement uttered out of the unfolding of the nature of cause and effect, as opposed to a statement by a free agent "if you deny me, then a pox on your house". Don't misunderstand me. Once again, the psychological turmoil of these poor souls is not to be denied. However just as any parent must aspire not to be simply the friend of their child, and certainly not an extension of the child's hand, any parent or physician qua parent object needs remember their role is to do what is best. What is best is not always what the patient thinks or feels is best. And it is certainly not to do what one is coerced to do by another. By the same token, not every soul who says it is tortured is tortured in fact. Sometimes the most raging of waves sit above the shallowest of reefs. I have had the patients who, when incidentally asked, will say that they had a good time on leave from the ward for a morning excursion. When asked to describe the events of the morning, their thoughts and feelings, what is reported back is overwhelmingly positive. "So then…", I say with a sense of the opening to a shared celebration, "…..it seems you have reached a readiness to leave us". The reply then is, if they wish it to be, that such is not the case at all, and that if discharged they will surely kill themselves. The narrative then changes to all the awfulness that was the morning, this to legitimize what they want me to believe unto the ends they desire. Yet there is, in all of these exchanges, the unspoken conversation. Both of us give the small slight smiles at just the right times to acknowledge the move well played, that she/he is playing the move on what s/he perceives is my fear of suicide. And stay on in the ward they do until they grow bored with the world inside and curious about the world outside. They are cured only by their caprice, this being part of what ails them. Sometimes I have some moves of my own. Many a time I have encountered the a very suicidal patient who has decided not to be suicidal when I show them the ward list (identities of patients names covered) proving that all beds are occupied. When they see I am caring, honest and not rejecting them so much as us both being a victim to larger forces of finite resources, i.e. when they see that Mummy and Daddy have their hands full and really cannot drop tools for the metaphorical hug that is the hospital admission, then many of these adult children change the narrative from "I will surely kill myself if let go" to "well I'll just have to live on until a bed is available". And if one can survive a day without being in hospital, then why not a second, and a third, and so on. The reader can contrast this with the patient who has had a bone broken or a heart attack. The consequences from lack of action lay outside the choices of the patient involved.

Now many a psychiatrist reader will have the heckles raised at a description that has them standing cowardly, castrated and perhaps foolish before the threat of suicide. They will recall those unusual times they did discharge a patient who vowed to kill themselves if politely shown the door. Contrary to propaganda, the fact however is that suicide is a rare event. Far more than any casino the odds are without question on the side of the house (i.e. psychiatry), and most patients will not attempt to end their life, much less succeed, no matter how great their threats. Granted there have been many hanging attempts which have come my way, only saved by the branch breaking or the loved one who unexpectedly came home early. Yet there are also many more patients about whom it is said they have had several hanging attempts, though each one was made only when the suist could see the paramedics coming through the door. And I have seen countless patients for whom it is said they tried to jump off the cliff or building several times, being it seems miraculously pulled back each and every time. Apparently they don't make tall places like they used to. And though certain diagnoses are said to inflate the risks of suicide (e.g. bipolar disorder a 20-40 fold risk vs the population norm), when viewed through the lens of the actuary this is a very low risk indeed in the here and now (e.g. if the baseline suicide rate is 10/100,000 persons per year, then a 20-40 fold figure of 200-400/100,000 persons per year would still equate with a greater than 99% chance of survival within the given year). Ergo, psychiatrists can afford to bet on what courage they have, and ought to place the bet far more often than they do. I've seen such allegedly courageous psychiatrists also. But they don't exercise courage typically. And never ever have I seen them hold their ground to the end when the would be suist digs in and ups the ante. I have seen teams of psychiatrists sign documents as to the eternal futility of hospital admissions for a given patient, even its counter-productivity, then only to admit anyway when the newspaper writes the damaging article or the patient climbs the crane and demands their time inside. Surely psychiatry never attempts to withhold admission out of any principle of granting the patient a radical responsibility and radical freedom come what may. And if a suicide does come to crash into the orbit of a psychiatrist's career, their meagre courage is lost and they return to being agents of the therapeutic state, very unlikely to say no to a patient who would insist they say yes and depriving many a patient of liberty for even marginal risks who may even deny having thoughts to end their life. Who can blame the frightened psychiatrist, accustomed to placing pragmatism over principal? They never believed in personal responsibility anyway. Neither did their superiors (we all have superiors) or the whole psychiatric machine. They likely were only able to occasionally argue the case of forced discharge after observing "no pervasive mood disorder" or "no psychotic disorder", a direct appeal to the DSM to legitimise action in informing risks, this being the book they states is "just a guideline". And they only comfortably practice when they perceive themselves to be part of a collective opinion, i.e. the mentality of the herd. When a suicide does occur the fingers of responsibility are pointed not to the one who exercised autonomy to end their own life, often accidentally after a threat or gesture gone too far too fast or when too intoxicated. No the fingers are pointed at the practitioner who let them loose to do it. This finger pointing has consequences despite always buried by the smiling assassins in politically correct newspeak, of a culture of "no blame", of "incident analysis", of "quality improvement" and so on. Thankfully I never faced the inquisition after the suicide of a patient, probably more from good luck than good management. Yet I have colleagues not so fortunate. When the inquisitors say this isn't about you, then you know you're on trial.

Now you may say "yes but these are selectively chosen cases dramatic people, added to cases from history and mythology, and also the so called rational suicidality of the authors clinical experience. Am I perhaps implying we ignore all suicidal threats and gestures, even judging them all as bad behaviour"? What about the "real" mental illness such as major depressive illness or psychosis as earlier alluded to? Are there not any who are melancholic with the "disease" of depression, this in turn feeding their thoughts with irresistible temptation to suicide, driving in turn their behaviour to shuffle off the mortal coil as the only conceivable way to escape the pain, when other options remain unseen and unfelt until forced upon them by psychiatric drugs, shock therapy and psychotherapeutic indoctrination. Are there not also those whose voices tell them to kill themselves, with suicide being behavioural manifestation of the schizophrenic disease? And besides, ought not even those persons with infantile or dramatic personalities be afforded the unwanted protections of the state, perchance that they then avoid the misadventures that stand between them and future maturity and a life worth living? Am I not being terribly cruel, sadistically cruel, in implying to turn these victims over to their mental illnesses to kill them by their own hand? Am I not even projecting out my own sense of therapeutic nihilism after too many times hearing the same old threats?

To this I have several retorts, all the while informed by the cases I have seen, along with an initial call to clarity

Let us first consider the turn towards the zero suicide movement as a replacement for what came before, which was risk assessment with a view to prediction of risk and treatment accordingly (coercive treatment included).

Current practice in psychiatry is finally coming to the grudging realization that its crystal ball was useless, along with hierarchies of low, medium and high risk of suicide as similarly useless (years after I and many others realized the same). Instead they now say that whilst they may not be able to predict if the patient will or will not actually kill themselves (or even try), what we can do is intervene to prevent the same events. Pray tell how one even aspire to accomplish this save by measurement and manipulation of the very variables they rightly acknowledge are unhelpful in prediction? Lung cancer has a chance of being prevented if curbing smoking, as this behavioural variable is also predictive of risk. It's not so clear we have any fighting chance of establishing the predictive/ preventative symmetry with suicide. The turn from prediction to prevention is a cynical rebranding of the prediction calculus whilst looking to the same variables as if enlivened with new potential. It is deluded in it being any different. Surely the imposition of an illogical public health campaign upon a person is cruel, and neither my ego or purse profits from my alleged nihilism as the suicide prevention industry profits upon its own ideology.

Next, it is not piggish pedantry to note that the zero-suicide movement has made of suicide per se a disease, a public health problem, and an event in the world to which we must aspire to have eradicated (i.e. not the behaviour of a rational agent). They effectively equate a suicidal person with a malarial mosquito or an aquifer poisoned with cholera. If its goal was zero irrational suicide this might be acceptable, though I would then ask how the zero-suicide movement can discern the rational from the irrational when they fail the basic test of coherence to the extent they have attempted explain suicide on one hand, and dodged the issue of rationality on the other. This failure cannot be excused and may even be deliberate. Perhaps they pretend this question does not exist, hoping we will all be similarly ignorant, when it is crucial. To some, there is forever and always sound reason not to suicide, from which may be concluded all suicide is a priori and always irrational and/or immoral, depending on how the argument is formulated. For example, most, but not all, readings of Kant would have us arrive at this conclusion. Kant and others might say that our bodies, as Gods property, are not our own property, and so we categorically do not have the right to end the life of the physical body. Insomuch as the physical body is the vehicle within which moral life and duty is made possible, only under extraordinary circumstances where the grave corruption of the moral life is certain and imminent might we be permitted to end the life of the physical body (e.g. the turn towards being rabid, as symbolized in film as the turn towards being a zombie). At least we can take a deep bow to such a philosopher for having approached the question and to have formulated an answer. It remains another matter entirely if the answer is correct, let alone if another individual or state ought to intervene against an act simply in virtue of it being irrational and/or immoral as some might say suicide is in the vast majority of cases.

Then there are those who believe suicide is a sequelae of a disease rendering the diseased body or psyche so tortured as to leave them no other choice. Take the archetypal example of the cancer ridden patient with intractable pain who shan't survive long anyway. If so, the Epicurian or Utilitarian avoidance of pain is exceedingly rational. Might this not include those in emotional pain if the person determines to their own satisfaction that even psychiatry cannot serve their needs and they choose to reject what is offered? Whether the utilitarian basis of the belief upon which one acts is correct or not, whether it be moral and whether the state ought to intervene to prevent (or facilitate it) suicide are once again entirely different questions. It is rational to avoid emotional pain and maximize collective utility. And suicide is, rationally speaking, a way of avoiding pain for the individual and a way of reducing collective burden on the other. Though I happen to believe that a utilitarianism that places in individual values in jeopardy is monstrous, this is a question psychiatry is ill equipped to answer to the measure they have the authority to try. One utilitarian will run roughshod over the person to kill them. Another will run roughshod over the person to save them. The greater sin is that the cult of zero suicide fails to even venture into the question of suicide as a personal utility.

Then there are those radical materialists who believe suicide is the direct outcome of a psychological disease, only the psychological self to share identity with the brain. If true, then to speak of some behaviour being irrational is a category error projected upon the suist from another (meta) irrational agent, two brains pumping salts and other chemicals around and doing what brains do, one brain interacting with the other via stimulus and response. Only minds and mental phenomena can potentially be rational. Minds can have rational understandings of diseases, brains and moral speculations about the same. Yet diseases and brains themselves cannot be rational. And if everything is material then nothing is truly rational. It is simply what it is. As it so happens most of psychiatry is wedded to either the notion of mind brain identity (leaving rationality without sense) or deals with the functional sequelae of what is assumed to be brain disease (bodily lesions fail to mechanistically explain almost all suicidality, thus placing suicide a choice outside that of medicine, a choice that just may be rational).

You see it is not so easy to locate, define and argue the rational vs the irrational suicide. Such a notion is entangled with deep philosophical assumptions and problems. The praxis of use of the word has little to do with rationality anyway, and we need not labour too much trying to defend the rationality as an a priori for the critique against psychiatry and its excesses to curb suicide. Instead we ought to look at the use of the word "rational", as perhaps emerging from an empathy with the decision to suicide, and a word that is proxy for arguing, or being on the road to arguing, the political permissibility of suicide in the given case, i.e. when not to deprive persons of their liberty to kill themselves. Once again the onus is on the practitioner, zero suicide practitioners included, to defend both their formulations of suicide and their motivation to prevent it. This is but a taste of the depth to which the question might reach, and ought to reach, before anyone can even begin a claim to knowledge and before anyone can judge another's formulation of what suicidality is or is not. Certainly this is a question that ought to be asked and dialectically defended before anyone can have the audacity to intervene in what is the relationship between an individual with what is ostensibly their own bodies. It is not callousness to recognize that what is yours is not mine. Nor do I have the licence to be Kants God over the bodies of his creation. Those who wish to ride roughshod over the person to prevent their suicide have simply decided as a fait accompli that the suist is a victim. I disagree.

Rationality and irrationality aside, if the goal were a tighter fit for psychiatry, e.g. "zero depression", this might be arguably more appropriate, though not necessarily a moral justification to coercive practice. But then the zero-suicide movement would cease to be, replaced instead by the zero depression movement. The question might then be asked what the disease of depression is as opposed to a time of low mood, and why we ought to try to eradicate it, as if low moods never even conceivably served any salutary purpose and that it is reason enough to deprive persons of liberty. This is a very difficult question and I would argue "clinical depression" to be almost entirely a social construct, the boundary between it and garden variety low mood being necessarily arbitrary. Then the grounds to medicalize low mood so as to deprive a person of their freedom may be on account of the risk of suicide, in which case we would be back to smuggling in the zero suicide movement and placing suicide centre stage once again. One has visions of Huxleys Brave New World; let's spray the SOMA into the crowds until every man, woman and child is in blissful euthymia and anergy against the state. Great works and great revelations have been born from melancholic rumblings, and low moods at times are part of the human condition. Where do we draw the line? Depression is not a disease that kills the person via suicidal idea as its symptom and the attempt as its sign. This is scientistic nonsense. Suicide is a choice that someone freely makes within many contexts, mood state included. It makes little difference to say that person X or person Y later thanked us for intervening to prevent that suicide attempt they might have made in the past. Changing one's mind logically does not prove the existence of a disease, nor the rightfulness of our imposition any more than would be the case if we prevented another from the vote, and they later changed parties. Would not such an action be a crime against both person and democracy, and the change of mind be an explained on many axes to be sure, least of which would be the remission of a disease.

As for voices, delusions and such, these are addressed in the previous chapter, for voices and other so called psychotic phenomena are not the alien happenings they are commonly thought to be. Hearing voices commanding us to kill ourselves too sits upon a spectrum within which distinguishing the normal from the "pathological" is incredibly problematic, not the least given that such distinctions are again necessarily (and empirically) arbitrary. Voices of course cannot always be ignored or escaped, especially those generated from our own mind, which sometimes follow like an annoying shadow wherever one walks. Yet to the extent to which a patient exercises choice to take neuroleptic medication, these can often curb the voices if s/he wishes, as can entertaining the hypothesis that they (i.e. the voices) may be a product of one's own mind. To the extent they cannot be curbed, voices need never be obeyed. *******stoic quote******. Those of us who only hear the voices of flesh and blood people (i.e. persons who actually exist and stand before us) know this choice to be self-evidently true. To the extent to which a voice cannot be curbed and a persons decision is to end their life rather than listen to it, this too is a choice, however tragic it may be. Suffice to say for now, if suicide qua suicide is not disease or even a symptom, then it ought not be a variable that over-informs what we do as clinicians. It is not some way in which depression or schizophrenia is expressed through, as it were, the person with the person dissolving away as if they never had agency. To say it is a symptom, sign, public health issue etcetera are misplays of metaphor. Suicide is a choice a person makes, informed of course by their mood and many factors besides, yet not determined by it.

Next in the defence of the charge of cruelty and indifference that might be arraigned against me, we must examine the potential for the ever present rule of unintended consequences to rear its ugly head not against me so much as those who would like to consider themselves kind. The rule of unintended consequences makes fools of us all. Elsewhere in this chapter I have alluded to the fact that suicidality varies cross culturally according to the emphasis placed upon it and so it is a social idiom of distress as much as personal choice. And there is simply no denying that social idioms are necessarily contagions and gather strength by the response they engender in others. Taking bona fide objective medicine as the metaphor, were there to be an outbreak of severe influenza the likes of which occurred a century ago this would objectively be very contagious. Physicians would mount immediate responses, hospitals would have in depth protocols and histories would be taken from patients with the ear tuned to certain significant aspects of history, symptoms reported and signs observed. The amplified responses of the physician reflect the amplified nature of the threat, both becoming known to the community.

Now when we have a) psychological or physical distress and insecurity, e.g. the lonely old person, the wounded child within, the homeless person looking for shelter, the patient in chronic pain for whom inadequate analgesia is being provided etcetera all looking for recognition and b) the physician is looking for something to be recognized and happens to focus a la mode' upon a particular social idiom or representation of distress such as suicidality and c) the psychiatrist is crytpo-egoistically looking to be the saviour of the person as an object afflicted with a serious disease beyond the persons power to heal themselves, i.e. to be a real doctor, then we have the ingredients of d) the emergence of a transaction including expressions of distress such as suicide at far greater levels than would naturally be the case. These expressions are not just found to be expressed as in the physician discovering something already within nature and heretofore underdiagnosed, though this may be the case. No, such excursions of psychiatry into the world of suicidality leads to suicidality entering into the mind of the patient more than it otherwise would in the first place and with a greater intensity and frequency. The psychiatrist literally acts in this metaphor as some mad scientist inventing a more virulent strain of flu then becoming the vector of transmission. Psychiatry breeds the suicidality it seeks to cure.

In the above paragraph I refer to suicidal thoughts sincerely held. Insomuch as the mental world is not an objectively observable thing in the sense of which psychopathology is of a different category to physical pathology, we also must admit to the politically incorrect truism of the human condition, people can and do lie! Indeed they lie with such a great prevalence that pathological lying (i.e. pseudologia fantastica) is to date not part of the DSM, though factitious disorder is and is underdiagnosed. Why lie about suicide? Because expressions from which more intense care responses follow are naturally more likely to be also used by the malingerer. As was the case with psychosis and Rosenhan, outside of having made an unambiguously near fatal attempt, just how can the psychiatrist know when suicidal ideation expressed is suicidal ideation sincerely held and when it is not? How can psychiatrists know what the potential suist wants to get out of the disclosure? They want to believe they can know, though wanting, believing and knowing are three entirely different things. For the psychiatrist who remains a true believer in the sincerity of most if not all suicidal threats and their own power to treat the underlying disease I propose a thought experiment. For those who have had an established history of multiple threats and/or attempts, they get to choose either psychiatric care as currently provided them, or a 5 day stay at a luxury resort every couple months when they feel suicidal, this without possibility of extension, accumulation or transfer (this will be less expensive than standard psychiatric care). I predict such an option may be taken up in droves, the participants reliably become suicidal so as to avail themselves of the resort and more likely to survive so as to use it in future. A tiny fraction of these whom the psychiatrist would be utterly unable to identity in advance will end their lives, just as there will be those who take their lives and never announce an intent to anyone.

Next, we must consider the subtle dynamics in the exchange between the psychiatrist and the patient so far as suicide is concerned. These are the dynamics I have witnessed again and again not simply with psychiatrists yet mental health practitioners of all stripes, along with police and emergency services, mental health phone lines etcetera. The superficial psychological layers of the psychiatrist may believe he/she is focusing compassion and their empathic laser straight to the centre of the person, and they would take great umbrage at my suggestion that their over focus on suicidality is their act of cruelty, not mine. But this, to be frank, is insightlessness at its worst. Allow me to cut through this apparent contradiction and explain. With such a great focus on suicidality as we have, and such great consequences in terms of responsibility placed upon the practitioner to save the patient from acts of their own hand, what inevitably follows is that suicidality itself becomes the object of therapy and the patient as person recedes into the background. There is a world of difference between approaching a person in crisis where the beneficial outcome of the exchange might be that they decide not to kill themselves, vs the approach that we treat the suicidality (as primary therapeutic object) through talking to the person about their problems, and the person becomes nothing more than a vehicle through which the objective is achieved. Once again mine is the voice of experience. I know what clinicians care about by the focus of their behaviour and the dominant themes in their speech, which is not what they say they care about. Suicidality is a monster that has been elevated to such a great height by psychiatry and the whole social milieu that all else is just political lip service. Moreover, the matter is deeper than a direly needed turn towards a direct engagement with the person, something made impossible until we place suicide in the background. No. The subtextual layers become deeper still, for the psychiatrist and other mental health clinicians (and services) are driven not simply by suicidality itself as the primary therapeutic object. They are also driven by the preservation of themselves as the practitioner who does not have a suicide on their hands, the avoidance of questioning of their capability as a practitioner, and even the preservation of their career. The focus on suicide has all the appearance of being salvific to the patient, when instead it is much about the narcissism and professional life of the psychiatrist. Placing suicide back into the hands of the person themselves is one of the greatest act of respect and love we can give another, for it recognizes the precious qualities we have (or ought to have) within ourselves, i.e. free will and personal responsibility.

And finally, to defend the charge of cruelty, ironically I need to become crueller still. After the suicide of a loved one may ask "why"? In fact, the significant other usually asks this very question, and well they should. But what they don't realise is that they are not simply asking why their loved one marched before their time into the arms of death. No, they are also asking the necessary complement to this question, i.e. why did he/she let go of life? What they are therefore asking is the significance of life in general, including the significance of their own lives even as they live on in their mourning. This is existentially confronting stuff. A life affirming answer can only be found and expressed affectively and ceremonially in the lamentations at the passing of the one who would let go of life, and the regrets and guilt at not having saved them. Whom are they really trying to explain? Who are they really wishing could have been saved? Is it the life of the now departed loved one? Surely this is true in a sense, I do not doubt it for a moment after seeing years of tears shed by those left behind, enough to convince me thoroughly the most loved ones never ever "get over it", they never ever "move on" and rarely are "better off". This is partly the reason why I use the word "suist" when describing the one who takes their own life. Yet it is not just the departed love object about whom the one left behind seeks meaning and solace. It is themselves also. If the dearly departed can throw away life, then perhaps it is not so great a gift after all, not so great as to trump the option of returning the gift to its sender. Distasteful jokes can, in the final analysis, be true. Life really can be formulated to be an incurable sexually transmitted terminal disease. What is this life, a thin sliver of time sitting within transcendent eternity. If the loved one laments at the notion of the suist passing into hell this surely is a matter for religion, not psychiatry. The same can be said if God is so irresistible in love and forgiveness that even the suist is carried up into whatever heaven is, perhaps after a chastisement from the divine. This is a nicer ending to be sure, yet once again none of psychiatry's business what breaches of contract mankind has with his or her maker or, to return to the other metaphor, it is none of psychiatry's business if one looks a gift horse in the mouth. Similar is the case with reincarnation. As a consequence of suicide, what is a momentary karmic regression of a dozen generations or so against getting back on track towards the inevitability of a nirvana which is, ironically, the final blowing out of the candle of being, the greatest death of all. Finally, we have the bleakest metaphysical variant, that of the biological machine returning to the Earth from which it came, and that being the end of the matter of being in one form, and the beginnings in of being matter in another (perhaps a worm, perhaps a rosebush). From oblivion to meaningless absurdity to oblivion, in such a scenario the question of who cares ought not to be conflated with a metaphysical justification to cosmic tragedy, i.e. that there is anything to care about outside the act of caring itself which surely ought to be informed by the (in)significance of the whole cosmic circus. I don't subscribe to this latter view myself, though simply point out it's possibility and that its place also lay outside of psychiatry.

So what is suicide?

As previously described, currently in psychiatry the tide has taken us to a place where suicide or threatened suicide is rendered as a disease suffered by a person, and on the macro level a public health problem. Whether one is a traditional theist, a stalwart atheist humanist or of whatever other metaphysical stripe, I hope to have convinced that this is ridiculous, a category error, a metaphor gone malignant, and depends critically on the construction of psychiatric disorders to prop it up. And it is a ghastly confused position, for the disease is seen as morally neutral, displacing the morality to the attitude of all and sundry apart from the mind and choices of the suist themselves

So what is suicide? Suicide is, like many behaviours, simply the outcome of a choice made by a person. The gravitas of an act does not make of suicide any less the outcome of a choice than that of homicide, armed robbery of walking away from ones work and family and joining a commune or the life of a sadhu, all of which have been behaviours that at one time or another in one individual or another might have been described as acts of desperate necessity or an aligning of the will with fate. True, we may imagine that the vast majority of persons would rather not be placed in whatever situation besets them such as to be making this particular drastic choice, and to write or have written differently the final chapter of their life. They would rather have claimed victory in war, or to have avoided a collapse in stock prices, or to have been born into a better body, or better family, or any family at all, or to see a world sunnier than they perceive it to be. They would rather not have the flames at their back against which the only perceived choice is the leap from the balcony of life. And obviously they are often deeply ambivalent and pained, even terrified, at the decision and approach it with weakened knees, as if hoping that something or someone would deliver them from their own private Gethsemane. Only a fool would trivialise suicide and ignore this to very often be the case. And what of it? Does not the woman who might give up the child for adoption, or the one who might walk away from years of a commitment to a failed marriage or a thankless job often arrive at a decision reluctantly. Yet rightly or wrongly they arrive at a decision nonetheless. Even Socrates might have wished the tide to have turned otherwise, and rather not to have raised the hemlock to his lips. The lists of "would rathers" defies typology except by a fool, and so I would not put it past psychiatry to try. None of these regrets ultimately take an agent out of the world of choice and the liberty to decline what passes for alternate choices, or to disbelieve in their existence or relative value. Even the one who might, as one of my patients did, believe that the shape shifting lizard creatures will kill their family if they don't kill themselves, even they must make the choice of how to nobly act in a world of their own beliefs. Whether or not a behaviour driven by a choice is driven in turn by a false belief cannot possibly squeeze the place of choice out of the picture.

The suicidal literature from time to time attempts to make an issue of the temporality of thought to action, as if to imply this means anything substantial. Some say it is a myth that suicide is impulsive, stating that the suist lays out ample clues as to their covert or simply poorly detected ideation for perhaps months before the apparently impulsive event. Other will say that most suicide attempts are almost preconscious impulsive acts within the heat of the moment. Whatever ideation that they may have had before, the attempt/act comes all of a sudden without apparent "triggers" any different from the day before or the day before that. The answer is, of course, suicide is neither and both. As with any choice/behaviour dyad, some make the decision hastily (i.e. impulsively), and some deliberate and plan for quite some time, years perhaps. There is no valid objectification of suicide such as to say that it is or need be either impulsive or planned. The want to delineate the impulsive from the well planned attempt exists more within the pragmatism of the psychiatrist than a recognition of what suicide is, or as having informed the risk calculus. Just as any choice may be long considered or hasty, suicide can also be a choice made from deep consideration of the reasons to live or die, or the decision made by one whose capricious mind only fleetingly skims the surface of all that might be considered. Once again, the temporality of the decision does not take suicide out of the orbit of the category of choice made by a person with personality. If the decision to suicide is long considered we may argue therein is the evidence of a deeply entrenched chronic mental illness. Or we may conclude in the deliberation that it is hyper-rational and well considered, a choice to be respected. If it is impulsive we may claim that the person need be saved from an action they did not give due consideration, and we ought to attempt to capture and contain the wind almost before it blows (that is to say psychiatrically jail them always on account of the unpredictable). Or we may instead conclude that in its impulsively that there is no enduring or foreseeable risk, and so nothing that ought to be done at all. Once again, the argument is pragmatic. The goal is first defined, and the argument comes after.

So what might we do about suicide?

As with any moral question that enters into the political fray, with suicide the issue is the is/ought fallacy; what right does one have to X vs the question if X is right in itself.

The legal right to suicide is, prima facie, easily addressed, though not nearly as easy as might be imagined. It is contingent on whatever the state wishes it to be, and writes into legislation. To answer this question is simply glance at the calendar, note the year, orientate oneself to the location where one lives, and look at the local jurisdictions criminal and mental health legislation. The matter becomes tricky when addressing specific context (e.g. the displacement of physician's personal responsibility called physician assisted suicide) along with the question of the degree of vigour in application of law. We live in a time and place where, by and large, completed suicide is decriminalized, and fair enough. No corpse ought be thrown in jail. Yet insomuch as any mention or attempt towards the act of suicide might result in home invasion (forced entry into premises without need for judicial warrant), arrest (detention for assessment), trial (involuntary mental health assessment at the nearest authorized hospital) and corrective incarceration (further forced hospitalization and forced treatment), suicidality most certainly remains quasi criminalized. Why? Because the response of the state involves a deprivation of liberty, and so comfortably finds it's analogue in the penal system which in recent times has been formulated to be more rehabilitative than retributive in its justice. Jails claiming to be benevolent are jails all the same. None can argue against this basic fact open to all who might see, to those minds who don't allow themselves be intoxicated by the euphemisms they use against others. Moreover, I have also worked within legislative frameworks where arrest for a criminal charge justly requires evidence and a warrant, whereas one can be involuntarily detained, drugged, dragged out of one's house and transported for suicide risk assessment on nothing more than hearsay and accusation, without the police necessarily having heard or seen the would be suist say or do anything at all. Police and paramedics then document hearsay as if this was heard by their own ears and witnessed with their own eyes. Even when credible witnesses are present contradicting the charge of thought crime and conspiracy to suicide and the person themselves denies having made the threat, this also will probably not deter the police and paramedics from prejudicially insisting on a mental health assessment. They do this daily and with absolute impunity. Or alternatively the individual may confirm having made the threat, be thankful to receive help, and involuntarily detained and transported anyway without any hope of legal recourse of their own were they to pursue a complaint for being treated like a criminal. Why involuntarily detain a person who is willing to seek help? The police officer can only answer that the individual is ostensibly mentally ill, for that is taken to be reason enough. They may be erratic in behaviour. They may alight from the vehicle. They may change their mind and attempt suicide on route to the hospital, and so on and so forth. Or in quieter conversation the police and emergency services admit to their true motivations, i.e. that they will do anything and everything necessary not to be hauled up and have their career threatened for failure to prevent a suicide. Once again, the suist is assumed to be void of personal responsibility. All too often their senior officers have been instructed from on high to in turn instruct the paramedic or police foot solider to detain and transport no matter what, and the rank and file fall into step and deprive persons of their liberty using excuses that disguise reasons that vary from unprincipled personal interest to the Eichmann defence of following orders. Why are the police not as terrified and authoritative over the would be criminal who might have had merely an ideation towards real crime? The answer is that to do so would be to immediately reveal we live in a police state, the police patrolling against thought crime. Where other liberties find themselves perched upon the precipice of remaining unmolested for the time being, patrolling against thought crime is permitted under the rubric of psychiatry and mental health legislation. This is but part of the reason why the machine of psychiatry is best dismantled altogether, for the problem becomes more pernicious still. Mental health services might acknowledge the short comings of police and paramedics. Their solution? To create task forces of mobile mental health outreach teams, with ominous job titles such as "behavioural health technicians" and "mental health technicians". Naturally this is extension masquerading as substitution, for these services have it written into legislation that they may conscript police and paramedics to aid them in involuntarily detaining and transporting the person who wishes to end their life or for whom it may be said their eccentricities take a step too far. Can anyone not see in this the whole odious Orwellian infrastructure falling into place? The ethos hiding in plain sight, for the use of words such as "technician" is to engineer. Such an ethos would not change were the name to change tomorrow. You are form upon which the engineer places his stencil to craft a unit of the utopia of the therapeutic state. Your home is not a gulag. No, rather it is simply the ward of lowest acuity in the therapeutic state. Your neighbour is not the secret police and your children not Pavel Morozov. No these are deputized nurses. If the totalitarian state arrives in its full flourishing in the 21st century in the western world it will come not in brown shirts but white coats, not with the butt of a rifle but a smile with a syringe.

However even if the law were rendered perfectly transparent and a more robust due process put in place for alleged suists, the question arises what the individual morally ought to have the right to do with themselves, irrespective of the laws of the state. To this I would personally be inclined to the Kantian conclusion, albeit from an overlapping though not identical elaborate line of reasoning, along with an article of faith. That is to say, I personally view suicide as an almost universally immoral act, with the few exceptions proving the deontologic rule. Stated briefly, the religious regardless of stripe have the answer to suicide already at hand, and ought to be true to their faith. Yet even in a secular world, one can take a Burkean outlook and suggest at least the possibility that any individual has a duty to the preceding generations for the life they have been given and to future generations for the legacy that they may leave behind. Granted the suist may have had abysmal parents whom they wish to punish by punishing the parents creation and out of hatred and loathing of the creation itself (i.e. themselves). Their suffering is not denied. That having been said, there are plenty of innocently disenfranchised and lonely parental and grandparental figures about whose hearts and souls cry out to mean something to someone. These persons in their own indirect and small ways contributed something of good to the world of the potential suist. Why not be that needed person for them? Similarly, almost every would be suist has the wherewithal to be a meaningful source of kindness to some child somewhere, enough to make both lives worth living and pass onto the child a baton of the good, the beautiful and the true that the child in turn can carry on into future generations. Dare I suggest then that even a secular suist can find themselves by losing themselves, in the end perhaps this being the closest thing to mental health any of us can hope to achieve. It is difficult to ignore such a suggestion of duty without either being radically narcissistic or radically nihilistic, these also being descriptors of mental illness.

That short paragraph aside, to the reader gracious enough to have ventured so far this book is not a sermon. The question is not what I ought to do with the preservation of my life or you ought to do with the preservation of yours. The question is what I ought to do with yours and you ought to do with mine.

So what ought I morally have the right to do with the would be suist? Surely there is no greater exemplar of personal property than ownership over one's body and one's life. From Locke and Mill to Hayek and Mises or Szasz, a reading of the literature of the so called classical liberal and libertarian movement won't give a defence of why this is the case, for such a right over the body is assumed a priori and part of the foundation of further argument on private property rights and civil liberties. How can I even begin to approach the question of how my liberty might be exercised in the world and if the fruits of my labour be mine, or the question of land ownership via aboriginal propriety or free contract of exchange, if I am not absolutely a free and separate actor to you, and you to me. The starting point must be the body as a private property. My body is mine. Your body is yours. My labours are an extension of myself, as is potentially the soil I till that you do not. Only the almightly might be said to have a greater claim, this irrelevant in the secular state. It is this sort of thinking that in part undergirded the abolitionist movement. Only with these basic axioms can conflict over who purports to own me can be averted by the complete negation of the possibility of slavery. To imagine otherwise can mean that I am partly yours, or fully, for a moment or for a time. Only in the most extreme of cases; the unconscious, the demented, the delirious, the temporarily panic stricken "hysterical" patient and so on can we even countenance taking someone's choice of what is to be done with their body away from them. It is, after all, their personal property. Moreover, in the above examples, it is only under the justified presumption of what we reasonably predict they might have wished us to do to them, that we can manipulate the body without permission. And just as it is immoral and even logically incoherent for someone to make of themselves a slave (slavery being by definition involuntary servitude), the individual can never give away their responsibility over their own body except by voluntary contract, which is to say it remains subsumed within the fact of having made a choice and ongoing freedom, which is just as it should be. Now this giving over can only ever be done in contingent and indirect ways. I can choose for the welfare of my body to be placed into the hands of the pilot or bus driver. I can relax the body for the physical therapist or dentist to move it as s/he thinks best or the anaesthetist to insert the line. Yet when my unforced hand moves it is I who move it. Whether the act of the unforced hand is either to grab the gun to turn on another or to turn on myself, this is never, and can never, be seen as the responsibility of any but myself. I can form a voluntary contract with another to assist me in times of crisis, so that I might seek after a mental state where I might be less inclined to decide death over life. This courting of death versus life is like a courting in the romantic life, also a matter of choice and contract. But at the end of the day, which might be the end of all days, in suicide as in marriage, I have no one to blame but myself in saying "I do". If I am aggressive with another, that other (or agents/actors acting on their behalf) ought to have recourse to damage my own body if necessary in order to preserve the integrity of their own. Why? It is obvious. My aggressive act is impacting upon their liberty, and by extension their ability to act as moral agents to the furtherance of their own duties and potentials, with choices and their consequences. They cannot make of me a slave, even for a moment. And for the very same reason I ought to have no licence to molest their body and their liberty, even if to save the body, if they choose against it.

In my own practice, I see this war against this liberty and responsibility all the time. Often patients are asked "do you feel safe?" or speak of themselves in the same manner "I don't feel safe". Patients who have become well versed in this kind of exchange become quite perplexed when I first feign perplexity at hearing them say "I don't feel safe" or various permutations of the same. I ask them about their risk of being burgled, of domestic violence, of natural disasters, accidents and injuries in the home etc. When we together conclude the risk from all of these is low, or burglary etcetera not the business of psychiatry in any case, then I ask them how then they might possibly "not feel safe", i.e. in what sense might this turn of phrase have meaning. It is only then we can begin to deconstruct the perverse lessons psychiatrists and psychologists have taught them, as well as their own want to be a slave and a disintegrated self, or habit in being one. Only then can we have the discussion about free will and personal agency. For, as I challenge them, how can you feel unsafe from yourself, when it is you who controls the actions of your own hand, when your body is your personal property? And how can I, another person existing in a different phenomenological space apropos personal agency, control your hand for you when you are in possession of your rational faculties, or at least have the capacity to be in possession of them? Moreover, if you feel unsafe that implies a hostile force of nature or an aggressor. As we have concluded the aggressor is not outside of yourself or nature in any substantive way, then that aggressor is you. How can I prosecute and incarcerate the aggressor without also incarcerating the would be victim? Why I should I, a doctor, prosecute and incarcerate anyone at all, split internal objects inclusive. Would it not be better for the would be internal victim to decide within themselves whether to banish the internal aggressor or identify with them, for both are nothing more than different sides of a dialectic within the same person. And the person should be a single identity to themselves, and more importantly a single identity to the community around them. (This should be asserted at the outset to be the default. After all, we have dispensed multiple personality disorder in an earlier chapter). How can I conjecture on the diffusion of identity and ego as part of the psychopathology of a borderline personality whilst employing the language that someone is unsafe lest I take charge of their body, this in practice endorsing a diffusing of identity and self control? And with this conversational exchange I attempt a refusal from the nonsense notion of saving someone from themselves, when such an ostensive saving undercuts the very validity of their own agency and identity as the one who chooses which side within the self will win and integrates the choice within the greater self. For me to do otherwise is to breed psychopathology, indeed even to share in it. When I suggest it is not possible for someone to be unsafe with themselves, most of the time what I am then met with is not fear but a certain kind of frustration and confusion, this in turn borne from the dawning realisation that their idiom of divesting themselves of personal responsibility is neither convincing to me, yet more importantly, is not terribly convincing to themselves either. Disturbingly it is the patients more educated in psychobabble that present the greater challenge in this process. The more one is naive to psychiatry and the contemporary western infantilizing climate, the more they seem to comprehend free will and personal responsibility as a given.

But people are a complicated mix of competing drives you might say. What about those patients whose life preserving part of themselves is the weaker of the two? Ought we not tip the balance in our favour by imposing ourselves upon them and being a substitute for the greater self, to be an integrating principle that they can later hopefully introject and identify with (that is take control as an ally with their more sensible selves until the balance of power shifts)? To this I would say that a kingdom cannot war against itself. We should not lose our nerve, and our nerve should be true to principle. Slopes have a way, believe it or not, of fast becoming slippery. And a defence of personal agency and responsibility ought to be fought in the ever present now, never better than here in the space where we sit across from one another. No one ever crafted a legitimate adult by returning the adult to childhood, let alone the womb. In ordinary life, only children lack responsibility. It is no accident that this freedom from responsibility is complemented by an absence of liberty. Children are children until they are not. As stated above, except in cases of dire illness with gross unequivocal loss of cognitive function such as dementia, or temporary states such as delirium and extreme panic, adults ideally must never ever have the liberty and responsibility of their adulthood taken from them, even for a moment. Now I said that no individual can make of themselves a slave, and no state ought to sanction the same. You own yourself as a property and the state has no moral claim over that which you own prior to any contract, and what you wish to do with the body, even if it is to forfeit the body. If I can never force you to be responsible for me and what I might do in disposing of my life, then you have not the right to impose yourself upon me and prevent me from doing the same. As stated in the above and elsewhere, one of the greatest gifts of love and respect we might ever give the other is a recognition of responsibility, and the freedom to be.

LIBERTY. CLIMBING MT SZASZ.

"Of all tyrannies, a tyranny sincerely exercised for the good of its victims may be the most oppressive. It would be better to live under robber barons than under omnipotent moral busybodies. The robber baron's cruelty may sometimes sleep, his cupidity may at some point be satiated; but those who torment us for our own good will torment us without end for they do so with the approval of their own conscience. They may be more likely to go to Heaven yet at the same time likelier to make a Hell of earth. This very kindness stings with intolerable insult. To be "cured" against one's will and cured of states which we may not regard as disease is to be put on a level of those who have not yet reached the age of reason or those who never will; to be classed with infants, imbeciles, and domestic animals."

CS Lewis

Writing about the thoughts and ideas of another is, of necessity, an interpretive enterprise. The only remedy to which we might turn to avoid the dangers of (mis)interpretation is to fill a book with quotes that, if placed in context, would inflate to be a reprinting of the whole book to which we refer. The greater problem is when we are dealing with a prolific author whose whole corpus of work we may have not read, and whose ideas may have evolved over time. In my own little book, I have included a whole chapter revolving around the ideas of one person not as a hagiography from a disciple. Thomas Szasz was a man I never met, and I suspect I would not agree with him on everything, religion especially, along with his almost deified formulation of libertarianism and laissez fare capitalism. And yet our opinions are similar enough to each other viz a viz psychiatry, and so very different to the main, that it would be an injustice to write this book without giving due credit to the one who came before and probably said it better. All the more so as Szasz's star rose high in the 1960's and 1970's, then burned dim long before the man himself reposed, this on account of psychiatry finally succeeding in making him disappear by the end of the twentieth century, and many a patient preferring his message not exist either. Indeed, it seems we moved from the 1960's call to liberty from medicalized labels to a current infantilized want to be respected and cared for with or as a label, mental illness variously held as excuse, a fashion or some twisted masochistic badge of honour. Like Rousseau, man everywhere is free and everywhere in chains, to which I would add all the time seeking both despite the contradiction. And so for all the asylum walls which were torn down, as many as were liberated then built their own. We even see the same in the otherwise brilliant 2019 cinematic take on 1980's life, "Joker". The character is downtrodden and deeply troubled, and even his reality is placed in question. And yet in a crucial climactic scene he asserts himself not as a downtrodden man, yet rather as the downtrodden sufferer of a "mental illness", taking it on himself as a radical identity as opposed to being a man with problems and understandable responses to the same (any good psycho-dynamically minded practitioner will likely not make of one of his problems an organic pseudobulbar affect). His was thus never to be a freedom from psychiatry. He took it to his heart as himself. Ergo he can never escape his asylum and neither can the audience who agrees with his self-identification. The joke really is on an audience who leaves the cinema believing in mental illness of the protagonist more than a sick world in which he lived. Returning to the conspired forgetting of Szasz, in my own psychiatric apprenticeship, his was not a name included on any prescribed text, and the sum total devoted to him was approx. 15 minutes in a single lecture where his arguments were straw manned, mischaracterised and irrationally bundled up in a quasi-diagnostic category known as "antipsychiatry". Actually, though Szasz was a brilliant and witty polemicist, my own opinion is that he became lost in his own Ivory tower and partisan arms of the likes of the Cato institute, all too often failing to enter empathically into the minds of the swinging voters he wished to persuade. But that may just be me. Additionally, I find that even posthumously some attacks against the man still do persist. Even as an octogenarian he was fighting virtually the entire psychiatric establishment more or less single handed and in a way not shared by those who came to label or be labelled as "anti-psychiatry" or "critical psychiatry", as he rejected both. Championing a man outnumbered and who is no longer around to defend himself is a cause noble enough. To this end I will try and be faithful to Szasz's own thoughts in the earlier parts of this chapter. The reader will forgive if I drift into my own ideas in places, and hopefully will discern the difference if or when it arrives.

As a final preamble, in this chapter as in others I'll be faithful to not burdening the text with references. If the reader wishes to explore the matter further, I commend to them the excellent work "Szasz Under Fire" edited by psychologist and Szasz fan Jeffrey Schaler, along with of course Szasz own books (approximately 30 in number, I have read but 3) and also the published work of his key opponents, e.g. Robert Kendell, Edwin Torrey and, especially, Ronald Pies. These latter works are predominately to be found in the specialist journals, where each article will cost the lay reader more than this entire book and a lunch to read it with. Such is the sharing and caring socialist spirit of disseminating knowledge in science and medicines fourth estate. It is yours if you can afford it.

Thomas Szasz; a Brief Biography

Tamas Istvan Szasz was born to wealthy atheist ethnically Jewish parents in Budapest April 15th 1920. Had his father not changed the family name a generation earlier he would have likely been born Tamas Schlesinger. By all accounts the home was a harmonious one, with much love shared between Tamas, his parents, his older brother and the beloved Nanny, herself essentially a de facto member of the family and not the only member of staff. There is no doubt that he did have recurrent serious infections as a child, this being an era before the antibiotic golden age, and he could well be stereotyped as the sickly homebody child with the precocious intellect. Szasz himself admits on reflection that the lessons he learned as a child he transferred into his later reflections on the psychiatric patient. For having been doted on when ill, he would later embellish symptoms and malinger in order avoid the gymnasium. The uncharitable formulation would then have Szasz as the consummate child liar, later projecting this negative character trait out into the world of the "mentally ill" in accusation and a callous call to make them responsible for what was obviously beyond them. The more charitable, and I would submit more realistic, formulation is that lying is a thing many a child does, and many an adult also, and that lies can be so subtle as to be hidden even from the one who makes them. Anyone who works in psychiatry comes to see this as a pervasive fact of human nature. We cannot blame Szasz for his confession to introspection and observation of others. Inferences from our own minds is a time honoured technique in psychology.

Like many a continental European product of high learning in the Gymnasium, by the time of graduation Tamas was fluent in Hungarian, German, French, Latin and (I assume in virtue of his contact with the rabbis whose faith he saw as superstition), Hebrew also. Just as there is no substitute for interviewing a patient in their mother tongue and sharing an intimate knowledge of their cultural mores, Szasz was able build up a critical metanarrative of psychiatry from a reading of original psychiatric works in the authors mother tongues, availing himself of not simply the psychiatric literature itself, yet also the political and philosophical discourse of the time and place. And he was a voracious devourer of it all. With the rising spectre of Nazism, Szasz left Hungary in 1938 as part of the Jewish Diaspora, arrived in The United States as anglo Thomas, added English fluency to his arsenal in an immersive couple years and managed graduate in physics with highest honours before attending medical school where he continued to excel. His claim to have topped the class has never been contested. Szasz chose medical studies even prior to leaving Hungary, not as a route to a vocation so much as a want to understand the body as the property in which his person lived. A walk through the body was a walk through his own most intimate backyard, and example of just how attuned he was to the body as a bio-political object, a first point to explore and embark upon the philosophy of liberty and private property. Despite Szasz never really intending on practicing medicine, he did flirt with becoming a physician before deciding on psychiatry, as was always going to be his fate. Szasz completed much of the training in an internal medicine residency in Harvard and Ohio before jumping ship to psychiatry. This was still the golden era of the asylum, and Szasz needed plan assiduously and use his all his guile to avoid being placed in a compromising position of forcibly hospitalizing and treating another human being. He chose a psychoanalytically orientated training program in Chicago with this express goal in mind and threatened to resign when they sought to seconder him to the state psychiatric hospital. He may quite well be the last psychiatrist to be able honestly say never used coercion. Of course some may see this as his Achilles heel, never being confronted face to face with someone so mad as to require the straight jacket and the like. How does he know what he would not have done, or know it ought not to be done unless he is there? I do think it is fair to say that Szasz did see his fair share of madness and his principled objection was not to avoid a confrontation with hypocrisy so much as the upholding of principle for its own sake. After all, he had been honest and acted against any putative selfish interests when turned down from numerous ivy league medical schools for admitting he was a Jew. Nonetheless such a manoeuvre of ducking and weaving the asylums were also strategic and to avoid being placed in a conflict of revealing his hand against the state until his strength was up to the occasion. He had wisely taken stock of history and lessons learned, e.g. of a fellow Hungarian Semmelweis for example who became a pariah for speaking the truth about hand hygiene. By the late 1950's, Szasz had arrived. He was a staff academic with stable income and time on his hands at the State University of New York. Now he could turn that time and those hands against psychiatry. For the next half century he would dig in, defend his tenure against sometimes ferocious attack and launch a salvo of a few dozen books and articles aimed at undermining psychiatry. Taking from the old adage that the enemy of the enemy is my friend, Szasz with atheist even sidled up with the anti-psychiatric cult come official religion scientology (made official religion when it barraged the IRS with complaints such that the IRS relented and granted it tax exempt status). The outcome was the founding of the scientology front group, the citizens commission on Human Rights (CCHR)

I said earlier that Szasz was trained in and incredibly well versed in psychoanalysis. He received his own analysis by fellow Hungarian Jewish ex patriot Therese Benedek, who in turn received analysis by Hungarian Jewish Sandor Ferenczi, who in turn received analysis by the unanalysed (or self analysed) master himself, the secular Jewish Moravian Sigismund Freud. Such is the way classical analysis was practiced and taught, a predominantly secular Jewish enterprise similar in some respects to the Kabbalah, requiring two adults to dive into the gnostic territory of the unconscious, and pulling out truths to set the world aright. Christian readers will see in the requirement for the analyst to be analysed a metaphor of catechism and baptism, or alternatively the anointing of priests. Yet it would be a mistake to assume that Szasz saw psycho-analysis as Freud did. Rather he saw it simply as a conversation.

The Myth of Mental Illness

Szasz basic argument was aimed philosophically and practically at containing medicine to the matter of physical pathology of the physical body, and mental phenomena only if directly causally related to the pathology in question. All else that resides in the mental life and behaviour of the person is not medicine, and better left to be discussed as part of psychology to be sure, along with rhetoric, law, philosophy, ethics, politics, theology and plain old village life. Should we fail to observe and defend this boundary he warned, we run the risk not only of many a logical transgression, yet also one where the doctor becomes a political actor, a tool of tyranny if not a tyranny itself.

This was the gist behind the title of the article "The myth of mental illness," in the Feb 1960 issue of American Psychologist and followed up with the book of the same name, just as importantly subtitled "Foundations of a Theory of Personal Conduct". The subtitle has much to say about the theory and is often ignored by critics.

A simple example of the proposed demarcation is as follows. A man attends the doctors rooms, and may be subsequently diagnosed with emphysema. That such a pathology relates to smoking is a given in his case. Insomuch as the pathology is causally related to the behaviour, the doctor may advise the person to cease smoking, and even scale this up to mass public health campaigns encouraging the whole population to voluntary change. To be sure Szasz would endorse a certain compassionate attitude be had by the physician for his/her patient, as the diagnosis is delivered to a human being with a mental life. But Szasz would point out that the behaviour itself is a choice and outside the province of medicine beyond its limited scope to advise the one seeking the advice, or an invitation to change for the one or the many alike. To say that smoking involves the inhalation of chemicals with biological effects is also a given, as has been already recognised in the pathogenesis of the emphysema about which the doctor could elaborate and is expected to be expert. And all would acknowledge that the nicotine has certain psychotropic effects and a whole pharmacology that, within the narrow technical terms of art that the pharmacologist might use, is a substance which we might describe in terms of "tolerance" and "dependence", though "addiction" is a different notion altogether. And yet whilst smoking might cause an illness and emphysema is usually a smoking related disease, there is no reality to the claim that the patient suffers from a smoking illness or a smoking disorder or tobacco use disorder, etcetera. Smoking is a choice, however much it might be a poor one. The disease is nowhere to be found except as a metaphor! And medicine has no place in forcing or coercing the smoker to quit. The next step towards medical overreach is to speak of a "gambling disorder" explained using an illness model (another behaviour without a bodily pathology), an antisocial personality disorder using an illness model (a character or person without a bodily pathology) and so on. Now several years after Szasz death, there is likewise a call now for health care workers to be at the vanguard against so called intimate partner violence (previously termed domestic violence), the explicit call being that intimate partner violence is "a public health matter". When is assault more than a criminal matter, and how long until we pass from the victim being victim of a health matter to the perpetrator also a victim of an illness the psychiatrist will treat, perhaps a "domestic violence perpetrator disorder"? Or we might as well make divorce a public health matter also, and demand the nanny state step in and save us from what has become endemic. Surely there are symptoms (regret, sorrow, loss of sleep etc), signs and behaviours (visiting lawyers, arguments, scuffles over shared property) of divorce which may be descriptors of suffering, i.e. pathos. Is not suffering the province of medicine? And there may be attendant social and occupational dysfunction also. We could even develop a nosology of subtypes of divorce disorder and write them out on little gray cards a la Kraepelin. Presto, a new illness is born if we only want it to be so. But is divorce an illness? What place is the doctor in all this, and where will these incursions into good sense end? The psychiatrist may counter by condescending towards an explanation that the divorce can "trigger" a major depressive disorder, depression being something we are attuned to consider is a valid illness. But what is this major depressive disorder apart from its descriptiveness, it boundedness to precipitant and a turn of phrase for a divorce having passed an arbitrary threshold of what might be an acceptable impact upon the person and that which we wish were not the case (or what our values would morally proscribe as excessive). If one is excessively troubled by the divorce you will be diagnosed, e.g. with major depressive disorder for example. If glibly untroubled you may be diagnosed also, with narcissistic or other personality disorder for example. But why diagnose with anything, when diagnosis implies disease? And what of bereavement? Perhaps an urban myth, I've heard it said many bird species mate for life and have a response to a mate's death that may be said to be an equivalent of a severe major depressive disorder. And so what? Can no man or woman have a similar attachment without the psychiatrist's invocations of illness? The DSM criteria permit a human to mourn for a couple weeks and no longer. Are people not entitled to remain sad for life after the passing of a spouse without a psychiatrist saying they have major depression of the morbid grief variety? To all this and more madness Szasz would say a resounding "enough". Disease (or illness) involves bodily pathology, this being the place where the line is to be drawn lest it project into absurdity and tyranny. Neither sadness, badness or madness is disease.

Another example to illustrate the point is Nietzsche. Often prone to melancholy, one winters day in 1889 he simply became mad, flung his arms around a mistreated horse and from that moment his sanity never returned. Or did it, as after this fateful day he did continue to write for a time until he could write no more. Scholars have since read into his case the likelihood that his madness was neuro-syphilis, in this case the sequelae in the brain from an infection first acquired many years earlier in a brothel (pure speculation), or having been up to his elbows in syphilitic soldiers as a hospital orderly in the Franco Prussian War (a less likely means of transmission, and also speculative). Others have conjectured he had one too many strokes, a mercury poisoning or a slow growing brain tumour. Note that all of these conjectures hinge upon a catastrophic physical event in the physical brain. My own money is on the syphilis. But what if it wasn't and it were possible us prove this to be the case? What if it was just him? What if his brain, like any genius, appeared to the pathologist just like any of ours? What if he came to simply believe he was literally Dionysus, much as the Tibetan in exile to whom millions fawn believes he is the reincarnation of the Bodhisattva? And after Nietzsche's proto-PETA failed attempt to liberate the horse, when he then wrote (also in 1989 mind you) that the world should attack Germany and all anti-Semites be cast out, does this make him any more insane than the perfectly sane yet evil man who 50 odd years later attempted to do the opposite? And when Nietzsche elevated himself to the person of the Godhead himself above the minor Dionysus, why ought we see this as any different to Jung with his sincerely believed pseudo-divination a mere 24 years later, and countless other Antichrists of the fin de siecle then and since? At the sheer arbitrariness of it all should we throw out an objective biological criterion for disease?

Szasz was fond of the line, that when you talk to God it is called praying, when God talks to you this is insanity. So people have beliefs about themselves and the world, sometimes very strange beliefs. People have emotions, sometimes powerful emotions. People make decisions, sometimes stupid and poorly considered ones. And sometimes these thoughts, emotions and attendant behaviours become a nuisance to themselves, and sometimes a nuisance to others, a state of being "at risk of harm to self and/or others" or "at risk of harm to reputation". When such risk involves psychological suffering we might be tempted to use all the same language of medicine and disease with none of the physicality as its ontologically necessary requirement. If so, we are using the language of medicine metaphorically. We can talk until the cows come home of "signs", "symptoms", "behaviours" all of mental "illness", of psychiatrists "examining" persons whom they now refer to as "patients" to whom is administered "treatment" and so on. Yet this does not bridge the gap between real medicine (bodily disease) and counterfeit medicine (i.e. psychiatry). From the rubble of a fallen church and ministers to the soul who are disqualified from being ministers to the psyche, a whole new industry can breed these counterfeit medical specialists claiming to be experts over the mind and behaviour, along with guilds of these same individuals whose power is underwritten by the state, "hospitals" and "clinics" in which to "treat" the alleged illness of what people think, feel and do. It additionally acts as a filter capturing certain species of social deviance that does not obviously fit within criminal law. And when we believe these turns of phrase and use of metaphor, the belief elevates the new psychiatry to the status of tangibly real organic pathology that is the stuff of real medicine, of broken bones and tubercle bacilli. This bewitched belief, in the fallacy of its own misplaced concreteness, is the makings of a myth. In 2020 we now stand on the other side of many decades of sedimentation of metaphor into a superstructure of dissimulation that we believe is solid as a rock and yet crumbles when approached with a relentlessly critical mind. To those who would claim that the diagnoses in DSM 5 or ICD 11 are medical illnesses, Szasz would challenge them to prove the ethics and logic of the sense in which this is the case. To those who say they are physical illnesses in particular he would offer the same challenge. They had not in the late 1950's when Szasz launched his attack, and they have not now 60 years later. And the hubris has taken us all in the entirely wrong direction he would say.

His formulation of mental illness and the appropriate place of the physician is encapsulated in the fifth Act of Hamlet, Shakespeare being just one of many literary luminaries who understood the mind far better than the psychiatrist. In the play, Hamlet calls for the physician to attend to Lady Macbeth; "Canst thou not minister to a mind diseased" he says and continues his plea "Pluck from the memory a rooted sorrow", "....and with some sweet oblivious antidote". The physician rightly diagnoses that pain of a tortured mind and its voices is not the stuff of medicine. It is conscience. It is coming from, and remedied by, a conversation between lady Macbeth and herself, if not the divine also.

And Szasz himself writes

"According to pathological-scientific criteria, disease is a material phenomenon, the product of the body, in the same sense that urine is a product of the body. In contrast, diagnosis is not a material phenomenon or bodily product: it is a product of a person, typically a physician, in the same sense that a work of art is the product of a person called an "artist." Having a disease is not the same as occupying the patient role: not all sick persons are patients, and not all patients are sick. Nevertheless, physicians, politicians, the press, and the public conflate and confuse the two categories".

Now the contemporary reader will often see the word "medicalize" or "pathologize" and take it as a pejorative against more holistic care, suggesting that we ought to treat the patient already divested of autonomy and responsibility more humanely, with more than simply the "medical model" or "drug therapy". That is to say we ought to care about them as people and not biological machines. Szasz went further to say medicalization in psychiatry is a logical fallacy, thus rendering the question of the "medical model" not simply excessive or myopic, but irrelevant. In its pretensions to be medical it is, a priori, harmful. We cannot have a humane person centered medicine for something that is not medical! Even to see the person as a patient with a mental illness is medicalization, regardless of the model of care.

But what did Szasz, and yours truly, both think of so called "symptoms" of psychosis, these being the most confronting challenge to the claim that mental illnesses do not exist as illness, except metaphorically. I have covered psychosis elsewhere in chapter 9. He thought delusions were like any other belief. In these cases, the beliefs are more often than not incorrect to be sure, and often very idiosyncratic and strange. Yet wrongness as such is hardly the licence to medicalize. Although critical in some senses of classical psycho-analysis, he considered the belief to be psychologically constructed according to some inner need. The need defends the belief as a lie to the self against the reality of the world. And insomuch as so called delusions are a lie to the self or an error of thinking stubbornly held, it is a choice made by the person if to engage in a dialogue towards a flexibility to change their mind, where mind in turn is a verb and not a noun. I would see belief in less flexible, less libertarian, less consumerist terms. Some beliefs we simply have. Autochthonous or semi-autochthonous they are what they are and their fixedness is more fate than pathology. Some of us even have beliefs we would wish we did not have, yet cannot lie to ourselves and pretend we do not believe what we believe. Nonetheless and notwithstanding beliefs might have their mysteries, once again this is hardly licence to medicalise. Auditory hallucinations he saw as they are, conversations had with the self, disavowed and on an unconscious level chosen to be experienced as the voice of another. Even the voice of the other is the voice we speak to ourselves as from the other, what we think they are saying to us, or would say to us. And insomuch as the hallucination involves beliefs about the voice heard, on some level they are inseparably bound up with the so called delusion, which is an alternative belief. My own transcultural and trans-historical view is that the externalization of such phenomena (the ego alien aspect) makes of voices and such the latter day equivalent of demon possession, and the psychiatrist the priest who will perform the exorcism.

The Therapeutic State and Pharmacracy

The therapeutic state is simply the power invested in psychiatry by the organs of government to police and engineer the desired thoughts, feeling and behaviours of the citizenry, with the authority to force their engineering upon the person if, according to the metrics of psychiatry, the mental state is beyond the pale. Obviously the agenda of psychiatry must harmonize with the government in order for the state to run smoothly, and not be detected by the citizenry as averse to their own liberty. The project is aided by the cultivation of an attitude in the citizenry of actually wanting the shackles of the therapeutic state, as this will absolve themselves of personal responsibility, along with the burden and embarrassment of loved ones who are social deviants (or its euphemism "mental illness"). Psychiatry places all those parts of themselves they dislike as the other, the mental illness they suffer from. Though an international phenomenon, the therapeutic state could also be best historically formulated in that colossal ongoing social experiment known as the United States of America. Puritans and Masonic seals aside, the United States explicitly separated church and state. Nonetheless the same social unconscious was at work with the same needs for the same controls that the church provided in augmenting state power and providing meaning, just as it did in the old world. And so when God died in America as in Europe psychiatry acted to fill the void, a different kind of church with a different kind of priest, yet wedded to the state all the same. Where once the outcasts were managed by the Church, now we had psychiatry. Where once we had demonic possession now we had psychosis or severe neurosis of borderline personality structures. Where once we had inquisitions as forced therapies for the soul, now we had forced psychiatric treatment, for the patient's own good of course. As some might say, the content changed yet the form remained the same, a passing over of power from the papal ferula to the staff of Aesclepius (or worse still, the Caduceus of Hermes). Szasz neologism for this, dare I say, unholy collusion of (predominantly) psychiatry and the government he termed the Therapeutic State, or Pharmacracy.

In Ceremonial Chemistry, Szasz writes

"Inasmuch as we have words to describe medicine as a healing art, but have none to describe it as a method of social control or political rule, we must first give it a name. I propose that we call it pharmacracy, from the Greek pharmakon, for 'medicine' or 'drug' and kratein, for 'to rule' or 'to control'".

Szasz writes in the preface of his 1968 text Law, Liberty and Psychiatry" the following

"For the most part, psychiatrists are engaged in attempts to change the behaviour and values of individuals, groups and institutions, and sometimes even nations. Hence psychiatry is a form of social engineering. It should be recognised as such"

To which he added in the introduction to golden anniversary of the Myth of Mental Illness

"For the practice of pathology and for disease as a scientific concept, the person as potential sufferer is unimportant. For the practice of medicine as a human service, in contrast, the person as patient is supremely important. Why? Because the practice of Western medicine is informed by the ethical injunction, Primum non nocere! and rests on the premise that the patient is free to seek, accept, or reject medical diagnosis and treatment. Psychiatric practice, in contrast, is informed by the premise that the mental patient may be "dangerous to himself or others" and that it is the moral and professional duty of the psychiatrist to protect the patient from himself and society from the patient"

In this sense, psychiatrists might purport to care for individuals, yet to imagine that this is the boundary of their concerns would be a subtle error on their part and ours. They are public health clinicians working on individual instantiations of public health problems. The question ultimately is not what a person wants but what society needs and proscribes. The psychiatrist sees through the former towards the latter, and will incarcerate the person to achieve the goal. In a later interview Szasz spoke bluntly the obvious fact

"if you're in a building that you can't get out of, that's not a hospital, it's a prison".

Psychiatry as a substitute for religion and a quest to socially engineer the man (or woman) desired by the powers that be is a bold claim. Yet one does not have to look far for the evidence of this. In the few short years before the release of chlorpromazine, take also the keynote speaker at the 1946 William Alanson Memorial lecture in Washington DC, lamenting at the state of man in the wake of the second world war

"the only psychological force capable of producing these perversions is morality"....

"the re-interpretation and eventually eradication of the concept of right and wrong which has been the basis of child training, the substitution of intelligent and rational thinking for faith in the certainties of old people, these are the belated objectives of practically all effective psychotherapy"

The speaker later continues

"if the race is to be freed from its crippling burden of good and evil it must be psychiatrists who take the original responsibility. This is a challenge which must be met. If psychiatrists decide to do nothing about it but continue in the futility of psychotherapy only, that too is a decision and the responsibility for the result is still theirs"....

In calling for the mobilization of a 10 fold increase in the army of psychiatrists and conscripting other doctors also in the war against human nature, he states

"shock, chemotherapy, group therapy, hypno and narco-analysis, psycho drama, even surgery, can all be used..."

And later still

"Psychiatrists "should be trained as salesmen and taught the technique of breaking down sales resistance"

Things get ominous when he asks

"should attempts be made by the profession to induce governments to institute compulsory treatment for the neuroses as for other infectious diseases"

Such were the words of none other than Brock Chisholm, the first director of the World Health Organization, celebrated humanist and (not surprisingly) psychiatrist, who in a fervent attempt to avoid a repetition of the first two world wars calls for a one world government and psychiatry at the vanguard as explicit micro and macro social engineers. Such is the progressive mania seizing a reflective moment following the war, a wholesale hatred of the world and all it has held sacred the likes of which one might read in a Robespierre or unveiled Voltaire. One can hardly not feel in such sentiments the palpable potential for totalitarian evils, all opportunistically cloaked in the knee jerk sentiment to avoid another Hitler. Chisholm's speech was fawned over by powerbrokers in government and psychiatry itself. Present for example was Harry Stack Sullivan, one of the founding fathers of contemporary American psychiatry who described Chisholm as "a rarely wise man". Stacks tone was more cautious and his eye more widely and deeply scanned the psychodynamics of the situation, whilst retaining the same progressive drive nonetheless. As the dust settled after the war, psychiatry continued its aspirations, developed further its armamentarium and caked upon this layers upon layers of public relations and the language of care.

Psychiatry isn't the only participant in the therapeutic state of course. We have public health measures which might include seatbelt wearing and vaccination campaigns, and some coercive activities when persons drive intoxicated or mandatory notification or quarantine of persons infected with tuberculosis, plague or Spanish flu. Yet note these are usually either predicated on encouraging voluntary assent by the individual subject to the marketing, or coercion only when there is a clear and present danger to others from something beyond the control of the individual (no one individual can purify an aquifer and no willpower can resist the flu). What is under the control of the individual is potentially a crime and not a public health measure as such. Recklessly infecting another person with hepatitis or HIV can, for example, be rightly considered assault in my own, and other, jurisdictions. Another manifestation of the power of the state is as prohibitive nanny over what chemical substances the person wishes to take for their own private reasons, this the subject of another chapter. Nevertheless, it is in psychiatry that we arguably find the most pervasive, concentrated and contentious manifestation of the therapeutic state as running roughshod over autonomy. And we have metaphor heaped upon metaphor, from thoughts becoming illnesses to treatments and public health campaigns becoming a "war" on mental illness or a public health "campaign". And yet who are the invading forces? A person who may commit a crime on account of deviant thoughts? Do we not have a police force for that? A person who may harm themselves? Why not the right to be sick and damage ones own property, i.e. the body that is theirs? Tyranny always invent the solution first, and then the emergency to justify the solution. Each generation as psychiatric power grows its claims to catastrophe become greater. As the numbers treated with so called antidepressants increase, unlike with antibiotics or vaccination the cases of depression rise also.

Eventually even the jailors of the therapeutic totalitarian state become captives to its cause. As Szasz quotes Alan Leshner circa 1998, Head of the American National Institute of Drug Abuse involved in the majority of drug addiction "research"

"My belief is that today, in 1998, you [the physician] should be put in jail if you refuse to prescribe S.S.R.I.s [Selective Serotonin Reuptake Inhibitors, a type of so-called antidepressant medication] for depression. I also believe that five years from now you should be put in jail if you don't give crack addicts the medication we're working on now"

Strong words, yet hardly surprising or unusual. In my own practice, untreated "psychosis" and refraining from forcibly saving someone from the "mental illness" of suicidality can get the physician in hot water. But nurses, teachers, clergy and all public servants are being brought into the orbit of mandatory "duty of care". Even the banking officer on the phone will call the police or paramedic if you threaten suicide in response to them threatening to foreclose on your mortgage, for neither you or they are responsible for what you do. They are not responsible for taking your home and you are not responsible for taking your life. Indeed they might be fired for what you do with your body. The health sociologists say health is human flourishing, disease is anything that obstructs the road to health. The health socialists say your brother is public property and you are his keeper, you being one of the million eyes of the therapeutic state. And should you not keep your brother well you are a criminal or traitor. These are the makings of a Pavel Morozov. It is all around us. Don't believe me? Just start taking about hearing voices.

To properly understand the danger posed by the therapeutic state requires an understanding of, and more to the point an affective leaning towards, libertarian principles. It won't be to the liking of those red shirts of a more communitarian bent who believe that they are their brothers (or sisters) keeper and vice versa (or more accurately their brothers purifier using the state to re-educate). Liberty is not for those who wish to suck on the teat of the state and turn to the same at signs of trouble, expecting all facets of life to be politicized and the government to license approval, regulation and supervision. It is not for those whose naivety would lead them into excessive trust in their leaders simply because they are not liquidating their own citizens, and always pointing the finger at those foreign regimes who are. The libertarian in principle sees the adult as a private person, not a public property. And the libertarian in principle sees government as inherently dangerous to individual freedom. Any elaboration upon state powers agreed on by the citizenry is a necessary evil, say for taxation of emergency relief or the mobilization of an army. This always carries a risk of gathering gravitational mass and carrying us further towards the proliferation or more and more organs of government, regulation and oversight as we undoubtedly have today. Apart from possessing two eyes and two ears, why might any person have so strong a view? For the simple reason that just as I have defined the psychiatrist on the basis of the power to coerce, this is exactly the sine qua non of government, i.e. the rapacious power to control the individual, the power to control you. You may like the roads upon which you drive and the health care for the poor. Yet you do not like the tax that pays for them, and cannot choose either the amount taxed or its allocation. And in virtue of paying taxes you have less income available for your own philanthropy, though can always apply for a grant that nanny government will provide, and regulate, audit so on. You might finance via taxation the defense research programs from which smart phone and internet technology develops, yet pay twice over when the government gives the technology over to large corporations that charge you a fee for the product. And things get ominous when that same road that you paid for can carry you against your will to a technologized hospital which can admit you against your will, hold you down and inject state sanctioned drugs, all for the crime of thinking differently. Postmodern man can scarcely imagine a time or a possibility of things being otherwise. As George Washington himself stated

"government is not reason; it is not eloquence. It is force. Like fire it is a dangerous servant and a fearful master"

How can any open eyed student of history doubt the truth of this?

The purist form of libertarianism would imagine a rational agent stepping out of the Lockean state of nature into free assembly and voluntary contracts with other free individuals, voluntary contract being the atomic units from which even a national army may be assembled. You would pitch your tent or build your log cabin, fence around it, sell the tomatoes and prosper. Or you might worship the garden fairies if that was your pursuit of happiness. Alternatively, you could just drink yourself to oblivion. Every individual is free to do as they please up to the point of violence against another's life, liberty and property. And actions always carried consequences, with no one to blame but oneself.

When considering the danger psychiatry poses, let us neither overstate the case (say with puerile and cliché comparisons to totalitarian states of the previous century) or understate the case (by viewing psychiatry only through rose coloured glasses). But to state the ethical and moral case we need understand the gravitas of what deprivation of liberty is, along with the complement to liberty, i.e. personal responsibility. So as to apply this to the person whom we might be reflexively accustomed to believe deserves to have their liberties taken from them, we need also enter into the mind of the other in an act of empathy that few can achieve. We need be bravely open to a process of unlearning, dwelling in a place of sceptical tension, resisting the drive to foreclose on a greater knowledge by prematurely falling back on the comforting prejudice and bewitching language of our current selves (i.e. the myth of mental illness). Hopefully the bonds have already been loosened as I have addressed the matter of psychosis above and in a previous chapter. Hopefully the reader will forgive my repetitiveness. Here and there I've gone as far as I can to convince the reader of its arbitrariness, where arbitrariness is defined in terms of an autocratic system which operates according to power over persons, not having won the argument of either the moral warrant behind the power, nor the logical use of it. A similar case is made with respect to suicide and the myth of addiction, also in previous chapters.

So let us say for the moment that you have a belief, any belief, and this places you in a position of conflict with others (social and / or occupational dysfunction). If this belief is to cast aside your own personal property that is your choice is it not? If this belief leaves you in a state where you fail to flourish as the society would like, is it not your responsibility to take or reject what help may be offered? If this belief involves infractions upon others liberty this is criminal is it not? And let us take a leaf out of Rawls book and assume that you do not know what the ensemble of your beliefs might be before you are thrown into the stuff of life and the world, only that there is a state mechanism to take certain deviant beliefs from the street, hold the bearer of the belief down (i.e. you), forcibly inject you with medication and up the ante with forced hospitalization if it chooses for an indefinite period. This mechanism exists to augment the police and judiciary to capture and control the other fraction of social deviance that violates the criminal code. Are you comfortable with such an augmentation, simply because the odds are in your favor that your beliefs won't be the one arrested? Or might there be the faint stirrings of some principled qualms against even the existence of such a mechanism?

The reader might be interested to know that on the basis of psychiatry and its predicates existing (i.e. what Szasz would call metaphor and myth), that police and psychiatry act hand in glove in the service of the therapeutic state. All over the world police and paramedics have the legal authority to detain and transport a person for psychiatric assessment. Certain jurisdictions may even have instantiated into law that a psychiatric assessment will first need be a) available and b) provided in a timely manner for c) the police or emergency services worker to bring them in and hospital staff to keep them there. That is to say the emergency services worker's authority is bound up with the existence and function of the psychiatrist, the process analogous to due process in criminal law where a defendant has the right to a timely trial. Police and paramedics cannot function on their own with their own concepts of mental illness and what they do now legally depends on what is available later. They are essentially deputized by psychiatry and their powers to detain contained within acts of legislation that are explicitly health (not criminal) related. This first point of arrest and detention is underwritten by the law to be sure, and with use of legal terms of art that might not be entirely part and parcel of the clinical praxis of psychiatry. Actually my own experience is that emergency services workers actually exercise excess power, detaining people for trivial reasons or as a ready mechanism to dump the person (and responsibility thereof) into a substitute jail (hospital) for acts that do not obviously fall within the chapters of the criminal code (non criminal deviance). Nonetheless these observations aside, psychiatry is the pneuma of the assault to liberty from the outset.

The length of time the person may be detained for involuntary assessment is not trivial. Even an hour or a day may matter to the patient themselves as it may also matter to the reader, most especially the principled reader. What will follow is a paranoia against the state and ever more ardent attempts to evade psychiatric surveillance, this assuredly making a diagnosis of a psychotic illness more likely. But what happens next after the ambulance brings the person to the hospital is certainly not a trivial bite out of a patient's (qua ex person's) life. Depending on the jurisdiction, having been assessed by the psychiatrist as being a danger to self and/or others and this informed by a mental illness, patients might be detained for one to several weeks before having the opportunity to present their case for freedom to an independent tribunal. Such a tribunal always involves a legal professional of some standing, essentially a presiding judge who chairs the tribunal and who makes the final adjudication. It may or may not involve an alleged "independent" psychiatrist whose function is perhaps to question the "treating" psychiatrist claiming the person requires ongoing involuntary hospitalization and/or treatment. The proceedings may or may not involve independent state appointed legal counsel representing the patient, counsel who notionally plays an adversarial role against the designs of the psychiatrist come jailor. From all this there arises a sense whereby the psychiatrist might attempt to weasel out of responsibility for the incarceration of persons in psychiatric hospitals by deferring responsibility to the judge or more diffusely still, claiming they are simply part of a due process or dialectic. However, the judges in such cases, and also the state appointed legal counsel, are both supremely ignorant of psychiatry, and supremely trusting of the same. Moreover psychiatry is not itself on trial. The legal professions only role is to referee the correct application in law, of what psychiatry has decided is the reason to detain and/or treat according to the assumed reality of the psychiatric constructs. The myth of mental illness is itself not placed on trial and so is inviolate and beyond the law. One can imagine a counterfactual history where an independent court of arbitration were to sit between the witch and her executioner. A witch is one who dances, yes. And this woman was dancing yes. Ergo she is a witch. And so her soul is to be freed by a benevolent burning she, needless to say, does not want for herself. But what pray tell is witchcraft? It is what the witch hunter tells the legislature it is, and so is the principal determinant of her being declared a witch. The reasoning is circular with a linear outcome.

Now a minority fraction of those in psychiatric hospitals are there notionally on a voluntary basis, I say notionally as this too is the world of mendacious appearances. If I tell you that you can remain voluntary on the proviso that you agree to the admission and from this exchange you agree to stay, are you truly free? Have you freely chosen? Not at all! This demarcates the difference between an overt deprivation of liberty and coercion, between the fist of power that falls upon the patient and the first held high and ready lest it is needed. Ergo the voluntary admission in a great number of cases is fraudulent. In my own practice I always attempted resist the temptation to coerce. If I was not going to take no for an answer, I saw no need to ask the question.

We cannot understate just how powerful this collusion is between state and psychiatry. And I must parenthetically restate here the central point of the second chapter, i.e. that the necessary and sufficient variable that defines a psychiatrist is the power over persons freedom. Moreover, it is not possible for the trainee psychiatrist to become the specialist consultant without exercising the use of this power and endorsing the same on guild exams. Psychiatrists, especially inexperienced ones, may be anxious when approaching tribunals and even the rare independent lawyer who a patient may retain. Yet the psychiatrist need not be afraid. The power is theirs for the taking. They just need become experienced in what to say in addressing the criteria under law for involuntary detention and treatment. I once observed in my own jurisdiction that almost all tribunals result in upholding the designs of the psychiatrist to extend involuntary treatment / civil commitment. Why this massive bias in outcomes I thought, when the tribunal ought to serve an adversarial role and play devil's advocate in the service of the patient (or "mental health consumer") who was once a person? I compared this to data from the criminal legal system (which is often necessarily adversarial) and found similar numbers, most are found guilty. The prima facie conclusion from this would suggest psychiatric tribunals are doing their job well and psychiatrists playing their own devil's advocate. The allegedly unwell are unwell in fact, the allegedly guilty are guilty in fact. However, the devil is in the detail. The majority of "crimes", be they misdemeanors or felonies, are crimes to which the defendant pleads guilty. Take the fraction where the defendant "lawyers up", claims to be innocent and fights the case and the odds shift in favor of the defendant. Compare this to the case of our hapless psychiatric patient. To a man (or woman) they all want their freedom and all deny the crime of mental illness. They are all fighting the charges made against them and they all protest their innocence of the crime that their thoughts, feeling and behaviors ought to be separated out for persecution by drugs and psychiatric confinement. And yet despite universal protest they almost universally lose their case.

Insanity Defence

Szasz next concern was the so called insanity defence, and he was an expert witness for some high profile criminal trials of his day. Forensic psychiatry and the insanity defence is a huge subject beyond the scope of this book. Suffice for now to include certain of Szasz's key observation along with my own. I have worked in emergency room psychiatry longer than anyone else I know, and lost count of the number of times I've been called on to psychiatrically assess those who have made threats to kill another, simply on the basis that they have at some time in the past have attracted some kind of psychiatric diagnosis and involvement, whatever that may be. It is as if once labelled, be it with schizophrenia, ADHD, anxiety or PTSD or whatever, the person is forever more assumed not to be a rational actor. Or worse still, very often someone is brought into the hospital by police or paramedics as they have "thoughts to harm others" and "afraid they might act on these thoughts". Non-psychiatric physicians regularly make similar referrals. I invite the reader to let that sink in, that collectively these educated and ostensibly responsible highly intelligent professionals even countenance the idea, let alone introject it as a given of the human condition, that thoughts of violence suggest mental incapacity unless and until proven otherwise. It is as if the whole of society ardently wishes free will and personal responsibility not to exist, or rather wishes such quaint notions of free will to be real only up to the point where praise stops and punishment starts. Sanity it seems is a diagnosis of exclusion when someone may be violent. And no clearer an example of repression is this, that man does not wish to know that he personally is capable of evil. He wants the excuse for the other such that it can be held in reserve for himself. One hardly needs even approach the vexed issue of the forensic psychiatric patient to have learned the lesson, though forensic psychiatry is the most deluded psychiatric subspecialty of all.

Next of course we have the frank commission of acts of criminal behaviour. To the materialist, they may if they like turn the tables on Szasz. They might say that all mental phenomena of necessity must have a basis in brain activity. And so any dysfunctional behaviour is material in its basis. But then every single fact of the human condition can be vulnerable to being disease, and so no one can be blamed and no one can be praised either. Such would be a facile and fatuous argument, as there is not a basis of disease the likes of which is substantially discriminative from the normal anatomy (or physiology) of the brain. As was the case of the third chapter, this little catharsis of a book cannot answer the mind body problem. Nor can this chapter address the many problems in forensic psychiatry that remain veiled to a critical eye and especially veiled to a laity who actually believe there are experts into the mind of the criminal. Suffice it to say that criminal behaviour almost by definition has often violated the non-aggression principle of libertarianism, and this ought to be the basis of consequences that operate on a criminal axis. Ought these consequences ever be psychiatric? Szasz controversially would say no, never, and for reasons laid out towards the beginning of the present chapter. If the criminal act was not informed by a physical illness which removed from their person the capacity to do otherwise, then they ought to be respected with the responsibility to face the consequences of their actions, regardless of how strange the cooccurring beliefs and motivations. The argument of course is that in the absence of severe physical illness to provide an objective attribution and mechanistic explanation for the criminal act, then it was informed by beliefs and behaviours which were objectively antisocial in their manifestation, if not intention. In his time Szasz did, as I could, marshal example after example where expert witness psychiatrists would argue that the defendant was mad and not bad, these psychiatrists being little more than hired sophists oblivious to the obvious fact that the defendant knew exactly what they were doing contra the law. Consequently, there ought to be no place in law for forensic psychiatry and the insanity defence. In my own experience, it is very rare patient indeed who does not recognize the relation between their desired behaviour and the law and its consequences, i.e. it is exceedingly rare a person lacks the awareness of criminality (the mens rea) of the criminal act (the actus reus). Even rarer still is the individual who will not modify their behaviour (even psychotic behaviour) should they fear and have personal experience of a law actually applied against them by a willing police and judiciary. I've even personally observed a patient with a supposedly rare form of epilepsy resulting in explosions of violence have the trajectory of their "disease" radically altered not by anti-convulsant drugs, but by the police knocking on the door. It is worth pointing out in closing that much of the prosecution of insanity by forensic psychiatry rests not upon physical evidence, as opposed the mental state of the defendant at the time of the crime. The delay between the crime and the assessment of mental state may be delayed days, weeks or months, and is always inferred by what the patient tells the psychiatrist at the time of the review. Good jurisprudence is about evidence. How does a psychiatrist know the mental state of another in the here and now, let alone in the past? How can they know?

Contra Szasz

An honest psychiatry would be acutely aware that is has failed to find the biological basis of the vast majority of its diagnoses. It was so in the 1960's and 1970's, and remains unalterably the case in 2020 despite the propaganda to the contrary. Accordingly, psychiatry's only ham fisted lines of defence are philosophical and hermeneutic. It ought not to be lost on the reader that when they throw everything they have at Szasz, and they did throw everything at Szasz, this is not the work of dispassionate enquiring minds. Surely they must be motivated by a strong desire for his thesis not to be true, it being something they wish not to believe.

On the Historical Breadth of the Disease Concept.

Much of Pies and Kendell's attack relied on finding examples from antiquity where disease was defined as more than on anatomical and physiological terms, even suffering in the broadest possible sense. Consequently, they are arguing that if an historical quantum of precedents be found where the doctor was granted authority over more than mere physical pathology, then this ought to continue. Not surprisingly many examples are to be found, for there were not many MRI scanners or EEG suites found in the ancient world, to say nothing of sophisticated chemical pathology laboratory. Diseases might only have been known as constellations of signs and symptoms clustering together (syndromes), which might only have been known eponymously. And so for perhaps millennia Kendell writes that disease was

"...essentially an explanatory concept, invoked to account for suffering, incapacity, and premature death in the absence of obvious injury, and suffering and incapacity are still the most fundamental attributes of disease"

To which Szasz responds

"until the nineteenth century, and beyond, illness meant a bodily disorder whose typical manifestation was an alteration bodily structure" or "physicians distinguished diseases from non diseases according to whether or not they could detect an abnormal change in the structure of the persons body"

He is then stating that modern psychiatry invented the non-physical suffering as illness. His detractors state that this was not possible, as the epistemic question of what was known as to the organic pathology was not known, and yet these were diseases nonetheless.

There is no controversy and both are correct in their way. The question was not what was known, yet what was inferred. Hippocrates humoral theory was said to interface with the body and indeed constitute the body in the physicality of its pathology. That was Hippocrates account of all of mental life. All eponymous syndromes of continental and British medicine were assumed to be bodily diseases with yet to be discovered pathophysiology, however much matters might involve attendant psychological distress or social dysfunction. In the America's, Benjamin Rush was of the belief that mental illness would be explained as brain vasculopathy, this being his proposed road to legitimize mental illness as medicine. And as any medically minded feminist knows, hysteria in antiquity was the migration of a delinquent uterus around the body, perturbing the humours of the mind in its travels. Uterine expeditions could be cured, inter alia, by being grounded by sexual intercourse. Nowadays a hysterectomy would offer the most fulminant cure.

Szasz was a voracious reader of history. Though not having read more than a fraction of the corpus of his work, I trust he knew only too well all the uses and abuses of appeals to traditional thought employed against his own anachronism. He makes short work of such argument, in being dismissively incredulous to the journey down the memory lane of medical history. We live in modern times Szasz will say, and must have a modern measure of disease. To Szasz, Pies and Kendell both use the deficiencies and myths of primitive medicine to defend the myth making of the psychiatrist.

Or to put it another way; it ought not to be lost on the reader that at precisely the historical age when medicine was turning to biological roots for both its epistemology and ontology of disease, psychiatry was hoping to do the same of course. Though early and contemporary psychiatry also insured itself against failure by simultaneously seeking to shore up a definition of the disease concept that defined itself entirely in functional and phenomenological terms, this only increasing to the current day. It wants to eat its biological cake and have it too in ever more nebulous and inclusive, though ultimately disjunctive forms.

Psychiatry attempts claim legitimacy not simply from trawling the history of the disease concept, yet also to find examples of modern constructs of mental illness in antiquity, as if to imply that what has always been is part of the psychiatric triumph in having been discovered. Now there is no denying that such descriptions approximating schizophrenia or psychotic depression can be found in times past. So what? This will not challenge Szasz thesis one iota. No one would suggest that the kind of social deviancy and personal distress whose liberty he wished to protect had never been seen or documented in times past. This is obvious, for nothing is new under the sun and ours is a cycling through the human condition. Yet we must be cautious of just how dull our keen eyes can become when looking back through time. Time and again I have read of even Hippocrates himself describing the mania of bipolar disorder and melancholia of severe major depressive disorder. But beware. A commonality of terms does not an equivalence of diagnosis make. Actually what Hippocrates likely described was what we might call today noisy and quiet delirium. We would wish today to transport Hippocrates manic and melancholic patients over two millennia into the future of our intensive care wards, not into the arms of psychiatrists.

A finally "ought not be lost" ought not be lost on the reader, and that is that social deviancy, distress and dysfunction can also come to be defined and partitioned to the experts as disease and illness on purely utilitarian grounds. In other words, psychiatric illness comes into being and is said to exist when the psychiatrist can do something about that which might previously have been considered part of the human condition. This is pure pragmatism, and unashamedly Kendall fly's its banner high in his submission to Szasz Under Fire. If the dreamy or rambunctious child can be made docile and a good cog in the machine by stimulant medication, we have both the invention of ADHD and with it necessarily the disappearance of both personality as an attributing formulation, along with the deficiencies of the school system, if not the family system. ADHD exists if we can do something to control the behaviour, same for schizophrenia. The reader too might be inclined to define others mental illness on the grounds of the utility of controlling another's symptoms and unwanted behaviour. But beware that something in yourself does not go against the social grain, and you be the one for which psychiatry has the label and pharmacological answer. I can only be true to myself, to state and restate. Philosophical pragmatism is the privation of principle, the turning ones back to the will towards the good, the beautiful and the true. Ergo it is evil.

On Disease Only for the Living

The next line of attack is the definition of disease as made by the pathologists themselves. Pies quotes the pathologist Krehl for example, who in tones suggestive of a postmodernist social worker stated that there is no such thing as illness at all.

"there is no illness, there are only sick people. In principle, nothing biologically different happened to a sick person than a healthy one".

This is to say that illness is not an abstraction apart from the one who suffers it, and so cannot be found in the cell, tissue, organ or organ system without consciousness, only in the suffering person. Or when Szasz holds up his beloved Virchow and says that disease has its being in the anatomical lesion, this readily observable in the cadaver, psychiatry quotes Virchow to have said that disease can only exist in a living cell in the living person.

"Disease presupposes life. With the death of the cell, the disease also terminates".

Only cells (or organ systems) in their living state are functionally perturbed by the lesion, and only the living person is the one "suffering" the disease. Ergo dead men do not have diseases and none can be found in the cadavar. This is a small quibble, for what Virchow (and Szasz) were saying was that the basis and meaning of medical disease is its physicality. Moreover, this can often and in paradigmatic cases be ascertained posthumously, or in dead tissue obtained via biopsy of the living person. To be sure, it is a simple truism that there is no such thing as a sick corpse any more than there is a healthy one. Yet if disease were to cease to exist in an ontologically radical way upon death, then what need do we have for the forensic or anatomical pathologist? The cause of death and all that is of interest to Virchow writes its signature upon the corpse. You see death and disease is like a marriage. Though marriage is said to be until death do us part, death is neither divorce nor even a negation of the past, for the corpse still wears the ring. In pocketing the ring, even an illiterate grave robber could make the correct diagnosis as to what afflicted the living re their matrimonial state of affairs. But note that Virchow did not consider bad music or a bad marriage to be a disease either, though the music be obviously only played by a living human being, and music too ceases to be played upon death. Neither music or marriage were medical matters that ceased to be of interest to the physician upon death. They were never of professional interest to the physician when the patient was alive, and would not be of interest to the pathologist after. Virchow and indeed the whole triumphant metanarrative of pathology as Aesclepius vs Hippocrates was an implicit logical defence of Szasz, if not an explicit one. One needs be wilfully ignorant or a sophist engaging in great mischief to ignore the obvious. In their little quibbles the critics seek to charge Szasz with a fallacy of ignoratio elenchi, when it seems that this is what they themselves are eminently guilty of. But who can blame psychiatry in its feebleness. All over the world of mental health today we will hear not of patients with symptoms but of "clients" or "consumers" with "lived experiences". Well, to the best of my knowledge the dead don't have experiences do they? And so why the need to qualify the term as if to distinguish the lived experience from that of the dead? I could deliver my own petty little metaphysical blows against the notion of a lived experience (past participive) as opposed to a living experience, the latter being the better of what would still be a ridiculous tautological term. Regarding the "lived experience", this from an industry which might criticize Szasz for suggesting a corpse can have a disease, we might reply that his was the lesser fallacy. We might also ask ourselves if we have ever known of a consumer or client forced by the state to purchase a product or service? Why then call them consumers or clients?

On Dissolving the Boundaries of Disease Within the Body

The next line of attack is the distinction between anatomy (i.e. the structure of the body) and physiology (the functional dynamism of the anatomical structures). The metaphysical distinction between what something is and what something does could make for a whole book, though won't be required here. Suffice to say that there are pathologies of bodily function that are not conceived of in the same sense as an observably dead piece of organ or a fracture of a bone, or the pathogenic bug grown from the patient's sputum and the like. This manifestation of disease might only be said to have a material manifestation and be known to us in perturbation of concentrations of chemicals in the blood, or via the output on a machine that measures the dynamism of the body. And so if psychiatry thinks or implies Szasz (and Virchow et al) might argue that disease is anatomical pathology alone, pathological physiology is shown up as a common sense exception. I cannot speak of course for Virchow, having not read his work. But Szasz was not at all averse to defining disease in physiological terms, as his argument was to defend physicality per se. But Anti-Szazsians are more subtle here. They are arguing not simply that disease can be defined by perturbation of physical dynamics, yet also defined by abstractions and numbers that might seem prima facie arbitrary, and yet are sound markers of disease nonetheless.

Kendall for example is quoted in the Pies article in Szasz Under Fire as follows

"There is no single set pattern of either structure or function....even in health, human beings and their constituent tissues and organs vary considerably in size, shape, chemical composition and functional efficiency"

What Kendal is saying is that if Szasz cannot fix normality within certain boundaries, then Szasz is denied a reference frame from which to argue psychiatry violates the boundaries in the overplay of metaphor. But what he (Kendall) is also implying is that we can define disease by other means, by a holistic and pragmatic calculus of bodily (dys)functioning, suffering and other more diffuse arguments with which to appeal. There is no set pattern, and so anything goes so long as suffering and dysfunction are involved. This is to open up the cognitive door a little wider such that the mental world can, in its apparent non physicality be also considered pathological.

With a quote the likes as having been made by Kendall (vide supra), we could be forgiven for thinking that psychiatry does not care at all about the bodies physicality as the defining ground from which diagnoses grow and ultimately have their being. And this would be true. Yet psychiatry is desperate to find the brain lesion or pathophysiology of schizophrenia and bipolar disorder, of major depression and ADHD, or anorexia and PTSD. What they have found is essentially nothing. They do delude themselves about concepts such as "duration of untreated schizophrenic illness" leading to "brain damage, ironically oblivious to the fact that macaque monkeys treated with antipsychotics suffer brain shrinkage in the order of that which is thought caused by the schizophrenia itself, and against which the drugs are mendaciously marketed as "neuro-protective". Presumably these poor monkeys were not schizophrenic before the fact, though no one asked the questions. Perhaps they heard voices when no one was there. Perhaps the CIA had been stealing their bananas also. I doubt both. Likewise, we have had psychiatry peddling for decades the notion that depression and schizophrenia both were chemical imbalances in the brain. When no imbalance was found, the strategy was to wait one generation and then deny the claim was ever made in the first instance. Much have been written about this intentional forgetting. Pies himself began an article in 2011 with a (presumably) materialistic quote by Will Durant

"Mind and body do not act upon each other, because they are not other, they are one."

Pies continues…

" I am not one who easily loses his temper, but I confess to experiencing markedly increased limbic activity whenever I hear someone proclaim, "Psychiatrists think all mental disorders are due to a chemical imbalance!" In the past 30 years, I don't believe I have ever heard a knowledgeable, well-trained psychiatrist make such a preposterous claim, except perhaps to mock it. On the other hand, the "chemical imbalance" trope has been tossed around a great deal by opponents of psychiatry, who mendaciously attribute the phrase to psychiatrists themselves.2 And, yes—the "chemical imbalance" image has been vigorously promoted by some pharmaceutical companies, often to the detriment of our patients' understanding. In truth, the "chemical imbalance" notion was always a kind of urban legend- - never a theory seriously propounded by well-informed psychiatrists."

If Pies, qua an experience of loss of temper, is one with his limbic system, pray tell what/where/who is the separate subjective "I" that "experiences" limbic activity? And just who were these psychiatrists who believed the claim to be preposterous and railed against the big pharma companies, where big pharma (and doubtlessly also family physicians) are scapegoated as spreading the chemical imbalance lie. I'm all for a good bashing of big pharma when they deserve it. Yet here they are at worst minor accomplices, and perhaps being honest in a sense. Pharma was being true to themselves as profit orientated free marketeers as opposed to alleged promotors of scientific truth marching to the beat of the physician's ethical drum. It would be charitable to say Pies is playing the Scotsman fallacy. For he would have it that the minority of stupid ones who might have promoted the chemical imbalance myth aren't the real psychiatrists, the smart "well informed" ones, the ones like him. They are an urban myth he would say. Then why 32 years earlier in the landmark article of 1979 to which this chapter is largely addressed and in which he attacked Szasz did Pies write

"But now let us suppose that hallucinations and delusions are caused by an excess of dopamine in the brain-a thesis Szasz has never refuted. It would not be absurd, or silly, or wasteful to ameliorate these symptoms with dopamine antagonists".

Actually Szasz never bought stock in the chemical imbalance theory and was one of the few never found in bed with the pharmaceutical industry. And we might ask why Pies raised this particular supposition contra Szasz if Pies and his limbic system never took the chemical imbalance seriously? In point of fact, institutional psychiatry (yes the intelligentsia of psychiatry, the guilds themselves and their thought leaders) were up to their elbows in promotion the chemical imbalance theory. The remainder less biologically inclined psychiatrists were busy with other nonsenses such as psychoanalysis or the satanic panic, or stayed silent not rocking the boat of their industry. We might be reminded once gain by Orwell

"Who controls the past controls the future. Who controls the present controls the past".

Let us not let them get away with rewriting history.

We also have perinatal psychiatrists claiming, with a straight face, that depression in pregnancy (where depression by all accounts is a non-physical state of being) causes birth defects, the implication being that SSRI's will protect the foetus against the teratogenicity of its mother's mood. And yet why then are SSRI's (undeniably physical substances), associated with a doubling of risk of birth defects (undeniably a physical outcome), if they are so protective?

Returning to the matter at hand, many examples of nominal and statistical "diseases" can or have be provided by anti-Szazians. On the nominal side we have nominal examples such as "essential hypertension". When a physician consistently reads a blood pressure as 145/85, they might inform the patient of a mild hypertension. This is related to the patient in terms of them rightly having attended the doctor's rooms and not the bartender, of having the disease of hypertension and perhaps requiring medication and not the purchase of a new car. There is not necessarily any anatomical lesion diagnosed and none was looked for. In point of fact, what was observed was a machine, and inferences made about the body from the numbers on a dial. And were the medical student to ask the significance of a boundary between what might be called normal blood pressure of 139/79 and the systolic hypertension of 145/85, the answer would be "not much, the cut off is semi arbitrary and a convention informed by risks. We have to set a limit somewhere". Many other biological abnormalities are given medical labels despite being explicitly informed directly by convention or statistical norms. If your blood level of a chemical constituent falls in the upper or lower fifth centile, you might have "hypo"-this or "hyper"-that. This does not in any way negate the notion as to the physicality of disease a la Szasz and Vichow.

Even Kendells as quoted above (in the Pies article) is only true in the most superficial and inconsequential sense. Surely we shan't charge him with a relativism such that "there is no single set pattern of either structure or function.." can be used in turn to argue physical disease is anything we want, and that Szasz has no frame of reference whatsoever to define a disease as a physical abnormality of a specific kind. But then why raise the argument? The fact is that Szasz has every right to demand a firm objective frame of reference with which to label one as mad and deprive them of their liberty, and the onus is on psychiatry to provide it. As a former lecturer in embryology, I might say that some persons are born with several extra small accessory kidneys, this being a normal variation. Another common variation is the absence either unilaterally or bilaterally of a small muscle in the forearm called the palmaris longus. Neither are diseases. Yet compare this with the following little personal anecdote; once as a medical student one of our pathology professors spoke of a recent case he had, the case of the unexplained death of a child. The post-mortem had collected tissue samples, including brain tissue that had been processed to be observed under the most powerful of microscopy, the electron microscope (an instrument only found in large tertiary university hospitals articulated with large universities). And so one night he was up into the wee hours painstakingly scanning the tissue field by field in the darkened room. And then he found it, a single sarcomere, the functional unit of skeletal (and cardiac) muscle. You see even a single sarcomere in the brain is radically out of place, and pathognomonic of a malignant tumour from its source (a rhabdomyosarcoma). This an example that the exceptions prove the rule as a refutation of Kendals relativism in defence of psychiatric pragmatism. It is ok to lack a forearm muscle or two. It is ok to have a little third kidney (or even a fourth or fifth). It is never ever ok to have skeletal muscle growing in the brain.

Or think of plasma pH (a measure of acidity/alkalinity). Take all the therapeutic bicarb soda or apple cider vinegar one wishes, and the plasma pH will remain within a very narrow range indeed. Though one healthy person might have a plasma pH of 7.35 and another 7.45 (these being the boundaries of the normal range by common convention), and though we might reason correctly that one does not suddenly die when the pH is 7.34 or 7.46 (in fact there's a margin of error in the machines measure as to what the plasma level actually is), none would argue that a level of, say, 7.15 or 7.65 is compatible with life. Plasma pH is thus immensely informative as to the reality and acuity of bodily disease states.

Or let us return to the matter of hypertension. It is obviously true that physicians arbitrarily define high blood pressure as, for example >140mm Hg systolic and/or >90mm Hg diastolic, and these numbers relates to a physiological process which is not in and off itself a pathological anatomical state. In a sense pressure is an abstraction and only exists in circular relation to physical concepts such as force per unit area or in relation to flow and resistance. Nevertheless, it would be misleading to detach hypertension from even the hard Virchowian idea that pathology is anatomical pathology. The reason is very simple. For the numbers to have any meaning at all, they must inform a risk of developing an anatomical pathology that is conceptually linked in its physicality to the blood pressure itself. The endothelial lining of the vasculature is not like a sturdy wall of tiles so much as, on a molecular level, more like a delicate coral reef. This delicate reef, this complex ecosystem if you will, is pressure sensitive. And in a less subtly conceptual level, the walls of vasculature are sensitive to pressure in the same way that one could strip the paint off, and ultimately blast through, a plaster wall with a high pressure water cleaner. If one were to have a blood pressure of 225/120, death would be sooner rather than later. Elevated blood pressure relates in its physicality to all the sequelae that might result from it, be it stroke, renal failure, an aortic dissection, arteriosclerosis or whatever. And one can seamlessly link the conceptualization of the physicality of one process (i.e. hypertension) to all the others (e.g. the stoke). If we were to find tomorrow that we were wrong all along and blood pressure bears no relationship whatsoever to the matter of anatomical pathology, then hypertension would cease to be a concern to doctors. The argument must also be made what makes a state of mind a disease if not causally related in a strong sense to a disorder of the body.

We could say the same for blood glucose levels, calcium levels and countless other examples as we have for blood pressure and plasma pH. Even height is the same. Great height is only disease marker and only of interest to the doctor if it is a manifestation of a pituitary tumour for example. A healthy giant, if one exists, is none of the doctors business. Neither is the water supply the business of the doctor if not contaminated by Vibrio cholerae and the like.

Statistically abnormal, deviant and interpersonally (even intra-personally) distressing thoughts, emotions and behaviours in the absence of any anatomical correlate with strong causal inference sit within an entirely different category to the above examples of blood pressure and the like. Granted what is called schizophrenia indirectly impacts on physical health. Typically, this cohort of persons smoke and otherwise poorly attend to their health, dying prematurely from most of the diseases common to the western world. But schizophrenia is not like syphilis with its multi-organ manifestations and a pathophysiological narrative to link them all together. It is not a multi-organ disease manifest by emphysema or obesity (in the so called schizophrenic who smokes, is sedentary and who is administered fattening psychiatric medication).

On the Dissolution of Szasz Disease Concept into a Language Game

Pies, in his debate against Szasz (In "Szasz Under Fire") makes the surprising turn to use Wittgenstein. I too had my proto-Wittgensteinian revelation as outlined in a previous chapter, i.e. the shocking realization that psychiatry can only define delusion on the basis of the use of the term, without appeal to any essentiality, i.e. that the patient does not have a delusion before the psychiatrist gives it to them as its existence is bound up in the use of the word. An understanding of Wittgenstein is like Feynman's formulation of quantum physics. Those who claim to understand him (or quantum physics) are likely not to, and anything I write here is likely not improve on things. But one formulation of the so called latter Wittgenstein is to say that language does not directly point to anything in the world. It refers only to itself as its use in a "language game", i.e. a practical system between persons as to the use of a word. It is impossible to fix ourselves upon a definition that is impervious and a priori, of a word that represents a thing in the world the way we might aspire to being like Adam, when God charged him with naming things as they are in a strong sense. Pulling out Wittgenstein is Pies way of devaluing Szasz's biophysical definition of disease as a proposal to elevate just another rival language game. But does it escape the mind of Pies that that in using Wittgenstein as a weapon, he embarks on a philosophical suicide mission as the weapon also explodes onto himself. For Pies himself cannot escape being captured in the orbit of admitting his own psychiatry to be a language game, where Pies only claim to have the greater game could be in its having greater political power. Actually I suspect that Pies, as a philosophical pragmatist amongst pragmatists, is all too aware of the manoeuvre and could frankly not care less. His is a language game where mental illness is spoken of as existing, of being diagnosed as it is, of being treated as it is, this including deprivation of liberty. They would love for it to be reified as physical pathology, yet just as happy if they cannot. The game played is psychiatry's game. And that is that.

On Suffering and Dysfunction as Illness/Disease

In something of an extension of the use of historical notions of disease under which the doctor has authority, the anti-Szaszian might then say that any and all suffering and incapacity with a predominant (or exclusive) mental component could be termed mental illness. We might look at contemporary formulations of disease such as the World Health Organization which defines health as

"a state of complete physical, mental and social well-being and not merely the absence of disease or infirmity"

Such a definition appeals to sentiment and lofty aspiration, also had in certain quarters of clinical psychology where the absence of neurosis does not necessarily imply that one is living to the best of the psychological and social potential. It's a sentiment that has given rise to thousands of positive psychology practitioners and life coaches working with otherwise unremarkable people who are at least not cutting themselves or talking back to the voices they hear. And so the WHO definition is superficially sound enough and uncritically accepted by almost all medical students who hear it. Their reaction, if critical at all, will be simply a recognition of its tedium by the "health sociology" lecturer when all they really want is to learn the "real" medicine. Yet it should not be a definition considered only by tired and disinterested eyes. Lurking beneath the surface of the WHO definition is the potentiality of a medical overreach of totalitarian proportions. Is this health vs illness a spectrum or a dichotomy? If someone lacks disease, can they ever be teetering in a neutral state of lacking wellbeing either? That is to say, what do we call a state of falling short in the goal of "complete wellbeing"? If this is not health and it is not disease, what is it? Is it partial wellbeing or partial disease? And so we might argue that the definition implies what would be incoherent if formally stated, that the absence of complete wellbeing is a disease of a kind, for it is something that we wish to change and defined as disease by the WHO (not Szasz or I). In any case, this is the WHO definition. And who has responsibility towards the other in respect to reaching the goal of the health that is their right? Who has authority as advocate, architect (and enforcer) of the health of this new world order, where it could be argued that almost everyone falls short of it, particularly all in the developing world and the world of so called mental illness?

The American Psychiatric Association DSM and psychiatry in general avoids the use of the term disease, preferring the term disorder (which is synonymous with illness and equivalent in practice to that of disease), and defining a mental disorder including the following; "behavioural, psychological or biological dysfunction" manifest in terms of "social or occupational dysfunction" and excluding "deviant behaviour" or conflicts between the individual and society. This is also a muddle. Definitions or elements of definitions such as the above do nothing to resolve the matter of whether the individual in front of us is mentally ill/disordered and in what sense these terms might have meaning. Any conflict between an individual and their world necessarily involves some manner of dysfunction in social and/or occupational terms, this being experienced in any conscious person as a psychological phenomenon (collectively mind and behaviour). It places the individual in a place where the dividing line between the mentally disordered and the socially deviant is arbitrary and known only by the common customs. In "Szasz Under Fire", Kendall realizes this in outlining certain other definitions of disease, including to single out one by Scadding

"the sum total of the abnormal phenomena displayed by a group of living organisms in association with a specified common characteristic or set of characteristics by which they differ from the norm for the species in such a way as to place them at a biological disadvantage".

Kendall continues to suggest a disease concept meaningful to psychiatry might involve an impairment in fertility or life expectancy, both of which might be the case in the patient with schizophrenia. Collectively, Scadding and Kendall both seem to view disease (or illness or disorder) in some kind of neo-Darwinian frame where a human being, a person, is a function within a social whole, measured against a species norm. Presumably social functioning also is a Darwinian epiphenomenon. How to possibly escape the conclusion that the urban homosexual male and the ascetic monk in the Syrian desert are both, in their own opposite ways, as diseased as the one who talks to the green aliens in their roof crawl space? Both are exceptions to the norm. Both might well have reduced fecundity in serving the needs of the species or the tribe to reproduce its kind. Or maybe not. Maybe we might be eugenicists and see the value in their degeneracy dying out, if degenerate is what we decide they are.

In ever more expansive nebulous and protean definitions of disease, illness and disorder, many a psychiatrist seems to have a romantic and imperialistic notion of who the doctor is as physician over the mind and soul of person and village, for Psyche seems to have divorced herself from Eros and demanded her new psychiatrist bridegroom be worshiped in her stead. They imagine (or rather I imagine from their aspiration) the rural family physicians of some amalgam of all the clichés of a certain genres of fiction. And so up across the Victorian porch and under the hanging shingle of the M.D. walks the troubled teen who might get advice form the sage as to what life is and how to be. Why not receive some advice as to the sufferings of his unrequited love? Or maybe he is suffering some poor grades in mathematics and its attendant suffering drives him to the kindly family doctor, whose mathematical aptitude is the stuff of village legend. In between lancing boils and delivering babies the doctor might work towards ameliorating the other sufferings of the community such as organizing a grain depository against famine or running for mayor. Or he might take up with an amateur detective and tour around with Sherlock Holmes solving the suffering of murder and injustice. In an earlier chapter I described a time when psychiatrists battled the social suffering of Satan worship. Doctors today might take up their righteous place as "scholar", "expert" and "advocate" and preach who the people ought to vote for, and what their opinion ought to be in the fight against this or that social or climatic suffering that has usurped real bodily disease in the pages of any Pravda that was once a bone fide medical journal. Life is suffering and so the psychiatrist sage is the master over life on the way to its unsuffering perfection

Now we might say that such a fanciful vision of the physician (or psychiatrist) is a fiction. And in a limited sense it is, though not far from what the psychiatrist thinks they have the God given right to be and to do should they choose, given their infinitely plastic notions of suffering to which they minister. Currently we have the custom of leaving that kind of suffering that is known as burglary to the police and the judiciary. We leave that kind of suffering that is homelessness to the social worker, and kind of suffering that is educational underdevelopment to the teacher. We leave the kind of suffering that is the fracture to the orthopaedist and that kind of suffering that is the heart attack to the cardiologist or emergency physician. And we leave that grab bag of other kinds of suffering about which the village elaborates labels such as "depression" and "PTSD" to the psychiatrist. But what licence does the psychiatrist have to be master of anything at all? Is it because certain kinds of suffering appear to be better served by diagnosis and medication? This is the world of appearances only, and not enough to argue the case of reifying mental illness and elevating to the ontological status we might accord physical pathology unless wedded my own bete noir, i.e. philosophical pragmatism. We must come to see the dangers of a profession that considers itself to have expertise over undefined suffering, as this places the profession as masters over the human condition and all persons.

Really, we must challenge ourselves to the notion of how and why our psychiatric customs have developed, whether they be good or bad, right or wrong and what problems we have with them in the sense they represent an economy of power over knowledge and person's bodies, an economy within which certain power structures seek to expand or consolidate according to their own purposes.

Or what is next? We might formulate popular culture and art as informing health, and of being in the appreciation of the ugly (symptom) and manifestation of the ugly contemporary art (signs) an aesthetic forms of mental illness. Believing in the wrong political ideology (symptoms) and voting incorrectly (sign) is also a manifestation of mental illness, for this too can be interpreted as the furtherance of suffering about which the citizen (patient) lacks insight (symptom). And will loneliness (which is suffering) be the province over which psychiatry demands its place as the expert? What of the mystic who has the suffering of the dark night of the soul? Is Kierkegaards despair (supposedly shared by us all) an undiscovered mental illness? What of divorce as mentioned earlier and to repeat here, childhood temper tantrums, writers block? Choose your diagnostic definition where suffering is the necessary and sufficient factor and I can work any and all of these into it, and so much more besides. Moreover, I'll guarantee to find a functional MRI difference somewhere between those who suffer these pseudo-diseases and those who do not. These examples are not lexicographic or semantic ad absurdum to the notion of suffering and functional incapacity. These are always within reach of a psychiatry which might make opportunistic and pragmatic use of them if the political conditions ripen. The only means by which the individual can assure its own protection is by an in principled killing psychiatry first. And the individual has ample precedent as to the dangers it faces.

Szasz insight is in recognizing that the definition of a psychiatric doctor are the limits of the doctors power over persons liberty. His most consistent bulwark against all these slippery slopes of suffering = illness is the insistence that mental illness must be related to a physical disease as its antecedent and cause. Only then could medicine even consider to make a claim over the territory of the person. And so we now turn to the synthesis of the myth of mental illness and the therapeutic state.

Divide and Conquer; The Indivisibility of the Argument

Much of the problem with the anti-Szaszian lay in their reductively splitting at the outset his philosophy of mental illness on one hand (the myth from metaphor of illness), and use of psychiatric authority on the other (the therapeutic state). The critic of Szasz usually insists on first defending the flank of the construct of mental illness. Thinking to have resolved the answer in their own favour, this being a belief they held all along and were destined to "prove" one way or the other via various sophist manoeuvres, they then feign openness to humanely exploring the limits of coercion upon the mentally ill. Then and only then might they pay a trifle respect to Szasz as a misguided defender of patient's rights, all the while believing that curtailing the freedoms of the mad is self-evident, this being cloaked in the language of care and of course for the patient's own good. This token of respect is itself self-indulgent, for it is the granting to oneself the appearance of a peace maker, a condescending nod to that tiny piece of wisdom possessed by one whom we believe to be a fool. Szasz will have none of a compliment predicated on the myth.

In any case this reductive approach is a mistake, one of many made by the anti-Szasz camp, and inverse to the order the matters ought to be approached if to be separated at all. It is impossible to properly do justice to Szasz if to myopically cast him as a psychiatrist critical of psychiatry or as a philosopher of language wishing to peel wide open the analytic/synthetic divide. Although conversant in the practice and philosophy of science and medicine, he was instead a moral philosopher and political activist, and perhaps the most radical exponent of libertarianism specifically. Part historical accident and part his own choice, psychiatry was simply the city in which he built his church to liberty. Were life to have taken a different turn or were he incarnated in another form (if one believes in such a thing), he might well have been an American race liberator or anti-socialist dissident behind the iron curtain had he remained in his native Hungary. To be sure, "The Myth of Mental Illness" is his chef d'ouve. Yet it is his more political works such as "Faith in Freedom" that give us a better window to his project, and he is quoted to have said that were he to have succeeded in killing off psychiatry that he would devote himself entirely to political philosophy. His attack on mental illness as myth is robust enough. Yet always this question is viewed through the lens of liberty and the place of the state as matters of first principle, hence my earlier dwelling on the subject. And always the question is approached for Szasz also through a genealogical lens which, like Foucault, was to examine what diagnoses are as products of history. One needs to approach his argument in its totality or not at all.

And so when the anti-Szaszian contends that many illnesses have in times past been known only by their singular or collective symptoms, behaviour or pathos and not by their organic pathology (e.g. migraine and epilepsy), they will continue to contend that uncomfortable symptoms and abnormal behaviour alone are reason enough that what might be called illness ought to be seen as falling under the purview and authority of the doctor as an agent of the state. Such a non sequitur trades on three appeals to make it stick. The first is on the reader knowing what we know now, that these precedent example diseases are indeed pathophysiological events in the brain, and there no shortage of other examples either. I have lost count of how often the modern medical triumphalist parades out the corpse of that young man in the gospels allegedly exorcised of a demon as really having an epilepsy. Tourettes syndrome, like epilepsy, also has gone the way of the brain, as has migraine, albeit even in the 21st century migraine especially remains poorly understood. It not be lost on the reader that these and other discoveries of disease are deliberately chosen as historiographic tools of argumentation. From the matter of diseases once poorly understood or thought not to be disease, the anti-Szaszian attempts take the reader on a cognitive and affective journey to uncritically identifying all so called mental illness as also being biological pathologies, albeit with mechanisms yet to be discovered. And from here there are further appeals to the triumph of science and materialism. The reader, in their conscious or unconscious weddedness to materialism, is left in a position of not wanting to appear the fool when science one day finds that psychopathologies a la the DSM 5 or their criterion symptoms are found to be caused by anatomical lesions or pathophysiological processes.

The problem is that medicine in general and psychiatry in particular has a history replete with failed hypotheses masquerading as certainties. Psychiatry has invested literally billions without establishing the physicality of mental illness. Essentially all it has a grab bag of drugs found by serendipity and having largely non-specific effects to blunt emotionality, drives, initiative and attention. Unlike psychiatry, on balance internal medicine and surgery can certainly take a stance of optimistic verisimilitude, though even in these disciplines at the it is not entirely clear which medical facts of today will be disproven tomorrow. A knowledge of the history of psychiatry is not cause for even a guarded optimism, and the discipline lurches along either in stasis or quiet crisis.

The second anti-Szaszian hook is to assume he is proximally interested in whether a physician has ever considered migraine or epilepsy a disease before its pathology was elucidated. They assume that Szasz might have believed that medicine and surgery almost could and should not have existed before the days of Rokitansky, Virchow and Morgagni, of Leeuwenhoek, Jenner and Pasteur. They might even attempt to paint Szasz in absurdity, to imply he would be forced to admit that by the lights of own logic that before modern medicine and the pathophysiology we now know, there could be no disease. "if a tree falls in the forest and no one is there to hear it, does it make a sound", they would have it that Szasz would answer "no".

Both arguments would be a misreading of Szasz, who argued libertarian axioms of freedom and responsibility are a priori with the onus placed upon the illness monger to prove the case. However, Szasz is not a blind ideologue. He admits that if it were one day discovered that what we call mental illness is a physical disease in the way he reasonably defines it and which overturns free will in a way discriminating the brain of the ill from the masses, then he too would admit the same. And who wouldn't? But such a discovery is heretofore elusive and should it come to pass provides no vindication. Given that in science a hypothesis has at best meagre value until the day proof is found, there is no scientific sense in which one might speak of their cherished hypothesis "see I knew it all along", for the knowing comes into being only with the discovery. Even then, from Hume to Popper to Kuhn we would say our proof is provisional. Granted we might praise the one who makes the discovery as being intuitive or a skilled evaluator of the prior evidence in the formulation of hypotheses. Yet this praise does not amount to an acknowledgment that they knew, especially when freedom is at stake. In any case, it does not take a genius to hypothesize correctly that migraine, epilepsy, Tourettes disorder, Parkinsons Disease etcetera are brain (or bodily) pathologies in the broadest sense, and so we shan't inflate the value of those who claim the same, this especially when they stand on the right side of history looking back. The much more difficult hypothesis is to guess ahead of the game the precise pathophysiology involved, the devil of both meaningful hypothesis and knowledge being in the detail. And yet we ought to accept nothing less than solid proof when liberty is at stake. Then and only then would we possibly have licence to call mental illness a disease for reasons of using the therapeutic state. For Szasz, the question was not simply whether mental illness was a disease in and of itself or of the flexibility with which we might use the word if we wish to use it, a freedom underwritten by the first amendment of his adopted nation. No, the question is of illness in being an argument in favour of violating the libertarian non-aggression principle. It was to defend the person who might have their liberty and responsibility taken from them when they make the statements "I feel..", "I believe...." or "I desire..." or "I am going to do...". And parenthetically, notwithstanding the notion that the physicality of the disease might be located diffusely within the ecology of the body (body, brain and gut microbiome included), the newly discovered brain disease with mental manifestations would likely then be considered a new chapter within the neurology textbook, and find itself in good company with delirium, the dementias, central nervous infections and toxidromes. Accordingly, such a hypothetical discovery would not breathe life into a psychiatry that never could exist outside its use as a political tool for social deviancy. It would merely expand the borders of neurology and internal medicine.

I will make a claim that hardly ought to be seen as controversial to any who have read Szasz work, yet may be read with disbelief by most anti-Szaszians; i.e. that is he was extremely obliging of aberrant behaviours and alternative beliefs being referred to as mental illness, and even assumed to be bodily disease, though he believed these to be vastly different categories. He was also extremely obliging of the use of psychiatric drugs, as he was supportive of persons having the free market liberty to use drugs of all kinds, even if this were to place the user on the path of self-destruction. Insomuch as this is the case, he is not at all guilty of Pies imputation to having committed an exclusionist fallacy (i.e. that one cannot use the remedy of one kind of malady to treat a malady of a different kind). He repeatedly stated he was quite comfortable with two free persons coming together and involving themselves in a mutually consenting transaction where what troubles one is called a disease and the other assumes the role of doctor and seeks a cure by whatever means the patient assents to. The choice of language in such a case is a matter of individual taste in accord of the terms of the transaction, informed perhaps by science, yet informed also both by the prevailing ideologies and realpolitik of the time. As stated, Szasz even allied himself with scientology, all the while of the mind that Hubbard's pseudo religion was ridiculous and contra his own atheism. He would have had no bilious eruption against a free citizen of Greece attending a consultation with Hippocrates or Soranus, the subject being their humoral imbalances. That having been said, it is likely that he would have sat aside and rallied for a model of mind more in line with the Stoic school. Returning to the current day, though mercilessly scathing of so called complementary medicine, he had no objections to people spending their hard earned own money in a free market economy to receive healings by sitting under a wire pyramid with a crystal in their hand and a homeopathic tincture under the tongue. Caveat emptor and live and let live he would say, and more fool them. And so Szasz the radical libertarian protected the rights of people to do what they want within the limits of the non-aggression principle. He would have even gone so far as not to obstruct anyone seeking to take major tranquilizers (what are now misleadingly called antipsychotics) or be lobotomized if they did so voluntarily and having been adequately informed of the risks, taking personal responsibility for whatever follows. He thought these drastic interventions would be wasteful and destructive, though not to be prohibited amongst consenting adults. The problem as he saw it arises when the myth that is mental illness is coupled with infractions upon individual liberty and a means to avoid responsibility (the insanity defence much more pervasive than that which goes on in the court room). That was the myth he thought monstrous. In a sense we might then think of Szasz as attacking a triune myth of the mental illness/therapeutic state/insanity defence as a collective political outcome of an ethos.

Climbing Mt Szasz

Though I would argue all of the above to be critically important, quibbles over words and their meaning could be considered an exercise in intellectual masturbation missing the obvious realities of life. When confronted with the question if eccentricity in extremis is equivalent to madness, the Bard of Avon might have replied

"that which we call a rose, by any other name would smell as sweet"

That is to say, that the proverbial rubber hits the road when you or I encounter the other who sits across from us, and in this other is represented the extremes of social deviancy that might be described in terms of aberration of mental state and its attendant behaviours. What are the boundaries to liberty here when someone is obviously "mad"? Below are several examples, and a more radical Libertarian (i.e. Szaszian) ways in which they might be approached. Only in sitting comfortably with, or accepting the rightfulness of, such an approach might we claim to agree with the subject of our current enquiry. And if we shan't then Szasz's case, though perhaps correct, has failed to be convincing in advancing his cause towards liberty.

Firstly, we have the child with the various signs and symptoms that suggests perhaps a bacterial meningitis at play. The clock is ticking here, with life and limb dependent upon diagnosis and treatment which requires restraining the howling, hostile and obviously "noncompliant" young person who rejects the poking and prodding and the lumbar puncture. Even Szasz would have no compunction in doing what needs be done, for every child, in lacking adult responsibility likewise lacks adult liberty. The parent can conscript whomever they wish, whom if likewise acting in good faith can do what is in the child's best interests to diagnose and cure an illness that is by definition physical. The doctor, operating in parens patriae, has a proper place in this scenario to even usurp the authority of the parent in certain vexed cases. It is not a paradox that Szasz saw child psychiatry as a form of child abuse, as it trades on the myth of mental illness and treatment which the child lacks the maturity to assent to. Szasz prescription to troubled children was a loving gradual training into the world of adult responsibility, this by the parents or those appointed by the state if the parents are grossly inadequate for the task. Simple.

Secondly we have the adult patient. They have a modest elevation in white blood cells and certain other biological markers of inflammation, though all other investigations are normal. The previous evening, they were suddenly and uncharacteristically violent, "seeing things" and unable to attend to a conversation despite being notionally aware of where they are. Today they have a residual of the same perturbation to mental state, and they are unreasonably anxious to leave hospital. The most parsimonious conclusion is that there is something physically untoward informing both the deranged mental state and the physical markers, a delirium that in its nature they are not yet enduringly free of. It is just as likely as not that in the minutes to hours that follow they will succumb to the delirium again, as they have partially succumbed now. Given we infer a) that their mental state is affected by the physical illness and b) that in better times they might prefer upon a course of action maximizing their chance of survival and future exercise of rationality, we might c) detain them for a reasonable time to complete the observations, investigations and treatment. It is the physicality of the basis of their mental change and our not unreasonable optimistic hope that in future when their sensorium clears they will retrospectively assent to what we did that we feel justified in our strong paternalism. The doctor naturally has a proper place in this scenario.

In a similar vein, we have the elderly patient with a dementing illness (or those with either congenital intellectual disability or acquired brain injury). Presuming of course their faculties endure above whatever threshold is required to be the architect of their own destiny, they ought to be left to their own self-determination what is done with their body, whether the outcome be good or bad and even unto their own death. To be sure, the adjudication of where that threshold might be crossed is easier conjectured than identified, and is somewhat arbitrary. (It is the same with the very difficult question of when the child becomes the adult). Yet there would be a point where all agree that more of the mind is gone than can be trusted to make decisions in one own best interests, that in virtue of the diseases physicality the doctor might have right of place in these scenarios (alas often a futile role), and that liberty ought to be curtailed in the patients best interests.

Next we have the drug addled (usually) young adult. They may present to hospital disorganized in their behaviour and possibly in their mind also, raving nonsense and with some or all the hallmarks of what we might call "psychosis". After the storm of intoxication subsides, some strange and maladaptive beliefs and behaviours might persist. What to do if they wish to leave hospital and be left to their own devices, at the first or any other point along this journey? Undeniably, the physicality of the scenario is clear, insomuch as drugs such as cannabis and methamphetamine steer the brain towards a dysfunction that is manifest in what we call psychosis or intoxication or delirium or whatever we wish to call it. I'm not entirely sure what Szasz might say in such a scenario, though his response is likely be somewhat less conservative and medicalized than mine. And so I for one have no problem that the prison cell or hospital or other suitably containing environment be provided by the village or its up-scaled equivalent. Insomuch as the care may involve forced sedation, involving a doctor is a prudent inclusion in the response, though this is far from the makings of a pretentious argument that a special species of doctor is required (i.e. a psychiatrist). The more controversial question is what to do the next day, or the days after. Here Szasz and I walk a little way apart, yet relative to the rest of the psychiatric world still march in step. Suffice to say for the present that when the drug user has attained the barest modicum of the compos mentis and do not have obviously severely compromised ability to navigate oneself in the world, that Szasz would certainly argue (and I agree) that involuntary confinement in a psychiatric hospital and/or forced medication ought to be seen as a criminal act. Whether the police and judiciary are involved to prosecute the drug use is another matter and none of the psychiatrist's business any more than any other citizen. Yet what does psychiatry all too often do? It moves the goalposts of diagnosis. Where once there was first episode or recurrent drug induced psychosis, the shift is towards psychiatrists being called to treat "as if" the patient has schizophrenia, and now they are treated "as having" schizophrenia, potentially with loss of liberty and responsibility whether high or not. That or the psychiatrist will formulate the patient as having a mental illness that drives them to use the substances, the drugs receding into the background. Gone altogether are antiquated notions of free will and personal responsibility. Another manifestation of the insanity defense.

Now we have the final couple of patients. Each are adult and so, prima facie, liberty and responsibility ought to be recognized. There are no attributing physical illnesses for their aberrant behaviour. And they reject utterly our proposed interventions. The first, an extraordinary man who frequented mansion gardens under the fervent belief that these estates were his, granted to him by no less than her majesty Queen Elizabeth II herself. He was harmless enough. Despite threatening all and sundry with execution by Mi5 if they didn't acquiesce to his demands, he never did take matters into his own hands when Mi5 didn't show up. (As it happens they never did. Only once in my career did the real secret police show up when the patient claimed a connection to them, the secret police taking the patient away into the night never to be seen again). The previous psychiatrist refused to see him following these threats, I suspect more out of a fear of an extra patient on her list than out of fear of violence. He conveyed his fantastic entitlement with such poker faced sincerity (I believed his conscious mind to be sincere whilst the unconscious was lying through its teeth) that only I somehow managed to keep a straight face while the medical students in my charge quickly excused themselves from the room on account of laughter they could not contain. What struck me was that in every other way he was normal. His thoughts were coherent and articulate, his dress sense stylish, his manner debonair and aristocratic. It was never clear whether he was "hearing voices", though there were tell-tale signs that he possibly was. One Autumn day he managed to abscond from hospital, and off he ran. Szasz would have argued that he did not abscond at all, in the sense that there was no moral legitimacy to having been detained in the first place. From time to time I thought of our pseudo-aristocrat and his fate, until one night a few years later I was working the graveyard shift when the same patient was brought in by police for the same otherwise harmless trespass, a trespass for which I might add he was never charged, as why would a police force dissuade someone from nuisance behaviour using the rule of law, when dumping them in the emergency department saves them the paperwork on a charge that would never be prosecuted or convicted anyway (the insanity defence once again). What was sadly poignant in this story was that he was facially disfigured now, a shadow of his former self. You see in the interim years he took a gun to his head in a failed suicide attempt, an act that was documented as causally related to "schizophrenia". The problem was this; did he put gun to head for Queen and country? No. In the interim years he came under the clutches of another mental health service in another jurisdiction. They treated him with a medication causing a terrible sense of restlessness we call 'akathisia". And it was this terrible side effect that drove him to attempt suicide.

The first thought of the psychiatrist would be to lament that an alternative less troublesome drug had not been forcibly injected into our patient instead. So utterly committed they are to the therapeutic state, psychiatry would not dream for a moment of giving him his freedom to believe what he believed and face a criminal consequence for trespass. But my own thought then was as it is now. Here was a man with alternate beliefs. Startlingly alternate I'll grant you. And I shan't for a moment myself believe that his beliefs had a basis in reality, a reality in fact open only to a few in the British royal family. His isolation is probably more severe still, he being the only one in the whole world believing the story he gives others. We ought to take pause here at just how catastrophic might be the blow to the self if he ever attained the insight the psychiatrist wishes him to possess, such is the hazard of unintended consequences. After all, are all people at all times best divested of their delusions? Why are you so sure? How might you know the content of a delusion is a stochastic accident vs a choice by the person's unconscious that helps them get through the day? But whether fact or not, the question is whether a doctor ought to have the power to forcibly restrain, detain and inject powerful tranquilizers all for the sin of failing to agree on the facts of self and world. I invite the reader to first encounter the arguments made in the earlier chapter on psychosis. Enough to say for now that we all encounter persons with beliefs we do not share. And some will make claims that flow from these beliefs, claims even that imply a potential to infringe upon other person's comforts and freedoms. Our electoral podiums, professorial lecterns and priestly pulpits are full of people with views in part or in whole we do not share. And whether its taxation departments, terrorists, police states or possessive ex partners, they may want what we have and believe with all their heart that that it is their due. Arguing about the relative strength of argument of what constitutes strong evidence is a dead end about which even seasoned philosophers may not agree. And the psychiatric drugs we use to dull the fervour with which a belief is held can make a zombie of anyone and their drive to exercise beliefs if the dose is pushed high enough. They prove nothing as to the ontology of mental illness and so are only useful as domesticating chemicals to dull the deviant.

So what is the alternative you may ask? The alternative is a dialectic, an unforced invitation to challenge him as to the validity of his beliefs and how he might better live in the world. In the majority of cases such a dialectic will not budge the mind of the person with the so called delusion any more than that of engaging the strong political ideologue in argument. Hence psychiatry turns against the dialectical approach and makes many a non sequitur from it (the metaphor if illness and the construct known as insight lacking in virtue of illness). I hazard to add that challenging the so called delusional patient with a vigorous dialectic has surprised me with many victories also, even those written off as irredeemably psychotic. But even if the one with the deviant belief is not convinced, what the proverbial 99% of patients will grasp is that their truth is not shared by others, the police included. That is to say if we embark upon a learning process with repeated police involvement to extinguish the behaviour that is both criminal and "psychotic", this is often successful. As one militantly opposed to thoughts and feelings being considered crimes or pathology, I often advise a patient that if they manage to keep their beliefs to themselves and some trusted others and not attract from the wider world a suspicion that they are crazy, then who should care what they believe. The wider world, I tell them, has not developed the tolerance and "so what" attitude towards highly unusual beliefs that my experience has given me. Whether or not they take my advice will be theirs to make. Theirs will also be the responsibility come the consequences should they fail to heed it, and they fall into the clutches of a psychiatrist less tolerant than I who will drug them whether they like it or not.

Our final example case is that of a woman. She was raised in a more or less normal household, enticed into adolescent rebellion and minor drug use as a teen and cavorted with the "wrong crowd", a member or members of which more than likely at some point raped her. Fast forward to mid adulthood and she had the bizarre delusion of being raped by bikers even when in a locked room in the psychiatric ward, with no one around to touch her. She would claim other staff raped her also, even in the open area where the accused staff member stood at one corner of the room and her at the other. Naturally all this was quite distressing to all involved, and though "psychotic", hers were false beliefs echoing in her mind from traumatic events of the past that her mind could or would not shake. Hers was a case beyond PTSD, and though one could argue was continuous with it, a testament to the contemptable stupidity of the DSM project in carving nature at the joints. Needless to say, she was not living the life of a productive citizen. She had no need to work, as the state would support her for life as disabled with schizophrenia, this despite the fact that she could easily communicate, ambulate and navigate about town to her friends and cannabis dealer and to do the shopping etcetera. Despite her distress, there was no denying that our forced and very protracted psychiatric incarceration and treatment with clozapine resulted in a significant lessening of the phenomena, and with it what might be described as an objectively significant positive shift in her life. Readers who might be psychiatrists will not be surprised to be told however that our patient did not fall at our feet, wash them with her hair and worship us for saving her from the torments of her mind. Quite the contrary. She was bitterly opposed to the treatment program and the medication. She would attempt abscond and evade us as much as possible, not simply because of the events she believed happened to her in hospital as they happened much more so elsewhere. Rather she wanted freedom from hospital per se, and freedom also from our medications. And she wanted none of my Socratic conversation. How do we reconcile this? In a previous chapter I lament that as a younger man of lesser station in psychiatry my defense of the psychiatrist's conduct was that we were saving the patient from the jail that was their own mind, a jail worse than the walls and ceilings of our ward, worse than the regular forced administrations of medication. We were doing what caring experts do. I, like the rest of the psychiatric machine, objectified compassion, this despite knowing that "objective compassion" could only hope to have conceptual coherence as a transcendental from which I could not be its source. And I also had a practice of imagining this gnostic other person within the patient who wanted to be freed, a kind of iatrogenic multiple personality disorder that I projected into the patient, the healthy woman who wanted to emerge victorious over the schizophrenic one. Sure there is part of the patient who expressed their dissatisfaction with care and indeed wants none of it. But deep inside there is the other side of them which only the psychiatrist as seer into souls can see. She is (or they are) happier and perhaps one day will emerge and thank us. But such days rarely if ever arrive. In any case the conjecture is wishful thinking and doomed to failure in the arena of argument as to the evidence I can provide to defend it. There is only a single identity before us in the present. That much we know is true. And that identity insists to be free from psychiatry. That identity insists that our equally insistent compassion is disguised tyranny, ours a pale mirror of her past trauma, for it too was a deprivation of liberty. Now psychiatry will counter this and defend its benevolent tyranny with notions such as "she lacks insight" and so knows not what she does, or does not, want. We know better for her. We might even say she lacks "executive function" and has in theory the hypo-functioning frontal lobes typical of schizophrenia. Such science and psycho-babble are universal solvents into which we might place anyone who protests and disagree about anything, including every male under the age of approximately 30 years with unripe frontal lobes. Such appeals always appeal in turn to circular reasoning as to the relationship between the act of disagreement and the diagnosis we have placed upon the victim of diagnosis, a criterion being "lack of insight". Still the reality of the matter persists. The mind in front of us believes ours to be the greater torture and she wishes to be free of it. And part of my own mind (a part which I knew to exist as I was using it at the time, and long before I discovered Szasz), knew that psychiatry was wrong and that the danger in the power it held was contained only by custom. And yet I persisted in the moral fallacy that a) what I want for another, this being b) what they should have or want for themselves, mandates c) forcing this upon the person. Now for all the callousness we might accuse Szasz of, let us give him the benefit of the doubt that he also desires for this woman a life free of persecutory beliefs and distress. None of us should be comfortable with her pathos, though it ought not be our own sense of discomfort that we are treating using her psychiatric incarceration as a therapeutic object. But it is not from a place of callousness that we might grant people their freedom to hazard the dangers in the world, along with the world of their own mind. Dare I say it is even an act of love to grant people freedom and responsibility. And it makes little difference whether we add into the equation that the examples above might be hearing voices whose counsel they take before ours. Nor does it negate the argument if they wish to kill themselves for reasons we cannot empathize with as being reality based. It is their life to take for the reasons they wish to take it. If you have come this far and allow this woman walk out past the hospital gates to the life and fate of her choosing within the constraints of her person and past, be that life sweet and long or bitter and short, then you too have climbed Mt Szasz.

POSSIBILITY. WHAT IF IT ALL WENT AWAY?

"He who speaks of revolution without living it in their daily life speaks with a corpse in his mouth."

Raoul Vaneigem

"I suspect that our own faith in psychiatry will seem as touchingly quaint to the future as our grandparents' belief in phrenology seems to us now"

Gore Vidal

Now I'm surely no Socrates, no not even his sandal strap. But like Thrasymachus you may ask when I am going to stop criticising and offer something positive by way of a solution to the problem. I would hardly be an amateur philosopher worth my salt if to not give it at least give this a try, though the problem would not be as great as it is if solutions were easily found.

That having been said, some solutions are non solutions, or rather a problem erected on a fallacy requires no solution. Taking a leaf out of the book of Szasz, it is not as if we have abandoned medicalized mental illness as myth only to solidify it, via negativa, in another form. No, our project is more radical still. We must take a pause now, a measured breath even, and avoid falling into the "social justice" trap of looking for humane or more logically consistent alternatives to standard diagnosis and treatment whilst our fallacious premises remain ensconced in our minds as ever, forever perched atop the patient sits looming shadow of the therapeutic state of which we are one of its organs. The absurdity is reminiscent of one of many similar conversations with senior colleagues when I was more junior in psychiatry. When I asserted that so called antipsychotics were entirely inappropriate for a number of reasons in a particular patient with an emotionally unstable and antisocial personality (tax payer funded medication mind you), the response was that it was then incumbent upon me to arrive at an alternative pharmacological solution as part of a "package of care". What was I going to do with, and give to, the person labelled patient, that was the question. What I wanted to recognize in the person was her de-medicalized autonomy, responsibility and the rule of law hanging over her head as it is over my own. What I wanted to offer her were frequent empathic reminders to grow up and some advice on how this might be achieved. To this I could add all the appurtenances of psychotherapeutic psychobabble, though anyone's wise grandmother could identify the basic fault in her developmental history, her psyche and recognise also the necessary adult behaviour that would be a both a therapeutic exercise and a realization of recovery. Naturally such good sense anathema falls on both the deaf ears of the patient who does not wish to grow up, and the psychiatrist whose affirmations to mental illness and the need for medication assent to the same. The psychiatrist's ego wants the patient to pass through a process of confession of being sinful (insight into mental illness), acts of contrition (medication etc) and only in passing through this ritual is absolution (recovery) and partial freedom to be found (partial, as freedom is always conditional in the therapeutic state). When, to use an extreme analogy, we are to purport to be abolitionists of slavery and free the slave from chains even sometimes of their own making, our mendacity and incoherence would be betrayed by then asking "but what do we do with them now?". The answer of course is there is no "we", no "them" and no "doing with". When the one who sits across from me is a free autonomous citizen under the rule of law and assumption of adult personal responsibility, they are none of my business and I am none of theirs save for whatever free transactions we voluntarily choose to make amongst ourselves. After the twilight and just before the passing away of the slave / slave master dyad, "we" may go so far as to give our erstwhile slaves the plantation upon which they have laboured. Should free citizens choose make it into a productive endeavour the profit is theirs. Should they choose to raise it to the ground they face the consequences of their own ruin and famine. In the latter eventuality, the slave master cannot a posteriori claim licence to re-enslave the free citizen or claim the folly of an emancipation which is a moral a priori. And so it is with imagining a death of psychiatry and any transitional alternative objects we may employ en route to its death. The point is not to argue whose system of care results in greater performance outcomes re suicide, "morbidity" from depression and anxiety, untreated psychosis etcetera using existing psychiatric metrics and case control studies. The people who would argue such things are, to quote Wilde, those who know the price or everything and the value of nothing. I could easily argue in favour of some monstrous Huxleyan brave new world where autonomy is effectively abolished altogether, the polis is wrapped in proverbial bubble wrap, drugged into blissful oblivion and suicide as rare as a blue moon. But how would it profit the world if the psychiatrist engineers this utopia at the expense of the person's soul?

Naturally I am not so naïve to believe that were psychiatry to vanish overnight the next day would be smooth sailing. Every major change against that which we have adapted is a revolution of a kind. And every revolutionary, for lack of a better term, must be careful what they wish for. They must ask themselves what is to happen the day after they seize the barracks and the post office, or the psychiatric clinic as the case may be. Quite the contrary, I have no illusions the immediate upheaval would be enormous and impossible to render immune from some quantum of tragedy, though not the catastrophe that the professions narcissism would no doubt want us believe. Besides, tragedy is the stuff of life and it is the medicalization of tragedy that is the greater sickness. Psychiatry's narcissistic delusion is that a society without it is pathological. Problems arising in the wake of its sudden death would be more the clash between the inertia of iatrogenic fostered expectation against the equally iatrogenic emergent vacuum created in psychiatry's absence, as opposed to problems revealing the indispensability of psychiatry in principle or in the mid to longer term. Such would be the birth pains of society growing up. If we are to reject utilitarianism, philosophical pragmatism, the myth of mental illness, the specialist class of the psychiatrist as the minister to souls, the involuntary therapeutic state, the whole menagerie of these hideous little creatures, the consequent inauguration of greater principles within which we may come to live is its own reward. All this having been said, and notwithstanding there is no excuse for failing to move swiftly towards essentially a complete abolition of coercive and forced psychiatric practice and the market expansion of alternatives especially, one needn't be rushed and reckless to do what is best.

Apart from a calling to a different principle, or principle as such (vs the sophistic mischief of an unprincipled pragmatic void), it occurs to me that the task is harder still, for even a salutary suggestion might be seen as something of a fantasy, if not my own delusion. Just as many a youth today could not imagine a world as possible without social media and smart phones, these being places within which their identity dwells and is diffused, many a psychiatrist is so indoctrinated as to believe it is impossible have a functioning world without SSRI's, let alone involuntary hospitalization, civil commitment, ECT, lifetime administered neuroleptics and the psychiatrist themselves. They have swallowed the idea that without psychiatry there would be just as many unwell people suffering, taking their own lives or chained in the attic by the family or dying in the gutter, as if that is the only way. What follows then is a collage of suggestions, impressions and proposals, not solutions so much as an invitation to flexibility and possibility.

Trieste

It is impossible to discuss the psychiatric history of 1960's-1980's Italy without running the risk of that which was warned in the introduction, i.e. some matters are so controversial that the historiography and what is taken for "evidence" becomes terminally divided and polar in its conclusions. Accordingly, one can find whatever answer one wishes to find if to ignore the accounts and arguments one wishes to ignore. And that is the prism which one is handed when looking back at Professor Franco Basaglia, the "Psichiatria Democrata" (democratic psychiatry) and the alleged secular miracle in Trieste at the San Giovanni hospital. Consequently, I shall restrict myself to what is undeniable in what mainstream psychiatry thought impossible before the fact of the miracle, this to be compared with the miracle itself.

Franco Basaglia, like Szasz and revolutionaries of many stripes, was born to a wealthy bourgeois family, in his case Venetian. Although driven and brilliant in his own way, he was a chain smoking iconoclastic who did not universally work well with authority figures, and so was banished by his psychiatric betters to provincial Italy. In a certain strictly limited sense, he shares the same character and fate of another University of Padua alma mater, Galileo Galilei. Province begat providence as outside Padua he could then work unseen and unfettered on his grand social project of reform and deinstitutionalization. Nonetheless he was not the first Italian "reformer", and others had come before. He walked more than a century and a half after, though nonetheless partially in the footsteps of, a Florentine alienist Vincenzo Chiarugi. Chiarugi's story is parenthetically of value, it being part of stepwise humanization of patients that began as early as the late 18th century, though several years after the state under Grand Duke Leopoldo had already legislated to involuntarily detain the mentally ill and other social deviants and misfits. The state first introduces itself as tyrant before seeking to disguise its tyranny under the language of care and reform. Under Leopoldo and, proximally, Chiarugi, the Ospedale di Bonifacio (Bonifacio hospital) expanded from what was essentially a place for the infirmed and elderly and those insane with syphilis to a larger insane asylum with some physically ill patients also. And so we go from a few in chains without a clear rule of law to many more bound with leather straps in legal perspicuity. Such is the victory of the enlightenment. And today psychiatry will consider themselves humanely victorious if the patient and millions of others place themselves in the ideological and chemical strappings of voluntary identification with illness and medication. Nonetheless Chiarugi ought to be given his due, as the one who came before even Pinel and did much good. Though before we heap too great a pile of laudation upon these two Latin children of the enlightenment, we ought to remind to ourselves also that Chiarugi was both alienist and dermatologist. Leather straps are friendlier to the skin than steel and iron, and a moral outcome need not be entirely the product of a moral intention in the way we might like. But that's not really the point is it?

Where Chiarugi would work with the state in the reform of practice within instantiation of earthly laws to involuntarily treat those labelled insane and then claim to do so humanely, Basaglia's leftist Marxist goal was the state sanctioned destruction of the asylum altogether, and he was to inherit the draconian child of the likes that Chiarugi shepherded. These asylums were in every city of any appreciable size inside and outside of Italy, and every one of them would have had their own Chiarugi. The reader's imagination would not be off target if to envision some places with grey walls, shackles or straps, people left alone in the corner to rock and rot and sometimes be abused or exploited in "rehabilitative" work programs. In fairness to my older colleagues around who worked through the end of the 20th century asylums, the system was never as good as it could have been, though not necessarily as universally bad as imagined or portrayed. Not every older psychiatrist we can tar with the same brush as that we might use against the agents of Ceauşescu's state hospitals for example. Such would be a grossly unfair caricature. Critique aside, we can extend the same grace to some individuals in previous centuries also, and even to the clerics who had original governance over the Ospedale di Bonifacio in the 14th century.

Returning to Basaglia, his first forays into deinstitutionalisation were in the far north in Gorizia near the Slovene border in the 1960's, though it was in the San Giovanni hospital in Trieste commencing 1971 that the project really flowered. Basaglia was his own man of course, though influenced by the works of Goffman and Foucault, and to a lesser extent Szasz also, as all three authors were publishing seminal works, a perfect storm of opprobrium against the asylum system of the early 1960's, and psychiatry more generally. Equally influential was Basaglia's politics, both he and his wife Franca were active communist party members and the latter at one stage a member of the senate. It would not be too simplistic to formulate Basaglia to have decided that the liberation of the proletariat was to be a drama played out symbolically in the liberation of the psychiatric patient. And he was to be their Lenin. In Gorizia he managed to publish two books; Che cos'è la psichiatria? (What is psychiatry?) and L'istituzione negata (The institution denied). Curiously neither were translated into English and though I do not suggest any conspiracy by the Anglo psychiatric establishment, others have. Naturally Basaglia had a great many establishment enemies in Italian psychiatry, the public and the local fourth estate. It did not help that the endeavour fell victim to a tragic anomaly early in on in 1972 when an ex-patient murdered his parents for reasons I have been unable to ascertain. This, it appears, was a one off. To counterbalance opposing forces, he was able to mobilize certain powerful demigods in Italian politics and the media to his cause, and Trieste became a mecca for counterculture revolutionaries, bohemians and fellow travellers of many stripes from inside and outside Italy also. These were (paradoxically) the makings of a criticism if the project were it to succeed, for it could be argued it was only on account of turning the isolated little city into a heavily staffed de facto commune with a charismatic leader that it could go as far as it did. Some would say therefore it could not be up-scaled to a Milan or Rome. In any case, life at San Giovanni was to change from locked doors and involuntary patients to open wards and voluntary "guests". The guests were given greater free reign to roam about and choose their own destiny. In this "Psichiatria Democrata" guests were involved in frequent discussions as to the running of the institution. Like other socialist utopias, certain sexual proscriptions of the Latin Church were seen as oppressive and the genders no longer segregated, though gender segregation was also practiced for secular pragmatic reasons back in time and place with Chiarugi in Florence. Despite reservations and horror at the notion of sexual beings doing what sexual beings do, San Giovanni neither turned into a Sodom and Gomorrah or a nursery of little babies with mythical schizophrenic genes. Work programs were replaced with more egalitarian co-ops where the patient workers had more managerial clout. San Giovanni also became a place of regular street theatre, art and Communist graffiti and politically charged slogans were painted on the walls and architraves. Some were more libertarian than communist

'la libertà e terapeutica' ('freedom is therapeutic').

By the end of 1977, by some accounts he had reduced the involuntary patient number from over 1000 to about 50. He announced that the hospital would be closed, this later officially effected in 1980, the year of his death from a brain tumour. Basaglia's law, or law 180, was put in place in 1978 and over the largely posthumous decade to follow its implementation it liberated scores of thousands of institutionalized patients from the asylums across Italy.

One interesting analysis of Basaglia movement was that of a study tour completed by psychologists Kathleen Jones and Alison Poletti. They embarked on the first tour in 1984, omitting Trieste and Rome from the itinerary yet finding in other centres outcomes from which the conclusions were resoundingly negative of the changes that swept across Italy, including those cities they did visit (Como, Milan, Pavia, Pisa, Lucca, Florence, Salerno and Reggio di Calabria). This work was met with the understandable charge of not having visited Trieste itself, in addition to other criticisms as to the authors bias. Consequently, they embarked on a second glorified vacation (sorry study tour) the following year to Trieste, Ferrara, Rome and Bologna. The second revised conclusion was, to their credit, more balanced and positive of law 180. Of Trieste, they praised the informal atmosphere and the spirit of carnival. Nonetheless the dominant critique was that the hospital did not, ipso facto, close and some patients still resided there, as if this somehow negated the endeavour and the fact of their freedom. Many of these were patients rebranded into residents of what effectively became lodge accommodation. Yet we cannot possibly see the four walls the same when the door is unlocked and the one who dwells therein is granted liberty. Just as a deconsecrated church is a gentrified little restaurant with quaint stained glass, an asylum converted to housing is no longer part of the same therapeutic state. Nonetheless some persons were admittedly still held as involuntarily patients, those being the senile dementias and younger patients with intellectual disabilities and acquired brain injuries. However, the closest equivalent to the previous psychiatric ward proper, the optimistically named diagnosis and cure unit, was reduced to a mere 8 beds, and these were empty when Jones and Poletti visited. It must be added that home based care and integration of care back into the family unit (if available) was a focus. Another critique of the authors was that less therapeutic activities were available in this quasi-commune, this also missing the point that to liberate the patient from the locked door is also to liberate them from the medicalized language of the relationship. Only patients need therapy. People need community. Finally, in the very nation of Cerletti and Bini, the founding fathers of electroconvulsive therapy, Trieste saw no need for what many a psychiatric service thinks an indispensable therapeutic modality. To this day Italy is a country which exported ECT only to largely abandon it.

Of course the contemporary psychiatric rebuttal to the Trieste miracle would be to say that this was the righteous end of the asylum era, something echoed all over the developed world. And what of it they might say. How can this apply to the humane psychiatry of the twenty first century when we, in our wisdom, only involuntarily incarcerate and medicate persons when necessity forces our hand? The lesson however is in what people assumed was impossible and what was readily achieved when the will was placed upon the gears of the problem and people were freed or forced from ideological commitments that deprived another of freedom under the rule of law. From this we might ask what evidence do we have that Trieste is the terminal horizon of what is possible? We might further ask why might psychiatry need be dragged kicking and screaming to each and every reform with which it feels uncomfortable, a Kuhnian break with each paradigm. Why the resistance to down-modulating its influence even further, even onto Basaglia's dream to do away with the system altogether?

I have learned my own little lessons in my own little career. There have been times when wards have been forced to substantially downsize, this despite bed availability being ordinarily strained and in perpetual crisis. But boost community resources and the sky did not fall down, patients were not left languishing in the emergency department awaiting a bed or dead in a ditch somewhere. When I suggested that this was evidence to take seriously the notion of closing the wards altogether the response was as if I suggested we could turn water into wine. Government services, like hot air, have a habit of expanding to fill the available space whilst the government worker, like a gas, seeks the lowest available energy state.

This might give a clue as what Basaglia really accomplished. I once heard it said, and (mean culpa) unfortunately cannot recall the quote to credit its source

"if suicide is a cry for help, schizophrenia is a cry for housing".

Any honest psychiatrist will see the ring of truth in this, i.e. that many a schizophrenic is not a person who necessarily cannot live in the world, so much as cannot live comfortably in a world of people distressed by them, or exploitative of them. The hospital is a periodic place of sanctuary for the patient and a respite for the others. They are people who somewhere along the path of life lost their way and could not find their way back. Schizophrenia is a name we give such a wayward soul, and medication is to domesticate their many and varied disjunctive eccentricities. Unfortunately, many patients still cycle in and out of hospitals, where hospital stay costs the tax payer far more than placing the patient in a five star hotel. The miracle of San Giovani and the

Szaszian philosophy opens the way to an imagining public housing blocks staffed by a nurse or two and frequently patrolled by police on the beat. Residents would have the option to stay there and the obligation to act civilly and soberly. There would be no coercive psychiatry, only autonomy and responsibility of free citizens under the rule of law. Ideally also would be the social inculcation of the value of connectedness and community. Give this a generation of adaptation and perhaps we could take the further step to do away with the label of schizophrenia altogether.

Soteria; from Berne to San Francisco

If the measure of success is symptomatic control, a patient not being a nuisance to self or others and metrics based on these outcomes, the asylum system has no peer in managing the variable of public nuisance and embarrassment. Simply lock up the patient and throw away the key, and only the conscience and imagination remains to bother the populace walking past the high fences and dark grey walls. A good dose of egocentric self-centred psychotherapy and an SSRI will cure them of a social conscience. Second best to the asylum in a post Basaglia world, assertive coercive medication centred standard psychiatric treatment with threat of hospitalization has no peer. Should I be asked to speculate on the best treatment to bring about public safety and symptomatic control in 95% of patients (of all diagnoses, not simply schizophrenia), it would be to medicate the person with x diagnosis with clozapine (an oral medication), with repeated cycling of involuntary hospitalization should they be non-compliant until they learn their lesson. The patient will then be fat and domesticated, the mood would be neither too high or too low, the voices but a murmur and the beliefs in the strange and fantastic still held, but they don't care as much about them anymore, and not much else besides. Should they not tolerate the clozapine I'd simply forcibly administer a different neuroleptic available in injectable form, once again with periodic coercive admissions as required.

All this is said to concede the obvious whilst resolving the necessary; i.e. persons un-medicated will likely be more "psychotic" or "manic" than drug free patients, though this approach is not value free. A radical Szazian will reject this on principle, and reject Basaglia also as even Italy never dissolved the threat of the therapeutic state entirely. Those 8 remaining involuntary beds were the stain on Basaglias cassock that would not go away, or so Szasz would say. The next step along the spectrum of liberty and responsibility is Soteria.

Soteria, a name charged with an almost religious calling, is derived from the Greek for salvation. The use of the name speaks of the optimistic counterculture within certain marginal (and marginalized) sectors of psychiatry in the 1960's and 1970's, Basaglia, Szasz et al being but two aforementioned others.

Psychiatrist Loren Mosher and social worker Alma Menn began the Soteria project in 1971. Not surprisingly this was in San Francisco, ground zero for some of the American avant-garde movements then and since, though Mosher wasn't as fringe as one might expect, as he initially moved within the higher echelons of the National Institute of Mental Health before being pushed out for his heresy. Like all but Szasz, Mosher bought into the myth of mental illness, though rather than writing it off as a neurochemical imbalance requiring a neurochemical solution, Mosher largely though not entirely eschewed the use of antipsychotic medication and drew upon his German Jewish phenomenological background to posit that psychosis in large part is a psychological lesion of "Affektlogik". Affektlogik is a mereological re-conceiving of the component parts of the mental state along with the persons experience in the world. It sees affect (qua emotion in this case) and thinking not as separate modalities yet rather fused into a conceptual whole different to the component parts. Thus there is a mode of being (feeling/thinking) that is context dependent and further contextualized by the wider life and individual narrative of the person. Specific context dependent mental states may include rage logic, infatuation logic, fear or anxiety logic and so on. The psychotic state is another logic of its own kind, even paradoxically logical in the sense that the phenomena can be objectively understood, explained, explored and rectified. Soteria and affektlogik would have it that schizophrenia arises from certain disturbing experiences and emotions triggering a reflection of amplified disturbance within thought and feeling leading eventually to the psychotic state. So, for example, the person may experience a sense of loss of agency charged with emotion, this leading to excessive self-reflection, a worry and existential doubt that viciously feeds on itself until the resultant is perhaps disconnection altogether with one's own ego, or even one's own inner dialogue and sensory experiences as being "mine". And so we then have the hearing of voices, the wildly strange misinterpretations, "otherness" and persecutory delusions and so on. The remedy, so says Mosher et al, is a comprehensive restorative therapy that even includes the architecture and furnishings. The patient ought to be in a place where the rules are less alien, and hospitals are as alien to persons daily life as the person has become an alien to the world.

The lay reader may be interested to know that originally the keeper of the asylum might have been called the alienist, this being synonymous with psychiatrist. Ergo Freud was technically never a psychiatrist as he never worked in, or managed an asylum. Similarly, Szasz was a psychiatrist in qualification only and a professor of psychiatry by academic title, and not classically speaking a psychiatrist at all.

Returning to Soteria, our phenomenological alien (i.e. psychotic patient) is encultured back into humanity by living as a human, in a harmoniously furnished and welcoming home. Attachment theorists, cybernetic theorists and occupational therapists alike will also appreciate the heavy reliance on, and ubiquitous presence of, volunteers and professionals to give the patient an experience of "being with" and "doing with" normality. The patient has access to a sane human being with whom they share their mental experience and daily chores. In the process the patient recalibrates themselves to reality and normal human praxis by a process of introjecting the sane other (taking within and becoming the sanity surrounding them). The distinction between thinking and doing is always arbitrary, as there is conversation and cognition even in the doing. What do I think about what we are doing, and what do you think and why? From this comes the synthesis of a dish sanely cooked, a house sanely cleaned, a conversation sanely shared and also a sane mind. The language of "being with" and "doing with", of the psychotic person made sane by practice, reflection and becoming, is evocative for me of the Heideggerian language of "unready to unhand" to "ready at hand", of clumsily learning only to later reflexively expertly do. Naturally as per affektlogik, it is critical that the emotional tone be soothing and supportive, the makings of a sane and calm logic. Calm logic requires extremely intensive and motivated staffing and support. It would not be possible within a disinterested workplace culture periodically assessing safety and mental state with pro forma questions, dishing out medications and generally providing no substantial psychotherapy, this being the prevailing ethos of the contemporary inpatient ward (especially those wards who would deny the charge).

Empirical evidence in favour of Soteria is equivocal, studies being methodologically poor and largely restricted to young psychotic patients who might well remit regardless the treatment or lack of it. Notwithstanding this critique, the results at least point to Mosher's relatively radical approach having outcomes not inferior to standard care (i.e. not worse than coercive medication and hospitalization) in similar patients, and, primum non nocere, without the harms. Todays crop of psychiatrists would not believe Soteria possible, these not being divided on the basis of how to treat the young psychotic patient for it is reflexively assumed standard psychotic care is necessary and withholding this to constitute medical malpractice. Such are explicitly the guidelines of all guilds, who have purchased the nonsense that time off so called antipsychotic medications (the "duration of untreated psychosis" or DUP) is a time at which the un-medicated brain is literally being damaged by the disease of psychosis. From the perspective of personal liberty, the medicated patient might only be fortunate enough to choose from a list of similar drugs they will be forced to take. No, rather the debate today is whether the psychiatrist can diagnose and treat the adolescent or young person at risk of psychosis, that is to say one can look across at the troubled teen (adolescence often being a para-psychotic state), look down into the crystal ball, reliably then predict the future onset of schizophrenia and prevent the thought crime before it arrives without serious adverse effects of neuroleptic medication or the diagnosis of "at risk of psychosis" being reified, the label in and of itself qua label placing the patient at risk of one day being declared schizophrenic.

From San Francisco, Soteria spread across the oceans to Berne, certain other European cities and Jerusalem where it remains to this day, though largely fell into stasis in the USA due to lack of funding and being ignored, critique being not unexpectedly bias in its the ideology (see Carpenter and Buchanans piece in 2002 in Schizophrenia Bulletin for example). Today it remains as fragmented and fringe as it was when it was founded almost a half century ago. A pity.

Open Dialogue

Just as the relative isolation from scrutiny in remote Gorizia afforded Basaglia the chance to experiment with what would become realized in Trieste, the necessities of economic contraction and lack of hospital beds in remote Lapland in 1990's recession Finland drove the beginnings of open dialogue by psychologist Jaakko Seikkula and colleagues at Keropudas Hospital in Tornio, Finland.

An adaptation of psychiatrist Yrjo Alanen's Need Adapted Treatment model and other Finnish initiatives and conceptually feeding on the ideas of the Russian philosopher Mikhail Bakhtin and English Anthropologist Gregory Bateson, Open Dialogue was preceded in particular by an enormous regional upskilling of mental health professionals in the psychotherapies, most especially a full three years training in systemic family therapy. In many ways open dialogue simply is a kind of assertive narrative family therapy where multiple authors co-create the language and the shared narrative. This is central to the treatment model.

Patients in a state of crisis or first episode psychosis are triaged as quickly as possible and assessed in home by a team that forms a dialogue around the patient as nucleus. The component parts specifically include the patient, significant others (family is always invited), a moderator and treating psychiatrist and other clinicians (plural). Each hears the perspectives of all others, with a deep exploration of the shared experiences and meanings of the what is considered the psychosis. I say "considered the psychosis", as open dialogue is philosophically grounded in social constructivism and the meaning of the symptoms are not taken for granted as connoting anything alien to normality. Rather the patient's experiences and their impact are seen to have their meaning only in terms of how this is perceived by the social milieu and what can be negotiated as mutually understood at the close of the dialogue/s. As Seikkula et al write and I wholeheartedly agree "many psychotic states can be interpreted as reactions to difficult life situations and/or traumatic events rather than as symptoms of biological disorders" and "Psychotic reactions should be seen as attempts to make sense of one's experience and to cope with experiences so difficult that it has not been possible to construct a rational spoken narrative about them. In subsequent stress situation, these experiences may be actualized and a way is found to utter them in the form of a metaphor". In this sense paranoid psychosis can be a displacement metaphor for many things, for power dynamics, for dilemma of personal agency and so on. Eating disorders may similarly be about relationships, about expectations and the dilemma of an ambivalence to maturation, and so on.

Psychosis can even be conceptualized as an isolation in self conversation and isolation from effective conversation with the others in one's life. Open dialogue itself is the aide to restore what is lacking, and additionally borrows on the ideas of attachment theory and of Lev Vygotsky's "zone of proximal development in the child." As Seikkula continues "This means the space between adult and child, wherein the adult's more developed functioning provides scaffolding for the child to reach beyond the current limits of his/her abilities. This idea can be used to describe the psychotherapeutic situation as well". The sense of what is said cannot be known to the speaking patient until it is reflected off the listener, who in turn cannot know the speaker until they themselves become the speaker and the original speaker the listener. This the flow of a dialogue which is, a Bakhtin realised, inherently unpredictable. Yet it is not chaotic. A certain faith is implied in the shared understanding finding its way towards the kind of sanity that is neither the sole imposition of the family or mental health practitioner, nor the sane becoming as insane as the patient. Together the knots are untied, the dilemmas resolved and the affect responded to in ways less vulgar than certain other therapies such as the grotesque torture porn that is ISTDP (see chapter 6). The therapist reader acquainted with the concept of active listening may see in open dialogue something assumed to be their regular practice, though this is not so. The usual psychiatric conversation and the phenomenology of the participants involves an exchange of monologue and no shared space. I hear what you are saying in response to my own questions and construct meaning within the space of my own analysis. You the patient do the same. Clarification qua active listening is a polishing of one own personal monologue even whilst the other is speaking. Open dialogue is about the meaning residing in the centre of the circle, then the participants take it in together.

Other components of the treatment include the building of rapport whilst all acknowledging the uncertainty of how the crisis or episode will unfold, this being an honest humble admission to the limitations of what mental health professionals can know and predict, along with a deliberate cultivation of an attitude to speak in plain language as opposed to psychiatric jargon. This ethic extends even to the remarkably deliberate practice of the therapists and psychiatrist asking permission to talk about the patient and family, not behind their back as something necessarily isolative and conspiratorial, yet right there in front of them as part of the therapy. The practitioners can themselves feel invited and open in talking about their feelings, thoughts, concerns about family dynamics, risks, patient beliefs and behaviours and what the treatment plan may involve. In so doing the non-professional characters have reflected back upon themselves an understanding from another perspective in the dialogical shared understanding of the group, the family therapy session being a microcosm also of the world of plural views and uncertain outcomes.

Of medication, Seikkula et al write that "neuroleptic medication should not be introduced at the initial meeting, and should only be started if other efforts prove insufficient". Open dialogue even takes seriously the heresy that...

"neuroleptic medication could block biological and mental functions that are essential for remission. In OD, the more selective use, and possible postponement of neuroleptic medication may give opportunities for the psychotic crises to progress along a more natural trajectory with an adequate sense of mutual trust and security, and this might have a favourable impact on the outcome. Our results are in line with other follow-ups, in which it was found that long-term treatment outcomes for the schizophrenia spectrum population were more favourable with samples receiving less medication".

Evaluating the results of open dialogue have been made somewhat problematic by the methodology being suboptimal, though the idiosyncratic features of Finlands comprehensive national health system are a methodologists dream and render the results of sufficient quality not to be dismissed out of hand. And these results are quite impressive, with open dialogue patients at 19 year follow up requiring less medication, less hospitalization and less reliance on disability benefits. Notably, proponents write that failure to maintain all patients care under the open dialogue "paradigm" often resulted from "more threatening behaviour", though it is not elaborated whether this was informed by psychosis or simply medicalized criminality and antisocial personality. This is an important observation by the Szaszian, that implies the gravitational role of psychiatry in social control as an adjunct to the police. Insomuch as open dialogue always contains within it the fall back option of involuntary hospitalization and treatment, it does fall short of the Szazian categorical imperative, but then does all of psychiatry outside Szasz.

Naturally the American National Institute of Mental Health is reluctant to finance research into Open Dialogue, as recent as 2013 declining to do so as "its paradigm is too different". This is too brazen a dismissal that in the fullness of time could come back to bite them. They should simply do what psychiatry is long in the practice of doing, playing lip service to the value of family, psychotherapy, recovery models and other fluffy notions whilst being faithless in praxis to anything but the drugs. And then if ever open dialogue becomes mainstream, mainstream psychiatry can simply say it knew it all along.

Open dialogue is to be commended for its ardent attempts to place the so called medical model into a place more subordinate to notions of the person within the community, and is a damning indictment of the crude medication focused management and medicalization of the youth in Anglo psychiatry.

The More Severe Psychotic Patient

Soteria and Open Dialogue are predicated on there being staff adequately trained and adequately motivated. Naturally these models of treatment also depend upon the patient and other stakeholders meeting a certain threshold of personal investment, all this collectively being easier imagined than realized. Nonetheless the open dialogue situation, as almost the only game in the town of Lapland, proves that such an approach can be the default first port of call and a refutation that more coercive approaches are required from the outset. Nonetheless I understand how difficult it may be for the standard Anglo hospital based psychiatrist to imagine this as realistic, a model of care coming literally from the home of Santa Claus. Much of my own career I too have managed more severe psychotic patients highly resistant to intervention, where successful intervention is defined as a shift to conformity. Accordingly, the question might be asked what we might do with such persons if psychiatry (which I have established is by definition coercive) were to vanish? Taking the lead from Szasz and to revise the thrust of the previous chapter, if these persons retain sufficient architectural integrity of thought to understand the proposed treatment and yet still decline the "help" offered, this ought to be respected. That is to say that regardless of their beliefs however so strange, and what voices may or may not be counselling them, the vast majority will have the capacity to understand how their own world conflicts with that of others, and what the psychiatrist is wanting achieve in dulling their deviant thoughts and the volume or frequency of the voices. And from this fact they may make their choice to enter into a voluntary psychotherapeutic process, take medication, see a doctor or wise elder or whatever. This is the basic transaction between persons if freedom is to exist at all, and our sentiment to save the person cannot be permitted to trump the others dignity in facing the consequences of their own self-determination. Such an adjudication of this most basic understanding of mental state in no way requires a specialist of any stripe, let alone a doctor trained in bewitching psychobabble, for the recognition of interpersonal disagreement is the stuff of ordinary human life and language. When society dumps the person in the lap of the psychiatrist, society cannot be permitted to divest itself of good sense without at least being reminded of its inhumanity in turning its back on the other. We may not be our brother's keeper, though there is no excuse in not being their friend or being brave enough to admit we are, in our indifference, their enemy. Nor can "lack of insight" be allowed to be reified and smuggled in, a medicalized substitute to wash away what is essentially someone's stubbornness to hold a contrary view. Yet all this having been said, I do take a modest departure from Szasz. There are those persons who retain the normal architecture of thought who might benefit from a conditional and time limited imposition of their freedom from to hear an argument that ought to be made, on the off chance their ear this time is receptive. Once again, this is a normal human impulse as a normal part of human life, requiring none other than normal humans who care for the other. One must be a casuist here in the best sense of the term, and dispense before we begin with the questions of who might have the authority to temporarily deprive a person of their liberty and who might police its excesses. Such reflexive concerns are held by statists and socialists and public servants who are terrified of freedom, good sense and who always wish to have ordinary human life instantiated into law, regulated, mechanized and sterilized of its proper place in the praxis of your relationship to me and vice versa. And so I refuse on principle to be drawn into such minutia and its traps, except to say that anyone in good faith who latches the door and insists on "the conversation" about how destructive the person's behaviour is to themselves and others and how divided their world is from the rest is to be forgiven for making the effort. This is the way spouses play out their last ditch pleas and grievances when on the verge of divorce, the bags are packed and one is heading out the door. This is what parents do when their adult child is about to marry whom they perceive to be the wrong person. This can also be the conversation held between the drug user or alcoholic and the concerned other who holds them until they are sober, then lingering the incarceration long enough for a brutally frank plea to change. And finally this can be the conversation between the one whom we might call psychotic and the one who cares, health professionals being entirely optional. But then as all things do, the conversation must end and the door must be unlocked. None of this requires the psychiatrist to ever have existed.

Then there are of course those, labelled schizophrenic or not, whose architecture of thought is in such ragged disarray that we cannot infer what they are thinking (these are far rarer than the propaganda would have us believe), or those whose mind is thrown into turmoil by some unambiguously somatic psychosis (more common) or drug toxidrome (these are very common) that has rendered them mad for a time. Naturally we might find due place for the doctor here, though any species of doctor ought to be up to the task. Naturally also the hand of care is extended in such an instance and the inference is made that the patient lacks the capacity to assent to what we assume they might retrospectively agree in time. That is unless and until they have regained the capacity for "the conversation" whereupon the conversation is had which, even with a modicum of logic, is one where we accept the choice of what the patient wishes to do with themselves. Or they may just as well tell us to go to hell and alight into the street, a transiently sane person seeking that maddening substance and maladaptive behaviour all over again. What is the doctor to do with these frequent flyers, to continue to stretch out the caring hand to the one who bites it with ingratitude, or might the doctor be able refuse to partake in what has become a sadomasochistic vicious cycle? This is an ethical question, and ought to be an individual one. We must admit for now that just as every trapeze artist is more daring when the safety net is under them, sometimes one has to be cruel to be kind. Remove the net the one who may recklessly climb the pole may think otherwise. And no trapeze artist ought to have the right to compel a whole industry of potential net manufacturers. So let the person go.

The Classical Neuroses

A book such as this is not the place for an extended review on what depression and anxiety are, or personality and the personality disorders for that matter. Suffice to say for now that medication (especially SSRIs and SNRIs and off label use of so called antipsychotics) are rarely anything but glorified placebos and/ or with non specific emotional or drive blunting effects and unacknowledged adverse effects in my opinion, and coercive psychiatry has no place in the vast majority of patients who are described as depressed, and never in those who are anxious or with so called personality disorders, regardless of whether they threaten to kill themselves or others. There may then be that class of non-coercive doctor who, along with nurses, psychologists and allied health workers become trained in one of the other psychotherapies. These can compete with pastors, gurus and wise grandmothers within the marketplace of ideas inhabited by rational actors and rational consumers. The secular mindfulness practitioner can compete with the practitioners of the contemplative schools of the major world religions, with my humble advice being to choose the latter over the former. The doctor might additionally compete with the local bartender and drug dealer in leveraging their own unique talents as potential experts in psychopharmacology, if that is their interest and the interest of the patient to use what is offered. And the voter and government can negotiate what therapies are to be tax payer funded to these voluntary patients, or not as the case may be if gadflies such as I win the day (which is not at all likely). Nevertheless psychotherapy is nothing special. It is not something you do to the person, as in they take two tablets or ten sessions of psychotherapy. Let us please not be mystified. Psychotherapy is a conversation. After all the empathic hooks and rapport building (i.e. so called therapeutic alliance) are put to one side, it all boils down to a confrontation with choice. The past we cannot alter. The world presents us with constraints. Our thoughts and emotions emerge from a mystery. So what do you choose to do and be with what you have?

Suicide.

In an earlier chapter I imagined that certain readers may view my formulation of suicide and its (anti) management as cruel, a charge against which I offered some meandering defences. In that chapter also, as in this one, what will be repeated is a call for heeding the warning of the rule of unintended consequences. Herein I'll expand. Were we to completely turn a blind eye to suicidality qua expressed suicidality, then the mainstream psychiatric industry would predict that there would be an explosion of suicides and umpteen persons suffering in the silence of having their darkest thoughts unheard. There would, or so they would say, be countless cases of untreated mental illness and a core feature of the patients psychopathology (i.e. suicidality) would be stigmatized in being swept under the rug. They think that a constant focus upon suicidality is the recognition of a monster, whereas I claim that it is the creation of one.

Nonetheless I stand firm to the view that suicide is to be left as a choice and any discussion about it couched back in the context of all the persons problems, this in turn part of an entirely voluntary discussion between the person themselves, along with significant others.

With such a change as I propose I predict the following; were psychiatry to vanish some would suicide as they always have. I'm thinking here for example of the bankrupt farmer amongst other bankrupt farmers who quietly walks into the barn one evening and hangs himself. He never came to the attention of psychiatry and he was never to reveal any hints of what would be his final behaviour, even were he to be asked. Of course the retrospectoscope is a most powerful instrument, and beware those false prophets who give you the lottery numbers after they have been drawn. We will all be able look back and see the signs after our farmer departs from us, none of which could predict why him and why now any more than a thousand other farmers who will be found alive the next day. Or there will be the impulsive suicide from the drug addled mind previously not known to psychiatry, the only preventative remedy of which is to lock up all users and envelope them in bubble wrap. Such a preventative remedy will only last as long as the addict remains wrapped up or enjoying that particular high where they are not dysphoric, their mind somewhat organized and not inclined to kill themselves. In either of the above cases the only preventative remedy is the furtherance of a socialist nanny state under the guise of care and compassion. This I believe is axiomatically evil on one hand, and on the other will create in some of the populace, many thousands of state suckling infants with no resilience. In the case of our farmer and other liberty loving folk, the intrusions of the state into his life may be enough of an incursion as to actually encourage a desire to kill himself. I'm not joking. Deprivation of freedom by a nanny state is a stressor the likes of which may contribute in small or large part to death. Psychiatry get out I say.

Were psychiatry to vanish tomorrow I will grant that the marching brigade of suists would continue turn up at emergency departments. They would be drawing on the expectations and enculturation to what suicide was constructed as being up to that day, as would the emergency room staff themselves. Some may find it difficult to adjust to the change, and under the inertia of habit the patient may lead by playing the suicide card. Were the emergency doctor, nurse or psychologist refuse to play the game and instead empathically discuss practical issues, personal agency and insist suicide to be a personal choice, its currency devalued to purchase action or fear, the resultant would perhaps be a temporary spike in threats, attempts and even completed sincere suicides. But, or so I would predict, after this possible spike people would gradually adjust. They would talk suicide less, attempt suicide less and insomuch as suicide would lose its instrumentality towards other ends (shelter, medication, attention towards psychological pain not in proportion to the pain itself, the idiom of unhappiness and the social contagion, punishing others etcetera) we would see a radical stripping away of all these manifestations of suicidality that are constructed and perpetuated by the systems of psychiatry itself. Suicide would lose its sting. This temporary worsening of things I would not frame as the proverbial price worth paying. Such would be to imply I do not care about the loss of human life, this hardly being the case. Such would also imply that a change in strategy was towards some instrumental utilitarian goal and operating upon objects without agency, as opposed to being a strategy necessarily following from a recognition of what it is to be a human being with free will. Now I said in a previous chapter and here to repeat, placing suicide back into the hands of the person themselves is one of the greatest acts of respect and love we can give another, for it recognizes the most precious existential qualities we have (or ought to have) within ourselves, i.e. free will and personal responsibility. If psychiatry went away there would still be family physicians, nurses, pastors, spouses, lovers and grandmothers who, as humans, can hear and care about the lives and stories of others. They could work towards practical solutions and the mobilization of resources within the community with which to address the particular problems within and between people. And when the subject of suicide arises, as it inevitably will from time to time, the response ought to be that such an act would be supremely regrettable for sure, yet the choice of the potential suist nonetheless. Suicide as a subject of conversation ought to always be redirected into a recognition of personal agency. That is not to say that I am a radical libertarian completely against all deprivation of liberty made by caring others. If a loved one is about to reach for the noose then tackling them to the ground and conscripting the others in the village to action against liberty is a very human and very understandable thing to do. It naturally unfolds not as a response to a public health policy, a mechanization of morality or the constructions of psychiatry as an elite, which in such a world as I imagine would be no more. Neither would it be the business of police unless and until police get a grip on crime or the police officer were acting as a free citizen acting in good faith. But the question is not what to do in the heat of human passions and the impulse to save another. The question is what to do the next minute or the next day. What could or should follow is a frank conversation, human to human, a beseeching and petitioning if required, even perhaps a prayer or two. I commend the reader to Mccarthy's novel "The Road" (or it's film adaptation) for a conversation such as I describe, this between the character of "the man" and "the mother", the brutal conflicted tension between holding on and letting go. Nonetheless all conversations come to an end. And at the end of this conversation the potential suist would either take a step towards life or a step towards the noose. Surely it is their choice to make.

To Reform or to Dissolve

In the twenty 21st century there are of course those notional psychiatrists who dislike diagnosis a la DSM, dislike the "biological model", favour psychotherapy, dislike excess use of medication and personally eschew the wielding of coercive power that defines their profession. Often their heresy extends to being completely at odds with the guild machine. In the UK they call themselves "critical psychiatrists", a fitting name given the implication that the guilds are not critical enough of themselves, or not critical thinkers at all. One may find them at criticalpsychiatry.co.uk or clustered around the journalist Robert Whitaker and his madinamerica.com website. And yet I wonder why their psychiatrist members in particular do not take a leaf out of the book of Martin Luther. How far can one find oneself at odds with the guild and yet in good conscience or logical coherence still say "I am a psychiatrist", without tacitly endorsing the pragmatism and rather strange notion that a psychiatrist can be anything and everything they want to be? What would be the meaning and virtue behind Luther disavowing the legitimacy of the Roman church of his anointing and yet state he is a priest all the same? Better to break and create one's own church, this being what he did. Or better still join with the Greeks for they never indulged in indulgences. Speaking personally, though still behind the veil of pseudonym, I have certain qualifications sure. Yet I find the idea I could ever identify with the title of "psychiatrist" logically incoherent and dishonest to me as one radically critical of psychiatry, and a qualification would not be enough to redeem the titles meaning so as to be ascribed to my person in anything but the most limited sense. I would ask so called critical psychiatrists do the same. Cease involvement with their guilds. Cease identifying with the use of the term psychiatrist. Stop trading on the legitimacy of a title whose guild, history and current practice you so deeply critique and have so soundly discredited. Start over if you are truly progressive. Yet my challenge is hardly progressive, for mainstream psychiatry is hardly the product of the conservative mood either. But that I fear is part of the problem. I surely wish not to alienate myself from critical psychiatrists, whose virtue and brave honesty deserves commendation. But the danger may be in moving from one manifestation of a pernicious politic to another. Where mainstream psychiatrists are therapeutic statist socialists wishing to use force to liberate the patient from the clutches of their mental illness, in so doing engineering the new man of homo psychiatrus, the critical psychiatrists want to rescue the mentally ill from the guilds, and much more so the evil pharmaceutical companies and the side effects of the poisons they peddle. But who and what is ill and who and what are you to minister to them? Moreover, drug manufacturers only exist because there are drug dealers, that being the psychiatrist. And drug dealers only exist because there are drug users, that being the patient. And excuse makers only exist because there are excuse consumers, which may very well be all of us. Where is agency in this? Where is personal responsibility and liberty under a rule of law that sits outside psychiatry in whatever form it may take? Where is the cry that a person is only truly free if free from even the well intentioned reformer? Why not just dissolve all that is and might be psychiatry back into the world of person and family, or free citizen living in an (ideally) minimal state?

I wish to penetrate deeper here into a critique of the critics of psychiatry. Though not with blame and even with refrain from attaching to them the word victim, they are in danger of being like those characters of certain science fiction films, longing to wake from an unreal dream world only to be unwittingly find themselves in another, and the surface reality to be another layer still above. The problem is when we eschew the so called biological or medical model of psychiatry, the myths of chemical imbalances and the pushing of pills, the excesses of coercion and begin talking of the illness being more socially informed and constructed, and more amendable to therapies on the social and psychological axes. And yet what have we achieved and have we really escaped our prison, and by extension who else have we really liberated from theirs? We still place the person within the domains of functionality and dysfunction, of being the product of formal and efficient causes, of being a co-ordinate system of bio, psycho and social, of having an illness for which we simply have arrived at a different ostensibly humane formulation whilst still operating thoroughly within an engineering meta-schemata void of moral and real human life. We still seek to identify causal chains, classify, compartmentalize, formulate, plan, measure and act upon the problem to the ends of its correction. And were we to progress to an alternate psychiatry, the hue and cry would still be for the care of the mentally ill. And each year the funding would become larger, the mental illness disability pool would continue grow in disproportion to physical illness, the ranks of the mentally ill would balloon as they have done for each previous successive wave to address the mental health crisis in the past three decades. An end to all this! We can do away with ninety percent of the drugs and ninety-nine percent of coercive treatment. Psychiatry should consist of this. Two individuals situated in moral space, one ideally wiser than the other. What do you wish to be and what ought you to be? What is the life worth lived? No diagnoses. No talk of recovery. No promises. This should be the beginning and end of psychiatry, which is to say psychiatry would no longer exist as an arm of the state or a specialty of medicine. Time to work towards the dissolution of psychiatry. Time to work towards its death. Only then can the person truly exist and truly be free, and it is freedom, existence (and responsibility) I wish for you.

***

Lightning Source UK Ltd.
Milton Keynes UK
UKHW011557130520
363213UK00008B/1348